OLIVE OIL

Minor Constituents and Health

Edited by
DIMITRIOS BOSKOU

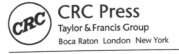

CRC Press
Taylor & Francis Group
Boca Raton London New York

CRC Press is an imprint of the
Taylor & Francis Group, an **informa** business

CRC Press
Taylor & Francis Group
6000 Broken Sound Parkway NW, Suite 300
Boca Raton, FL 33487-2742

First issued in paperback 2019

© 2009 by Taylor & Francis Group, LLC
CRC Press is an imprint of Taylor & Francis Group, an Informa business

No claim to original U.S. Government works

ISBN-13: 978-1-4200-5993-9 (hbk)
ISBN-13: 978-0-367-38714-3 (pbk)

Visit the Taylor & Francis Web site at
http://www.taylorandfrancis.com

and the CRC Press Web site at
http://www.crcpress.com

OLIVE OIL

Minor Constituents and Health

Contents

Preface

Olive oil has been used for thousands of years in the countries surrounding the Mediterranean Sea. There are many references to its use in the history literature and also in the mythology of the people of this area.

Virgin olive oil, a staple food for the people living in the Mediterranean countries, is extracted from the olives by gentle physical methods, the result of which is a genuine fruit juice endowed with a characteristic aroma and bioactive ingredients.

Epidemiological studies indicate that the consumption of natural antioxidants produces beneficial health effects and these substances are now considered potentially therapeutic. In the Mediterranean diet virgin olive oil represents the principal source of fat, but the oil is now becoming popular in many other countries all over the world, both near and far from the Mediterranean basin; thus, the role of virgin olive oil in the diet has become a topic of universal concern.

The protective role of olive oil in fighting certain diseases has been attributed to its fatty acid composition and the presence of minor constituents, mainly phenolic compounds and squalene. In the last 10–15 years a lot of research has been accumulated that links olive oil phenolics and other biologically active components with specific biological effects that may effectively contribute to the prevention of cardiovascular disease and certain cancers. This work is to a great extent scattered and not systematically discussed. Most of the experimental work was set up based on the knowledge of the composition of the polar fraction, but this knowledge has changed rapidly in the last decade; it is not clear if findings based on free hydroxytyrosol and oleuropein, two compounds found in olive oil in minute quantities, can be extended to actual major constituents, which, according to recent research, are the various aglycon forms of oleuropein and ligstrodide and also some lignans, flavonoids, hydroxy-isochromans, and various acids. Another typical example of the importance of the properties and also the actual concentration of minor constituents is oleocanthal, a tyrosol derivative whose anti-inflammatory role (similar to that of the drug ibuprofen) was recently discovered but has not yet been fully evaluated. It has to be stressed that the problem of the levels of individual bioactive compounds in olive oil (a natural product with great variability in composition) and the possible combined effects of various classes of bioactive compounds have never been properly addressed.

This book presents the current state of the art in the chemistry of minor constituents of virgin olive oil and their biological importance, providing information not covered by existing reference books. It also discusses aspects related to the development of technology to retain optimum levels of bioactive ingredients in virgin olive oil. The goals of the book are clearly defined. It aims at discussing critically accumulated knowledge and contributes to a more balanced understanding of pharmacological properties of phenols and other bioactive ingredients in light of new evidence for the composition of olive oil nonglyceride constituents. The task is distributed among authors who are pioneers in their fields and whose skills in this modern area of research (bioactive ingredients) can guarantee some answers to the remaining questions about the potential health effects of the many lipid and nonlipid minor constituents of olive oil.

The subject matter is organized into 10 chapters and an epilogue; there is also a brief glossary that elucidates some technical terms found mainly in the chapters discussing chemistry and technology aspects.

Chapter 1, "Culinary Applications of Olive Oil—Minor Constituents and Cooking," is an outline of olive oil culinary applications and the changes occurring in olive oil microconstituents during processing and cooking.

Chapter 2, "Traditional Mediterranean Diet and Health," discusses the traditional Mediterranean diet, common dietary patterns that prevail in this diet, and characteristics that stem from the fact that olive oil occupies a central position in this diet. Mortality statistics covering three decades that provide indirect evidence about the beneficial effects of the Mediterranean diet are analyzed. The results of major studies and assessment of the adherence to the Mediterranean diet, including those undertaken by the authors, are also presented. Why the Mediterranean diet could offer a healthy alternative approach to a low animal fat diet is explained.

Chapter 3, "Phenolic Compounds in Olives and Olive Oil," is an analytical presentation of the chemical nature of phenolic compounds present in olive oil, the levels of each individual compound in virgin olive oil, techniques to optimize polar phenol concentration in pressed olive oil, methods for the preparation of hydroxytyrosol concentrates, and antioxidant and antimicrobial properties.

Chemistry is a prerequisite for understanding the unique properties of this valuable oil and for correctly formulating experiments in the areas of nutrition and biosciences. Hence, the chapter covers a wide range of topics and contains recent information that is the result of the rapid development of analytical methods over the last decade concerning the nature, occurrence, and properties of natural antioxidant phenols in virgin olive oil and table olives. It also embodies information on techniques of isolating bioactive phenols from olive leaves and olive milling waste products that may be used in pharmaceutical preparations or functional foods.

Chapter 4, "Other Important Minor Constituents," is a short presentation of other biologically important minor constituents present in olive oil such as alpha-tocopherol, squalene, pentacyclic triterpenes, and sterols.

Chapter 5, "Detection and Quantification of Phenolic Compounds in Olive Oil, Olives, and Biological Fluids," covers recent developments in chromatographic and mass spectrometric analysis and hyphenated techniques. It also describes in detail novel approaches based on ^{1}H-, ^{13}H-, and ^{31}P-nuclear magnetic resonance spectroscopy for the analysis of phenols in olive oil as well as techniques for their determination in plasma and urine after ingestion of olive oil.

Chapter 6, "Bioavailability and Antioxidant Effect of Olive Oil Phenolic Compounds in Humans," summarizes very recent findings, many of them based on the authors' experimental work, related to bioavailability of olive oil phenols in humans. The authors indicate that after ingestion and metabolism phenols exert antioxidative activities. They discuss deposition in humans, ingestion in clinical trials and biomarkers, bonding with proteins, atherosclerosis, and postprandial studies on the antioxidant effect of olive oil phenolic compounds. They also describe future trends and key points for research on the antioxidant effects of olive oil compounds on humans that are related to oxidative markers, oxidative stress–associated processes, nutritional interventions, and selection of biomarkers.

Chapter 7, "Olive Oil Phenols, Basic Cell Mechanisms, and Cancer," reviews the epidemiology of olive oil consumption and cancer risk and addresses questions such as the role of olive oil in the prevention of certain types of cancer, attenuation of onset and progression, and inhibition of oxidation and inflammation. It discusses in detail research work in human cell lines and potential mechanisms involved, mode of action of olive oil constituents, interference with basic cell functions, angiogenesis, interaction with steroids and growth factor receptor-mediated functions, interaction with specific protein kinases and oncogenes/oncoproteins, and inhibition of enzymes related to tumor promotion and metastasis.

Chapter 8, "Antithrombotic and Antiatherogenic Lipid Minor Constituents from Olive Oil," includes information on theories for the pathogenesis of atherosclerosis such as inflammation and oxidation, the "PAF-implicated" atherosclerosis theory, antiatherogenic and antithrombotic properties attributed to olive oil minor constituents, and their effect on the hemostatic mechanism.

Chapter 9, "Olive Oil Hydroxy-Isochromans," deals with the properties of a class of compounds very recently identified in virgin olive oil. The biological importance of the presence of hydroxy-isochromans is little studied. The authors, based on the research work of their own group, describe the identification of these ortho-diphenols and levels in olive oil, their capacity to interfere with platelet function, and the relation of this ability to inhibiting platelet aggregation with radical-scavenging activity.

Chapter 10, "Mediterranean Diet and Olive Oil Consumption—Estimations of Daily Intake of Phenolic Antioxidants from Virgin Olive Oil and Olives," presents results of the estimation of antioxidant intake via olive oil and table olive consumption by the Greek population. The calculations are based on literature data for the content of olive oil and table olives in antioxidant compounds, and on consumption data of more than 20,000 Greeks in the context of the Greek cohort of the European Investigation into Cancer and Nutrition (EPIC study). The authors discuss difficulties encountered in existing approaches to assess the relative contribution of each of the entities to the overall antioxidant impact and suggest issues that need to be addressed in future studies of the magnitude of the contribution of olive oil antioxidant compounds to the overall positive health impact of the Mediterranean diet in fighting chronic diseases.

Chapter 11, "Epilogue," provides a brief discussion of conclusions from the various chapters and some of the suggested directions for future research work.

It is hoped that this book will be of special value to nutritionists, food scientists, dieticians, cardiovascular disease epidemiologists, pharmacologists, researchers, and professionals in the area of bioscience involved in research related to natural antioxidants, oxidative stress, and chemoprevention; and finally to companies and professionals promoting sales of olive oil as a health food.

I gratefully acknowledge the help of the renowned specialists who contributed to this book. I consider myself fortunate to have had the opportunity to work with so many knowledgeable colleagues from universities in Greece, Italy, Spain, and the United States, who prepared the monographs based to a great extent on their personal research experience. The acceptance of my concept of the book and of the editorial guidelines is highly appreciated. I particularly thank Prof. Photis Dais, University of Crete, for his enthusiasm and for preparing his valuable part of the work well ahead of schedule. I would also like to thank my daughter, Katerina Boskou, a graphic designer, for assistance in the reproduction of figures.

Finally, thanks are due to readers of any previous books on olive oil who stressed the need for a separate, more detailed publication focusing on the properties of minor constituents, because today more research is being carried out on phenolic and other minor constituents than on the triacyglycerol composition of olive oil.

—Dimitrios Boskou

The Editor

Dimitrios Boskou, Ph.D., earned his doctorate in chemistry from the School of Chemistry, Aristotle University, Thessaloniki, Greece; his Ph.D. from the University of London; and his Doctor of Science from the School of Chemistry, Aristotle University. He served as an assistant, lecturer, assistant professor, associate professor, professor, and head of the Laboratory of Food Chemistry and Technology, School of Chemistry, Aristotle University from 1970 to 2006. From 1986 to 1998 he was a member of the IUPAC Oils, Fats, and Derivatives Commission; from 1995 to 2005 he served as a member of the Supreme Chemical Council, Athens and since 1995 he has been a member of the Scientific Committee for Food of the European Commission and member and expert on the Food Additives Panel of the European Food Safety Authority.

Dr. Boskou has written more than 85 published papers and reviews and authored and edited 4 books (*Olive Oil*, AOCS Press, 1996; *Frying of Food*, Technomic Publishing Co., 1999; *Olive Oil*, Second Edition, AOCS Press, 2006; *Natural Antioxidant Phenols*, Research Signpost, 2006). He was lead author of more than 10 chapters in books related to heated fats, natural antioxidants, and olive oil chemistry. He has contributed to international scientific encyclopedias and the *Lexicon of Lipid Nutrition*, a joint IUPAC/IUNS work.

Contributors

Smaragdi Antonopoulou
Department of Science of Nutrition-Dietetics
Harokopio University
Athens, Greece

Dimitrios Boskou
School of Chemistry
Aristotle University of Thessaloniki
Thessaloniki, Greece

Elias Castanas
Laboratory of Experimental Endocrinology
School of Medicine
University of Crete
Heraklion, Greece

María-Isabel Covas
Lipids and Cardiovascular Epidemiology Unit
  and CIBER de Fisiopatología de la Obesidad
  y Nutrición
Parc de Recerca Biomèdica de Barcelona
Barcelona, Spain

Photis Dais
NMR Laboratory
Department of Chemistry
University of Crete
Heraklion, Greece

Rafael de la Torre
Pharmacology Research Unit
Institut Municipal d'Investigació Mèdica and
  CIBER de Fisiopatología de la Obesidad y
  Nutrición
Parc de Recerca Biomèdica de Barcelona
Barcelona, Spain

Vardis Dilis
Department of Hygiene and Epidemiology
School of Medicine
National and Kapodistrian University of
  Athens
Athens, Greece

Montserrat Fitó
Lipids and Cardiovascular Epidemiology Unit
  and CIBER de Fisiopatología de la Obesidad
  y Nutrición
Parc de Recerca Biomèdica de Barcelona
Barcelona, Spain

Marcella Guiso
Department of Chemistry
University of Rome "La Sapienza"
Rome, Italy

Marilena Kampa
Laboratory of Experimental Endocrinology
School of Medicine
University of Crete
Heraklion, Greece

Haralabos C. Karantonis
Department of Science of Nutrition-Dietetics
Harokopio University
Athens, Greece

Olha Khymenets
Pharmacology Research Unit
Institut Municipal d'Investigació Mèdica and
  CIBER de Fisiopatología de la Obesidad y
  Nutrición
Parc de Recerca Biomèdica de Barcelona
Barcelona, Spain

Tzortzis Nomikos
Department of Science of Nutrition-Dietetics
Harokopio University
Athens, Greece

George Notas
Laboratory of Gastroenterology
School of Medicine
University of Crete
Heraklion, Greece

Vassiliki Pelekanou
Laboratory of Experimental Endocrinology
School of Medicine
University of Crete
Heraklion, Greece

Giuseppina I. Togna
Department of Human Physiology and
    Pharmacology
University of Rome "La Sapienza"
Rome, Italy

Giuliana Trefiletti
Department of Human Physiology and
    Pharmacology
University of Rome "La Sapienza"
Rome, Italy

Dimitrios Trichopoulos
Department of Epidemiology
Harvard School of Public Health
Boston, Massachusetts, U.S.A.

Antonia Trichopoulou
Department of Hygiene and Epidemiology
School of Medicine
World Health Organization Collaborating
    Center for Nutrition
University of Athens
Athens, Greece

1 Culinary Applications of Olive Oil—Minor Constituents and Cooking

Dimitrios Boskou

CONTENTS

1.1 DOMESTIC AND OTHER USES

The olive tree is one of the oldest known cultivated trees in the world and olive oil has been used by man for many tasks since the days of antiquity. Modern historians consider the olive tree a cultural marker and a compass to explore the development of civilizations. Through the centuries olive oil has become one of the most widely accepted and used oils in culinary applications.

The olive tree possesses an amazing ability to survive with strong resistance to unfavorable conditions. On the other hand, it is a demanding crop if it is to produce well. Therefore, a suitable environment and proper cultural care are necessary for the full development of the agronomic characteristics and steady production conditions. The tree is cultivated today in many countries, including Spain, Italy, Greece, Tunisia, Turkey, Portugal, Morocco, Syria, Algeria, Egypt, Israel, Libya, Jordan, Lebanon, Cyprus, Croatia, Slovenia, Argentina, Chile, Mexico, Peru, the United States, and Australia.

Olive oil is a staple food for the people of the countries surrounding the Mediterranean Sea, but its use is now expanding to other parts of the world due to its unique flavor, high content of healthy monounsaturated fatty acid, and the presence of biologically important minor constituents. In the specialty food arena, olive oil is a dominant species that continues to grow in popularity. In the kitchens of consumers it is often the fat of choice for health-conscious people looking to extract the benefits of the Mediterranean diet. In 2004 the U.S. Food and Drug Administration (FDA) announced the availability of a qualified health claim for monounsaturated fat from olive oil and reduced risk of coronary heart disease (CHD) (http://www.fda.gov/-dms/qhcolive/html). According to the FDA, there is limited but not conclusive evidence that suggests consumers may reduce their risk of CHD if they consume monounsaturated fat from olive oil and olive oil–containing foods in place of foods high in saturated fat, while at the same time not increasing the total number of calories consumed. However, the biological value of olive oil is most probably due not only to its fatty acid composition but also to the nature and levels of minor constituents.

Edible olive oils are graded in six categories: *extra virgin olive oil, virgin olive oil, refined olive oil, olive oil, refined residue oil,* and *olive residue oil.* Extra virgin olive oil (acidity up to 0.8% as oleic acid), virgin olive oil (acidity up to 2.0%), olive oil (a mixture of refined and virgin olive

1

oil), and olive residue oil (a blend of refined residue oil and virgin olive oil) contain biologically important polar compounds such as phenols, in addition to alpha-tocopherol and squalene. Refined olive oil has the same glyceridic composition as virgin olive oil but contains less alpha-tocopherol and squalene. Refined olive residue oil is obtained by extraction of olive pomace with a solvent and refining. It has the same triglyceridic composition as virgin olive oil; it contains no polar antioxidant phenols but is richer in biologically active pentacyclic triterpenes such as oleanolic acid and erythrodiol.

Another form of olive oil is "cloudy" (veiled) olive oil, which is consumed before full precipitation in the tanks and filtration. It is an emulsion-suspension and can persist for months before full deposition of a residue. Small quantities of cloudy olive oil, the real fresh olive juice, are sold directly from the mills to consumers who consider this type "greener" and richer in flavor. This product is now gaining popularity due to findings related to the presence of secoiridoids such as *oleocanthal*, a *p*-hydroxyphenyl ethanol (hydroxytyrosol) derivative (the deacetoxy, dialdehydic form of ligstroside aglycon) and other minor components with pharmacological properties. Oleocanthal, which is related to the stinging sensation in the back of the throat, was synthesized recently and found to have the same pharmacological properties as the anti-inflammatory drug ibuprofen (Beauchamp et al., 2005).

Virgin olive oil has a remarkable oxidative stability. If properly stored, it can retain its characteristics for 18 months or more. This resistance to the development of rancidity, combined with a variety of flavors and distinct features, offers the opportunity for many culinary applications, many of which demand no or very mild processing (addition to salads, marinades, sauces, dressings, dips). There are also many applications of the oil in the preparation of fried and baked or grilled foods. Good olive oil captures the bright essence of fresh olives and can be drizzled on all savory Mediterranean foods. Traditional dishes are prepared with seasonal vegetables, pulses, and grains. In this case, "light" fruit aroma oils are more suitable. Olive oil imparts a peppery flavor to grilled meat. Pies, fried eggs, mayonnaise, and other products may require different tastes, but only by those who are experienced users and can explore sensorial differentiations more deeply. Like wine, each virgin olive oil has its own identity. Good oil, again like good wine, takes on different characteristics as it travels down your throat. It can be grassy or peppery. It can taste of apples or artichokes or nuts. The nutritional benefits of vegetables pan-fried in virgin olive oil following the traditional culinary practice have been discussed by Kalogeropoulos et al. (2006).

The biological importance of olive oil has stimulated the interest of the industry. Today in the market many patented foods, primarily margarines and cholesterol-lowering products, reduced fat mayonnaises, and chocolate products, contain olive oil. The justification for such products is obviously the result of many studies based on dietary supplementations with olive oil, suggesting that the replacement of other fats by olive oil reduces cardiovascular heart disease and other health risks (Sanchez-Munich et al., 2003; Rodenas et al., 2005) (see also Chapters 2 and 6–10). The level of replacement of other fats by olive oil is not well known because most of the applications are patented.

Muguerza et al. (2003) and Ansorena and Astiazaran (2004) suggested a new application for olive oil. To obtain better oxidative stability of fermented sausages they replaced part of pork fat with olive oil. This substitution resulted in a lower rate of lipid oxidation and a better balance of saturated, monounsaturated, and polyunsaturated fatty acids. Partial replacement of the animal fat by olive oil was also suggested to reduce cholesterol levels in meat products (Kayaardi and Gok, 2004).

In other cases the nutritional benefits of olive oil are combined with those of n-3 fatty acids. A typical example is the preparation of canned fish (Cuesta et al., 1998).

Medina et al. (1999) found that polyphenols extracted from extra virgin olive oil were effective antioxidants when added to heated tuna muscle in the presence of either brine or refined olive oil. The study aimed at evaluating effectiveness of polyphenols extracted from olive oil when added to tuna subjected to thermal autoxidation after canning. Among different oils, extra virgin olive oil, used as a filling medium of canned fish, showed the highest protection of the thermal oxidation of n-3 fatty acids induced during sterilization. This is probably due to phenolic antioxidants, which have a well-recognized antioxidant activity in bulk oils, micellar systems, and systems formed by minced fish muscle heated in oil or brine (Medina et al., 1998, 1999). The chemical modifications and partitioning of the brine of the major phenols of extra virgin olive oil were discussed by Sacchi et al. (2002). Sealed cans were filled with oil–brine mixtures simulating canned food systems in oil. The cans were sterilized and the partitioning of the phenols was studied by analyzing, using high-performance liquid chromatography, the fraction from the oil and brine before and after steriliza-tion. The hydrolysis of secoiridoid forms of hydroxytyrosol and the partitioning toward the water phase were used to evaluate the changes in the phenolic profile of olive oil after the oil had been used as a filling medium in canned food.

Olive oil–lemon juice salad dressing. Olive oil–lemon juice salad dressing is very popular in the Mediterranean countries; it is prepared instantly by combining two approximately equal por-tions of olive oil and lemon juice just before use. It is a rich source of biologically important com-pounds such biophenols, lipid-soluble vitamins, water-soluble vitamins, and squalene. A stable olive oil–lemon juice salad dressing was developed by Paraskevopoulou et al. (2005) using xanthan gum as stabilizer and gum arabic or propylene glycol alginate as emulsifier.

This dressing can be used in catering meals and convenience foods. Stabilization of the physi-cochemical character obtained by the polysaccharides also increases the oxidative stability (Para-skevopoulou et al., 2007).

Oils flavored with herbs. Dry herbs or their extracts may be used in olive oil to provide a more special flavor and to retard oxidative deterioration. Oregano and rosemary are the preferred herbs, which are rich in antioxidants such rosmarinic acid or phenolic diterpenes such as carnosic acid and carnosol (Exarchou et al., 2002; Boskou, 2006). Roasted garlic may also be infused.

The acceptance by consumers of gourmet olive oils containing dry oregano and rosemary and the pro-oxidant and antioxidant factors were studied by Antoun and Tsimidou (1997) and Damechki et al. (2001). The critical point in these herb-containing specialty oils is storage, since they contain more chlorophyll transferred from the plant material, and they are prone to more rapid photosensi-tized oxidation.

1.2 PROCESSING AND MODIFICATIONS

Olive oil is popular in its natural form (virgin olive oil) but like most vegetable oils, nonedible forms are neutralized, bleached, and deodorized to obtain a bland oil that is usually blended with virgin olive oil. The industrial process of refining is the restoration of a defective but still valuable product that retains its biological value as far as the fatty acid composition is concerned.

Alkali refining removes fatty acids, phospholipids, pigments, mucilage and resinous substances, and polar phenolic compounds. Bleaching reduces chlorophylls, carotenoids, and residual fatty acids and salts. If the oil is physically refined it first has to be degummed.

Hardening and interesterification. Olive oil is too valuable to be hydrogenated because even lampante (nonedible) oils are usually more expensive than seed oils. Thus hydrogenation is mean-ingful only in the case of surplus of raw material for the production of specific products. Olive oil is not rich in polyunsaturated fatty acids and to obtain a hard product it has to be hydrogenated under conditions that favor positional and geometrical isomerization (Boskou and Karapostolakis, 1983; Boskou and Chryssafidis, 1986). Interesterification of refined olive oil–tristearin blends yields zero-*trans* plastic fats with a higher percentage of polyunsaturated fatty acids than hydrogenated (Gavri-ilidou and Boskou, 1991). In two recent papers, Criado and co-workers (2007a,b) studied lipase catalyzed interesterification of virgin olive oil and fully hydrogenated palm oil and characterized the chemical properties of the semisolid product obtained. Enzymatic interesterification of olive oil with hydrogenated palm oil was first suggested by Alpaslan and Karaali (1998), who studied the induced changes and found that the interesterified blend had properties similar to those of package margarines with the additional advantage of high amounts of monounsaturated fatty acids.

Vural et al. (2004) prepared interesterified olive oil to be used as a beef fat substitute in sausages and thus obtain a better ratio of unsaturated to saturated fatty acids. Other attempts have also been made to use olive oil in the preparation of "structured lipids" (Fomuso et al., 2001; Tynek and Ledochowska, 2005).

1.3   HEATING OF OLIVE OIL AND MINOR CONSTITUENTS

In comparison to other vegetable oils usually richer in polyunsaturated fatty acids, olive oil has a much lower rate of alteration during domestic frying or other uses that require high temperatures. This stability of olive oil and its resistance to rapid deterioration at elevated temperatures are due to its fatty acid profile and the presence of natural antioxidants and sterols that inhibit oxidative polymerization (Boskou, 1999; Blekas and Boskou, 1999). However, when the oil is heated for repeated frying operations, its phenolic content and its antioxidant activity are diminished significantly. All the researchers who studied the lack of phenolics in heated olive oil indicated that these compounds deteriorate and the antioxidant capacity is partly lost. Andrikopoulos et al. (2002) determined the losses of polar phenols and alpha-tocopherol during successive pan-frying and deep-frying of olive oil under conditions applied in domestic frying. Brenes et al. (2002) subjected olive oil to simulated domestic frying and heating in a pressure cooker and microwave oven. Lignans were found to be very stable but there were significant losses of hydroxytyrosol derivatives (the main class of antioxidants) and alpha-tocopherol when the oil was heated at frying temperatures. Microwave heating caused lower losses, while in the pressure cooker a rapid hydrolysis of secoiridoidal aglycons was observed and the hydrophilic hydrolysis products were diffused in the water phase. In a recent report Carrasco-Pancorbo et al. (2007) investigated the deterioration of olive oil heated at 180°C. The concentrations of hydroxytyrosol, elenolic acid (not a phenol but present in olive oil), decarboxylated oleuropein, and oleuropein aglycons were reduced more rapidly than other phenols. Hydroxytyrosol acetate and ligstroside aglycon were found to be quite resistant to the treatment, but lignans were even more stable. Heating caused formation of new compounds from the oxidation of phenols not yet identified.

Losses of antioxidant activity of olive oil due to heating, measured by ABTS and DPPH radical decolorization, electron spin resonance, and other methods, were also reported by Carlos-Espin et al. (2000), Pellegrini et al. (2001), Quiles et al. (2002), Gomez-Alonso et al. (2003), and Valavanidis et al. (2004). Kalantzakis et al. (2006) studied the effect of heating on the antioxidant activity of virgin olive oil, refined olive oil, and other vegetable oils by measuring the radical scavenging activity toward the 1,1-diphenyl-2-picrylhydrazyl radical (DPPH·). It was observed that olive oil lost its radical scavenging activity in a shorter heating time relative to other vegetable oils much richer in tocopherols, but it reached the level of 25% total polar content (rejection point for a heated fat) after prolonged heating; all the other oils reached this upper limit in shorter periods. The results demonstrate that virgin olive oil has a remarkable thermal stability but, on the other hand, it should not be seen only as a good frying medium. If health effects are expected from the phytochemicals present, the number of heating operations should be kept to a minimum.

REFERENCES

Alpaslan, M. and Karaali, A., 1998, The interesterification-induced changes in olive oil and palm oil blends, *Food Chem.*, 61, 301–305.

Andrikopoulos, N., Dedousis, G., Falirea, A., Kalogeropoulos, N., and Hatzinikola, H., 2002, Deterioration of natural antioxidants species of vegetable edible oils during the domestic deep-frying and pan-frying of potatoes, *Int. J. Food Sci. Nutr.*, 53, 351–363.

Ansorena, D. and Astiazaran, I., 2004, Effect of storage and packaging on fatty acid composition and oxidation, *Meat Sci.*, 67, 237–244.

Antoun, N. and Tsimidou, M., 1997, Gourmet olive oils: stability and consumer acceptability studies, *Grasas Aceites*, 30, 131–136.

Beauchamp, G., Keast, R., Morel, D., et al., 2005, Ibuprofen-like activity in extra virgin olive oil, *Nature*, 437, 45–46.

Blekas, G. and Boskou, D., 1999, Phytosterols and stability of frying oils, in *Frying of Food*, Boskou, D. and Elmadfa, I., Eds., Technomic Publishing, Lancaster, PA, 205–222.

Boskou, D., 1999, Nonnutrient antioxidants and stability of frying oils, in *Frying of Food*, Boskou, D. and Elmadfa, I., Eds., Technomic Publishing, Lancaster, PA, 183–204.

Boskou, D., 2006, Sources of natural phenolic antioxidants, *Trends Food Sci. Technol.*, 17, 505–512.

Boskou, D. and Chryssafidis, D. 1986, Distribution of isomeric octadecenoic fatty acids in commercially hydrogenated olive oil, *Fette Seifen Anstric.*, 88, 13–15.

Boskou, D. and Karapostolakis, A., 1983, Fatty acid composition and trans isomer content of hardened olive oil, *J. Amer. Oil Chem. Soc.*, 60, 1517–1519.

Brenes, M., Garcia, M.C., and Dobarganes, M.C., 2002, Influence of thermal treatments simulating cooking processes and the polyphenol content in virgin olive oil, *J. Agric. Food Chem.*, 50, 5962–5967.

Carlos-Espin, J., Soler-Rivers, C., and Wichers, J., 2000, Characterization of the total free radical scavenging capacity of vegetable oils and oil fractions using 2,2-diphenyl-1-picrylhydrazyl radical, *J. Agric. Food Chem.*, 48, 648–656.

Carrasco-Pancorbo, A., Cerretani, L., Bendini, A., Segura-Carretero, A., Lerker, G., and Fernandez-Gutierrez, A., 2007, Evaluation of the influence of thermal oxidation on the phenolic composition and the antioxidant activity of extra virgin olive oil, *J. Agric. Food Chem.*, 55, 4771– 4780.

Criado, M., Hernandez-Martin, E., and Otero, C., 2007a, Optimized interesterification of virgin olive oil with a fully hydrogenated fat in batch reactor: effect of mass transfer limitations, *Eur. J. Lipid Sci. Technol.*, 109, 474–485.

Criado, M., Hernandez-Martin, E., Lopez, A., and Otero, C., 2007b, Enzymatic interesterification of extra virgin olive oil with fully hydrogenated fat: characterization of the reaction and its products, *J. Amer. Oil Chem. Soc.*, 84, 717–726.

Cuesta, I., Perez, M., Ruiz-Roso, B., and Varela, G., 1998, Comparative study of the effect on the sardine fatty acid composition during deep frying and canning of olive oil, *Grasas Aceitas*, 49, 371–376.

Damechki, M., Sotiropoulou, S., and Tsimidou, M., 2001, Antioxidant and pro-oxidant factors in oregano and rosemary gourmet olive oils, *Grasas Aceites,* 52, 207–213.

Exarchou, V., Nenadis, N., Tsimidou, M., Gerothanasis, I.P., and Boskou, D., 2002, Antioxidant activities and phenolic composition of extracts from Greek oregano, Greek sage and summer savory, *J. Agric. Food Chem.*, 50, 5294–5299.

Fomuso, L.B., Corredig, M., and Akoh, C.C., 2002, A comparative study of mayonnaise and Italian dressing prepared with lipase-catalyzed transesterified olive oil and caprylic acid. *J. Amer. Oil Chem. Soc.*, 78, 771–774.

Gavriilidou, V. and Boskou, D., 1991, Chemical interesterification of olive oil–tristearin blends for margarines, *J. Sci. Food Sci. Technol.*, 26, 451–456.

Gomez-Alonso, S., Fregapane, G., and Salvador Desamparados, M., 2003, Changes in phenolic composition and antioxidant activity of virgin olive oil during frying, *J. Agric. Food Chem.*, 51, 667–672.

Kalantzakis, G., Blekas, G., Peglidou, K., and Boskou, D., 2006, Stability and radical-scavenging activity of heated olive oil and other vegetable oils, *Eur. J. Lipid Sci. Technol.*, 108, 329–335.

Kalogeropoulos, N., Grigorakis, D., Mylona, A., Falirea, A., and Andrikopoulos, N., 2006, Dietary evaluation of vegetables pan-fried in virgin olive oil following the Greek traditional culinary practice, *Ecol. Food Nutr.*, 45, 105–123.

Kayaardi, S.E. and Gok, V., 2004, Effect of replacing beef fat with olive oil on quality characteristics of Turkish soudjouk (sucuk), *Meat Sci.*, 67, 249–252.

Medina, L., Sacchi, R., Biondi, L., Aubourg, S.P., and Paollino, L., 1998, Effect of packing media on the oxidation of canned tuna lipids. Antioxidant effectiveness of extra virgin olive oil, *J. Agric. Food Chem.*, 46, 1150–1157.

Medina, I., Satue-Gracia, M.T., German, J.B., and Frankel, N., 1999, Comparison of natural polyphenol antioxidants from extra virgin olive oil with synthetic antioxidants in tuna lipids during thermal oxidation, *J. Agric. Food Chem.*, 47, 4873–4879.

Muguerza, E., Ansorena, D., Bloukas, J.G., and Astiasaran, I., 2003, Effect of fat level and partial replacement of pork backfat with olive oil on the lipid oxidation and volatile compounds of Greek dry fermented sausages, *J. Food Sci.*, 68, 1531–1536.

Paraskevopoulou, A., Boskou, D., and Kiosseoglou, V., 2005, Stabilization of olive oil–lemon juice emulsion with polysaccharides, *Food Chem.*, 90, 627–634.

Paraskevopoulou, D., Boskou, D., and Paraskevopoulou, A., 2007, Oxidative stability of olive oil–lemon juice salad dressings stabilized with polysaccharides, *Food Chem.*, 101, 1197–1204.

Pellegrini, N., Visioli, F., Burrati, S., and Brigheti, F., 2001, Direct analysis of total antioxidant activity of olive oil and studies on the influence of heating, *J. Agric. Food Chem.*, 49, 2532–2538.

Quiles, L.J., Ramirez-Tortoza, M.C., Gomez, J.A., Huertas, R.J., and Mataix, J., 2002, Role of vitamin E and phenolic compounds in the antioxidant capacity measured by ESR of virgin olive oil and sunflower oils after frying, *Food Chem.*, 76, 461–468.

Rodenas, S., Merinero, M.C., and Sanchez-Muniz, F., 2005, Dietary exchange of an olive oil and sunflower oil blend for extra virgin olive oil decreases the estimated cardiovascular risk and LDL apolipoprotein AII-concentrations in postmenopausal women, *J. Amer. College Nutr.*, 24(5), 361–369.

Sacchi, R., Paduano, A., Fiore, F., Della Medaglia, D., Ambrosino, M.L., and Medina, I., 2002, Partition behavior of virgin olive oil phenolic compounds in oil–brine mixtures during thermal processing for fish canning, *J. Agric. Food Chem.*, 50, 2830–2835.

Sanchez-Munich, F., Garcia-Linares, M.C., Garcia-Arias, M.T., Bastida, S., and Viejo, J., 2003, Fat and protein from olive oil–fried sardines interact to normalize serum lipoproteins and reduce liver lipids in hypercholesterolemic rats, *Am. Soc. Nutr. Sci.*, 133, 2302–2308.

Tynek, M. and Ledochowska, E., 2005, Structured triacylglycerols containing behenic acid preparation and properties, *J. Food Lipids*, 12, 77–82.

Valavanidis, A.C., Nisiotou, C., Papageorgiou, Y., Kremli, I., Satravelas, N., Zinieris, N., et al., 2004, Comparison of the radical scavenging potential of polar and lipidic fractions of olive oil and other vegetable oils under normal conditions and after thermal treatment, *J. Agric. Food Chem.*, 52, 2358–2365.

Vural, H.P., Havidpour, I., and Ozbas, O., 2004, Effects of interesterified oils and sugarbeet fiber on the quality of frankfurters, *Meat Sci.*, 67, 65–72.

2 Traditional Mediterranean Diet and Health

Dimitrios Trichopoulos and Antonia Trichopoulou

CONTENTS

2.1 THE MEDITERANEAN DIET

The traditional Mediterranean diet refers to dietary patterns found in olive-growing areas of the Mediterranean region since the 1960s. Although different regions in the Mediterranean basin have their own diets, these may be considered as variants of a single entity, the Mediterranean diet. Indeed, the dietary patterns that prevail in the Mediterranean have many common characteristics, most of which stem from the fact that olive oil occupies a central position in all of them. Olive oil is important not only because it has several beneficial properties but also because it emphasizes the consumption of large quantities of vegetables in the form of salads and large quantities of legumes in the form of cooked foods. Other essential components of the Mediterranean diet are wheat, olives, and grapes, and their various derivative products. Total lipid intake may be high, around or in excess of 40% of total energy intake as in Greece, or moderate, around 30% of total energy intake, as in Italy. In all instances, however, the ratio of monounsaturated to saturated fats is much higher than in other places of the world (Trichopoulou and Lagiou, 1997).

From 1995 on, we and others have operationalized the Mediterranean dietary pattern by developing a score that captures the principal aspects of this diet. The score is very simple and has nine components that can be combined into a uni-dimensional variable ranging from 0 (low adherence to Mediterranean diet) to 9 (high adherence to Mediterranean diet). The components are: high olive oil and low saturated fat consumption; high consumption of legumes; high consumption of unrefined cereals; high consumption of fruits; high consumption of vegetables; low consumption of dairy products; high consumption of fish; low consumption of meat and meat products; and moderate wine consumption (Trichopoulou et al., 2003).

2.2 MEDITERRANEAN DIET AND HEALTH

In the Mediterranean region, there has always been a strong, albeit undocumented, belief that olive oil is the elixir of youth and health. It is intriguing that most centenarians in the Mediterranean region have been inclined to attribute their longevity to diet in general, and olive oil and wine consumption in particular — two key ingredients of the Mediterranean diet (Trichopoulou and Lagiou, 1997).

Mortality statistics from the World Health Organization (WHO) database covering the period 1960–1990 (WHO, 1993) provided indirect evidence about the beneficial effect of the Mediterranean diet. Even though health care for many of the Mediterranean populations was inferior to that available to people in northern Europe and North America, and the prevalence of smoking was unusually high among the former (Dalla-Vorgia et al., 1990), death rates in the Mediterranean region were generally lower and adult life expectancy generally higher in comparison to those in the economically more developed countries of northern Europe and North America, particularly among men. Cause-specific mortality statistics indicate that the health advantage of the Mediterranean populations is mainly accounted for by lower mortality rates from coronary heart disease, as well as from cancers of the large bowel, breast, endometrium, and prostate.

The first important epidemiological study to assess the postulated advantages of the Mediterranean diet was undertaken by Ancel Keys. This classic international study was launched by Keys and colleagues in the 1950s and involved 12,763 men, ages 40–59 years, in 16 sub-cohorts: 2 in Greece, 3 in Italy, 5 in what was then Yugoslavia, 2 in Japan, 2 in Finland, 1 in the Netherlands, and 1 in the United States (Keys, 1980). The results of the Keys study were interpreted as indicating that saturated fats could largely account for the variation of total cholesterol and, inferentially, the incidence of coronary heart disease. The argument of several scientists from Mediterranean countries, that the diet of their region is more than a low saturated fat diet and has implications for diseases other than coronary heart disease, was lost in the wider scientific community (Trichopoulou, 1988). From the late 1990s, however, a plethora of studies has provided strong evidence that the Mediterranean diet overall, as an integral pattern, and its central component, olive oil, are important components of a healthy lifestyle.

2.3 SELECTED ANALYTICAL STUDIES

Adherence to the traditional Mediterranean diet has been assessed in many studies, including those undertaken by our group, using the previously indicated Mediterranean diet score that incorporates the salient characteristics of this diet or variations of this score. The results of some relevant studies that have been published recently indicate the following:

- A higher degree of adherence to the Mediterranean diet in Greece is associated with a reduction in total mortality. A significant inverse association is evident for both death due to coronary heart disease and death due to cancer. Associations between individual food groups contributing to the Mediterranean diet score and total or cause-specific mortality are generally weak (Trichopoulou et al., 2003).
- The previously indicated Mediterranean diet score, modified so as to apply across Europe, was associated with increased survival among older people in most European populations (Trichopoulou et al., 2005c).
- Adherence to the Mediterranean diet in variable ways, chosen at will by coronary patients in the general population, is associated with a significant reduction in long-term fatality of individuals who have already suffered from a coronary attack (Trichopoulou et al., 2005a).
- Adherence to the Mediterranean diet and, in particular, high consumption of olive oil are inversely associated with arterial blood pressure (Psaltopoulou et al., 2004).
- The Mediterranean diet does not substantially affect body mass index and the high prevalence of overweight in Mediterranean countries is accounted for by the high prevalence of inactivity in conjunction with relative excess of energy intake (Trichopoulou et al., 2005b).
- Randomized studies and other major investigations in Spain, France, and Italy have provided powerful evidence in support of the beneficial properties of the Mediterranean diet

and have pointed out several of the implicated physiologic mechanisms (Esposito et al., 2004; Vincent-Baundry et al., 2005; Estruch et al., 2006; Fitó et al., 2007).

2.4 CONCLUDING REMARKS

It is not obvious that the Mediterranean diet can fully explain the relatively good health of Mediterranean people. It has been suggested that the pattern of eating and drinking may have elusive synergistic effects. Others have argued that the relaxing psychosocial environment in most Mediterranean countries, the mild climatic conditions, the preservation of the extended family structure, or even the afternoon siesta habit may play contributory roles (Naska et al., 2007). Nevertheless, it is highly likely that diet is essential for the good health of the Mediterranean peoples.

The Mediterranean diet may offer a healthy alternative approach to a low animal fat diet. Its expanded range of options could promote adherence, particularly over the long term. The Mediterranean diet is not sharply different from other recommended diets. Two elements, however, distinguish it from these other diets. It stresses the pattern rather than individual components and provides no restriction on intake of lipids, so long as they are not saturated and are preferably in the form of olive oil.

REFERENCES

Dalla-Vorgia, P., Sasco, A., Skalkidis, Y., Katsouyanni, K., and Trichopoulos, D., 1990, An evaluation of the effectiveness of tobacco-control legislative policies in European Community countries, *Scand. J. Soc. Med.,* 18, 81–89.

Esposito, K., Marfella, R., Ciotola, M., Di Palo, C., Giugliano, F., Giugliano, G., et al., 2004, Effect of a mediterranean-style diet on endothelial dysfunction and markers of vascular inflammation in the metabolic syndrome: a randomized trial, *J.A.M.A.,* 292, 1490–1492.

Estruch, R., Martínez-González, M.A., Corella, D., Salas-Salvadó, J., Ruiz-Gutiérrez, V., Covas, M.I., Fiol, M., Gómez-Gracia, E., López-Sabater, M.C., Vinyoles, E., Arós, F., Conde, M., Lahoz, C., Lapetra, J., Sáez, G., and Ros, E., PREDIMED study investigators, 2006, *Ann. Intern. Med.,* 145, 1–11.

Fitó, M., Guxens, M., Corella, D., Sáez, G., Estruch, R., de la Torre, R., et al., 2007, Effect of a traditional Mediterranean diet on lipoprotein oxidation: a randomized controlled trial, *Arch. Intern. Med.,* 167, 1195–1203.

Keys, A.B., 1980, *Seven Countries: A Multivariate Analysis of Death and Coronary Heart Disease,* Harvard University Press, Cambridge, MA.

Naska, A., Oikonomou, E., Trichopoulou, A., Psaltopoulou, T., and Trichopoulos, D., 2007, Siesta of healthy adults and coronary mortality in the general population, *Arch. Int. Med.,* 167, 296–301.

Psaltopoulou, Th., Naska, A., Orfanos, Ph., Trichopoulos, D., Mountokalakis, Th., and Trichopoulou, A., 2004, Olive oil, Mediterranean diet and arterial blood pressure: the Greek EPIC study, *Am. J. Clin. Nutr.,* 80, 1012–1018.

Trichopoulou, A., Rapporteur, 1988, The Mediterranean Diet and Food Culture. What, Why, How? Report of a World Health Organization (Europe) Meeting, Delphi, Greece.

Trichopoulou, A. and Lagiou, P., 1997, Healthy traditional Mediterranean diet: an expression of culture, history and lifestyle, *Nutr. Rev.,* 55, 383–389.

Trichopoulou, A., Costacou, T., Bamia, C., and Trichopoulos, D., 2003, Adherence to a Mediterranean diet and survival in a Greek population, *N. Engl. J. Med.,* 348, 2599–2608.

Trichopoulou, A., Bamia, C., and Trichopoulos, D., 2005a, Mediterranean diet and survival among patients with coronary heart disease in Greece, *Arch. Intern. Med.,* 165, 929–935.

Trichopoulou, A., Naska, A., Orfanos, Ph., and Trichopoulos, D., 2005b, Mediterranean diet in relation to body mass index and waist-to-hip ratio: the Greek European Prospective Investigation into Cancer and Nutrition Study, *Am. J. Clin. Nutr.,* 82, 935–940.

Trichopoulou, A., Orfanos, P., Norat, T., et al., 2005c, Modified-Mediterranean diet and survival: the EPIC-Elderly prospective cohort study, *Brit. Med. J.,* 330, 991–998.

Vincent-Baudry, S., Defoort, C., Gerber, M., Bernard, M.C., Verger, P., Helal, O., et al., 2005, The Medi-RIVAGE study: reduction of cardiovascular disease risk factors after a 3-mo intervention with a Mediterranean-type diet or a low-fat diet, *Am. J. Clin. Nutr.,* 82, 964–971.

WHO, 1993, Health for All — Statistical Database, World Health Organization, Regional Office for Europe.

3 Phenolic Compounds in Olives and Olive Oil

Dimitrios Boskou

CONTENTS

3.1 PHENOLIC COMPOSITION: CHEMISTRY, LEVELS, PROPERTIES

3.1.1 POLAR PHENOLIC COMPOUNDS PRESENT IN OLIVE OIL

Over the last 20 years most of the major polar phenolic compounds present in virgin olive oil have been detected and quantified. These phenolic compounds may be phenolic acids, simple phenols like tyrosol and hydroxytyrosol, secoiridoid derivatives of the glycosides oleuropein and ligstrodide, lignans, flavonoids, and hydroxyl-isochromans (Caruso et al., 2000; Owen et al., 2000; Tovar et al., 2001; Servili and Montedoro, 2002; Romero, C. et al., 2002; Brenes et al., 2002; Gutierrez-Rosales et al., 2003; Gomez-Alonso et al., 2003; Cerretani et al., 2005a; Boskou, D. et al., 2006; Parenti et al., 2006; Fregapane et al., 2006; Romani et al., 2007; Bendini et al., 2007). The term "polar phenolic compounds" is used to differentiate them from another class of phenols, the tocopherols. Olive oil polar phenol fraction, known for many years as "polyphenols," is in fact a complex mixture of compounds with varying chemical structures obtained from virgin olive oil by liquid-liquid partition with methanol/water (see Chapter 5).

In addition to the classes of compounds mentioned above, other phenols with different structures (e.g., vanillin) have been identified. Litridou et al. (1997) reported the presence of an ester of tyrosol with a dicarboxylic acid. The same authors demonstrated that total polar phenol and o-diphenol content was higher in the less polar part of the methanol extract. This part contains mainly the dialdehydic and decarboxymethyl forms of elenolic acid linked to hydroxytyrosol and tyrosol, hydroxytyrosol acetate, lignans, and luteolin. Brenes et al. (2004) identified 4-ethylphenol in all the oils intended for refining and particularly in the "second centrifugation olive oils," due to the paste storage.

Glycosides were also found to be present in olive oil but only in trace amounts (Garcia et al., 2001). Another class of compounds, hydroxy-isochromans, was identified by Bianco and co-workers (Bianco et al., 2001). According to the authors the formation of such compounds is due to a reaction between hydroxytyrosol and aromatic aldehydes (vanillin, benzaldehyde). The phenol present in olive fruit linked as an ester to the aglycon moiety of oleuropein is freed during malaxation of the olive pulp by enzymes. This hydrolysis process also favors the formation of carbonyl compounds and thus hydoxy-isochromans are formed.

Some of the identified secoiridoid compounds like the aldehydic form of oleuropein have stereochemical isomers (see also Chapter 5). The presence of such isomers was confirmed by coupling high-performance liquid chromatography with post-column solid-phase extraction to nuclear magnetic resonance spectroscopy (Christophoridou et al., 2005).

 The identification of the methyl acetals of the aglycon of ligstroside and of the β-hydroxytyrosol ester of methyl malate (Bianco et al., 2006), the study of oleocanthal by Beauchamp et al. (2005), a tyrosol derivative that has the same pharmacological activity as the anti-inflammatory drug ibuprofen, and other studies indicating an anti-inflammatory activity (Bitler et al., 2005) provide important new information for the forms of tyrosol and hydroxytyrosol derivatives present in olive oil and olives, some of which may be antioxidant and/or biologically active. Thus, quantification of some forms of aglycons may be important (in addition to the total polar phenols content) for the evaluation of quality, stability, and nutritional value.

The polar fraction may also contain nonphenolic but related compounds like cinammic acid and elenolic acid. The main phenolic and nonphenolic compounds reported to be present in the polar fraction of virgin olive oil belong to the following classes (see Figures 3.1 through 3.7):

Phenolic acids
  Hydroxybenzoic acids
      4-Hydroxybenzoic
      Protocatechuic
      Gallic
      Vanillic acid
      Syringic acid
  Hydroxyphenylacetic acids
      4-Hydroxyphenylacetic
      Homovanillic
  Hydroxycinnamic acids
      o-Coumaric
      p-Coumaric
      Caffeic
      Ferulic
      Sinapic
 Phenolic alcohols
    (*p*-Hydroxyphenyl)ethanol (*p*-HPEA, tyrosol)
    (3,4-Dihydroxyphenyl)ethanol (3,4-DHPEA, hydroxytyrosol)
    Homovanillyl alcohol
Derivatives of phenolic alcohols
    4-(Acetoxyethyl)-1,2-dihydroxybenzene
    Hydroxytyrosol ester of methyl malate
Glycosides
    Oleuropein (an ester of hydroxytyrosol with β-glucosylated elenolic acid)
    Ligstroside
Aglyconic derivatives of oleuropein and ligstroside
    Dialdehydic form of elenolic acid linked to 3,4-DHPEA (3,4-DHPEA-EDA)
    Dialdehydic form of elenolic acid linked to *p*-HPEA (*p*-HPEA-EDA)
    Dialdehydic form of decarboxymethyl elenolic acid linked to 3,4-DHPEA
    Dialdehydic form of decarboxymethyl elenolic acid linked to *p*-DHPEA
    Oleuropein aglycon (3,4-DHPEA-EA)
    Ligstroside aglycon (*p*-HPA-EA)
    Methyl acetal of the aglycone of ligstroside
    10-Hydroxy-oleuropein
Lignans
    (+)-1-Acetoxypinoresinol
    (+)-Pinoresinol
    (+)-1-Hydroxypinoresinol
    Syringaresinol
Flavonoids
    Apigenin
    Luteolin
    Taxifolin
 Hydroxy-isochromans
    1-Phenyl-6,7-dihydroxy-isochroman
    1-(3′-Methoxy-4′-hydroxy)phenyl-6,7-dihydroxy-isochroman
Other phenols
    Vanillin (4-hydroxy-3-methoxybenzaldehyde)
    4-Ethylphenol (not found in virgin olive oils but in oils of "second centrifugation," intended
      for refining)
Nonphenolic compounds
    Cinnamic acid
    Elenolic acid
    Elenolic acid glycoside
    11-Methyl oleoside

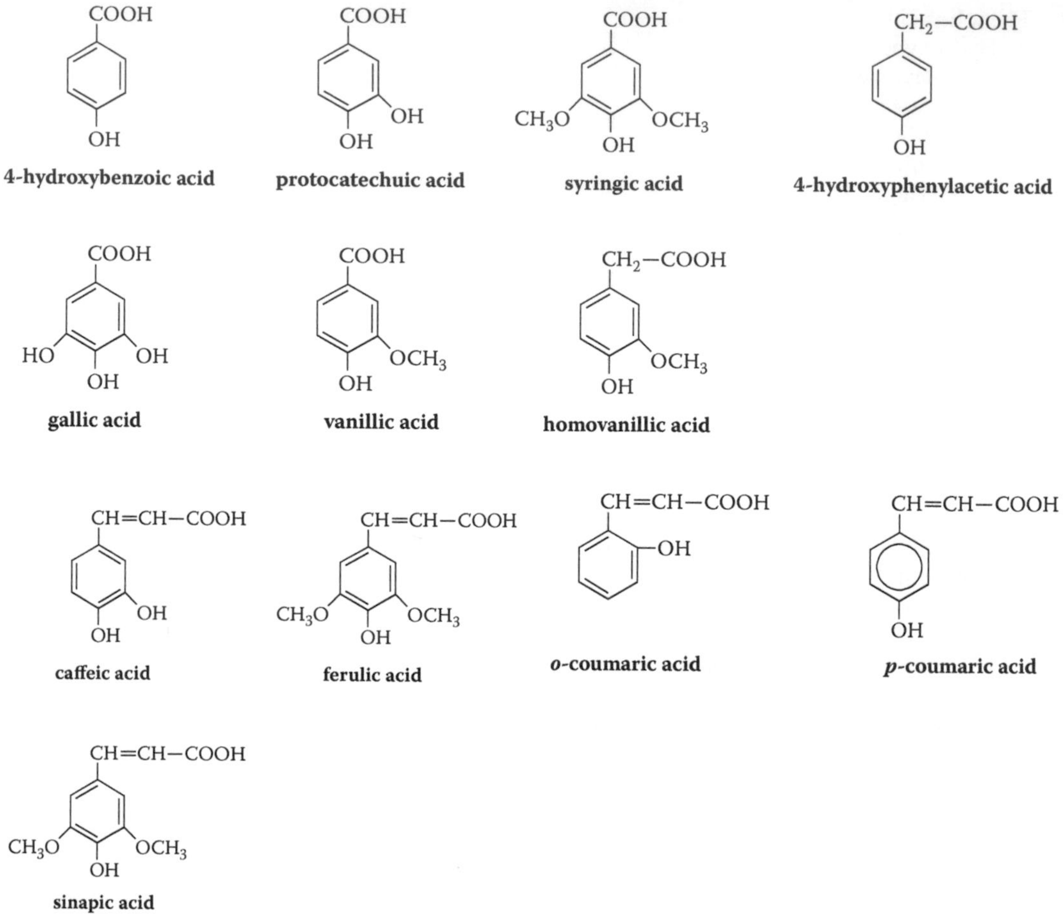

COOH
4-hydroxybenzoic acid

COOH
OH
OH
protocatechuic acid

COOH
CH₃O   OCH₃
OH
syringic acid

CH₂—COOH
OH
4-hydroxyphenylacetic acid

COOH
HO   OH
OH
gallic acid

COOH
OCH₃
OH
vanillic acid

CH₂—COOH
OCH₃
OH
homovanillic acid

CH=CH—COOH
OH
OH
caffeic acid

CH=CH—COOH
CH₃O   OCH₃
OH
ferulic acid

CH=CH—COOH
OH
o-coumaric acid

CH=CH—COOH
OH
p-coumaric acid

CH=CH—COOH
CH₃O   OCH₃
OH
sinapic acid

FIGURE 3.1   Structural formulae of phenolic acids.

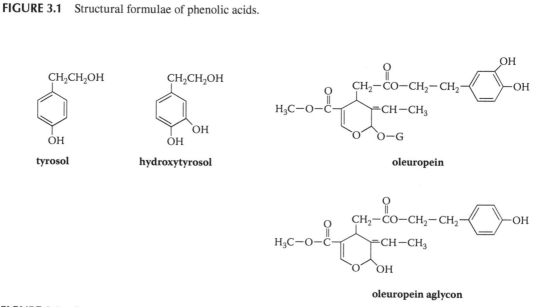

tyrosol

hydroxytyrosol

oleuropein

oleuropein aglycon

FIGURE 3.2   Structural formulae of tyrosol, hydroxytyrosol, and derivatives.

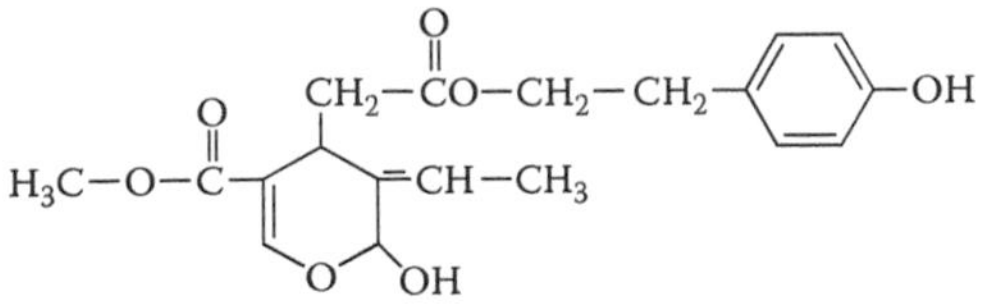

ligstroside aglycon

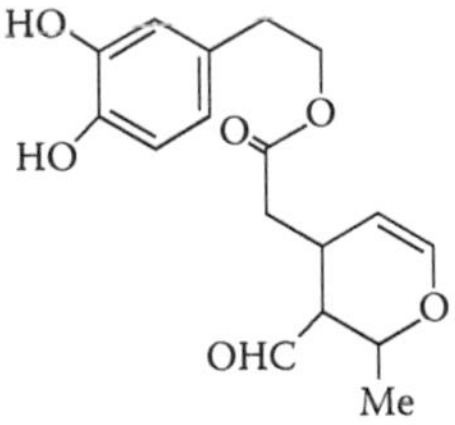

decarboxymethyl form of oleuropein aglycon

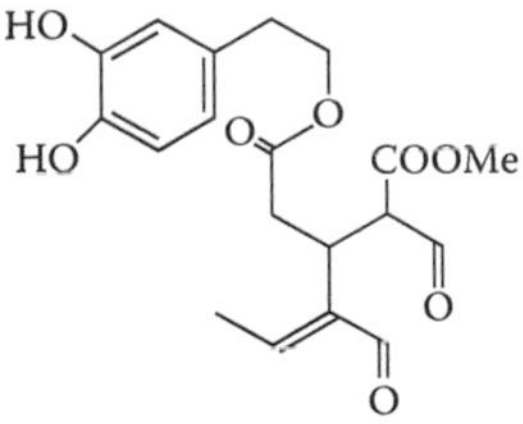

dialdehydic form of oleuropein aglycon

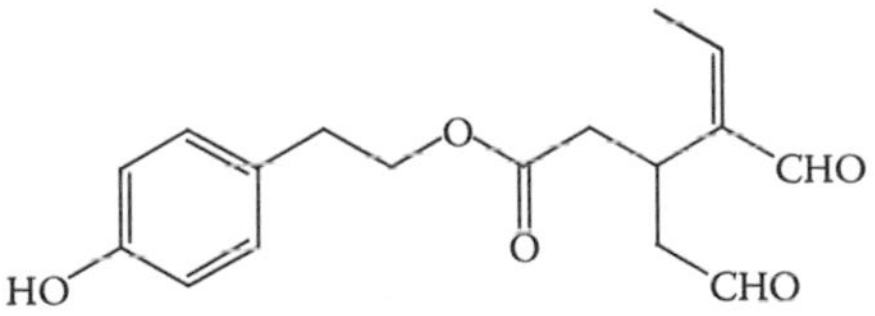

oleocanthal (the decarboxylated dialdehydic form of ligstroside aglycon)

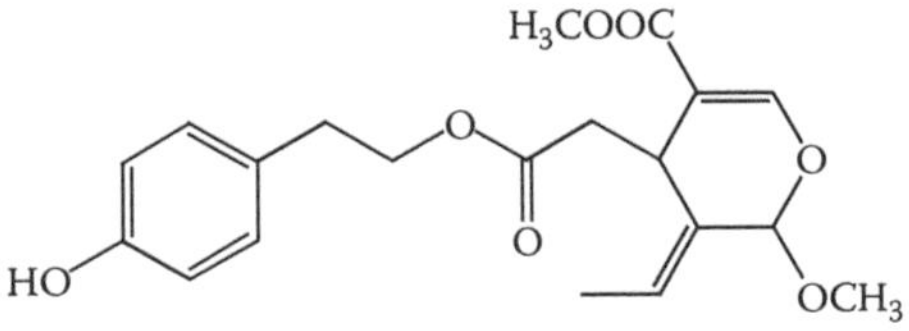

methyl acetal of the aglycon of ligstroside

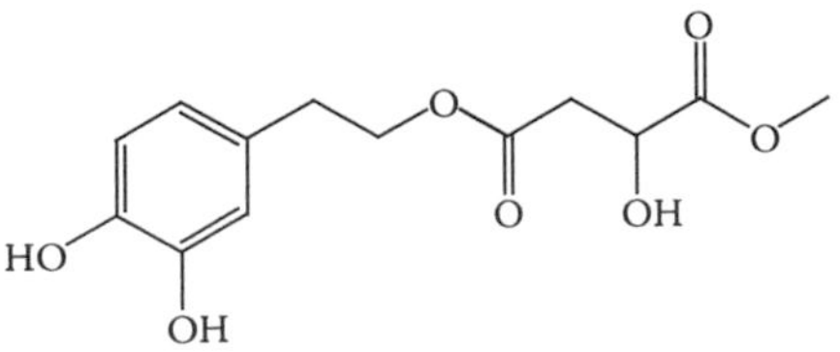

hydroxytyrosol ester of methyl malate

FIGURE 3.2 (continued) Structural formulae of tyrosol, hydroxytyrosol, and derivatives.

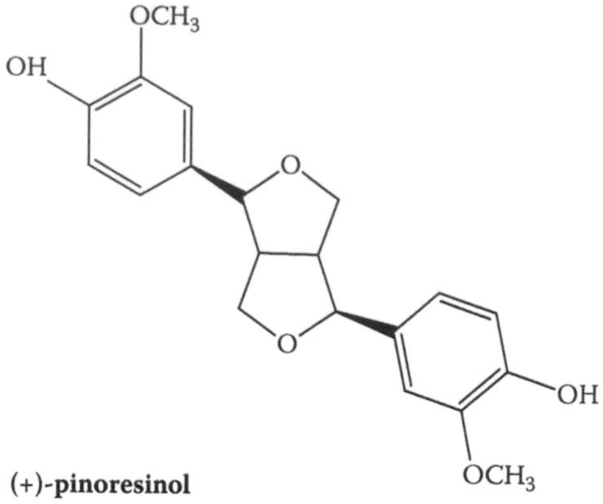

(+)-pinoresinol

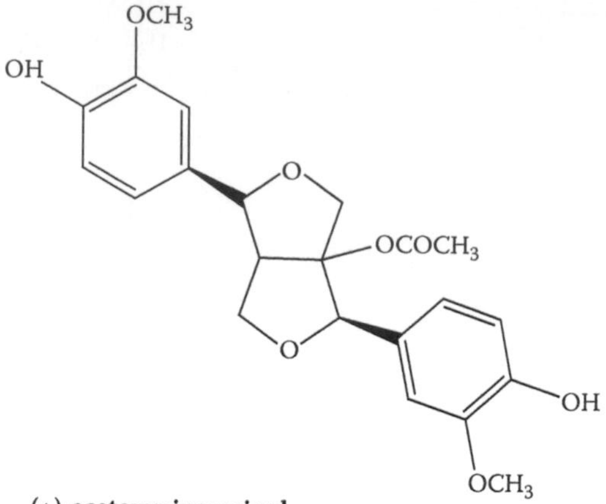

(+)-acetoxypinoresinol

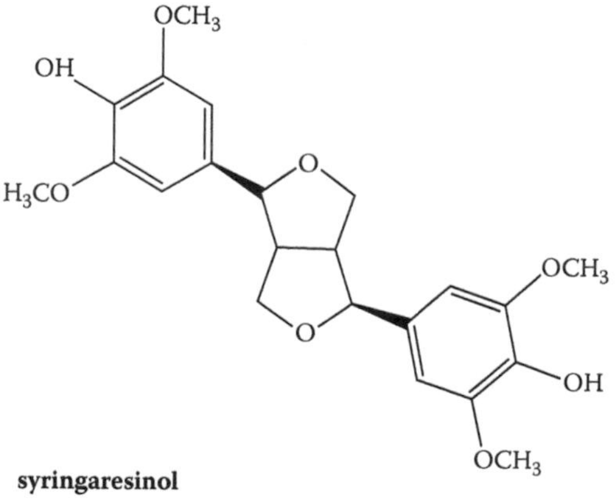

syringaresinol

FIGURE 3.3 Structural formulae of lignans.

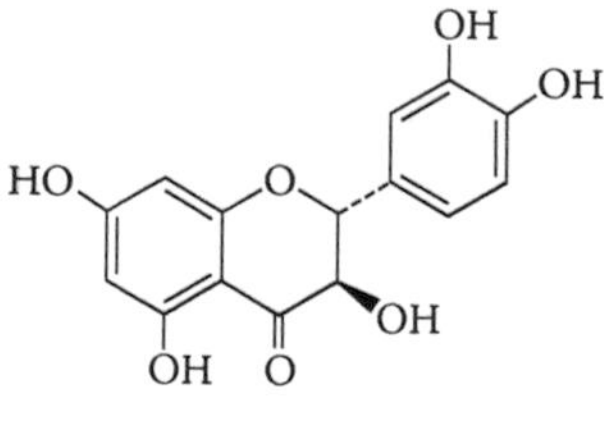

(+)-taxifolin

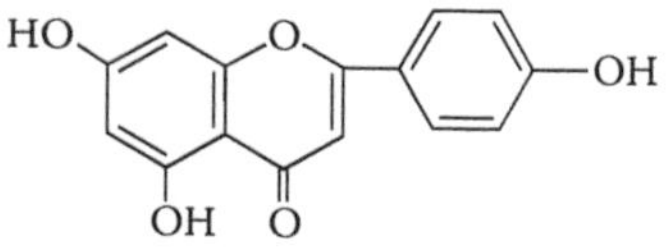

apigenin

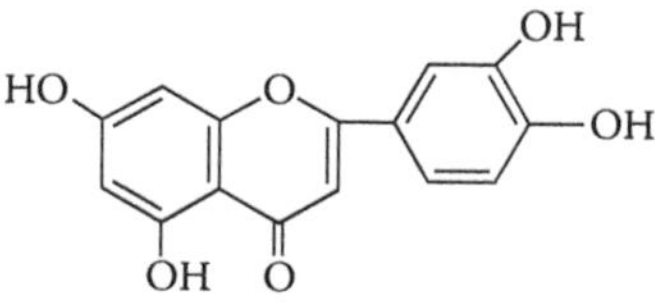

luteolin

FIGURE 3.4 Structural formulae of flavonoids.

hydroxy-isochromans

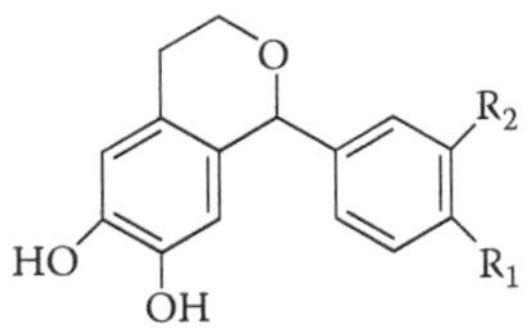

1-phenyl-6, 7-dihydroxychroman R$_1$, R$_2$ = H

1-(3′-methoxy-4′-hydroxy) phenyl-6, 7-dihydroxychroman R$_1$ = −OH, R$_2$ = −OCH$_3$

FIGURE 3.5 Structural formulae of hydroxy-isochromans.

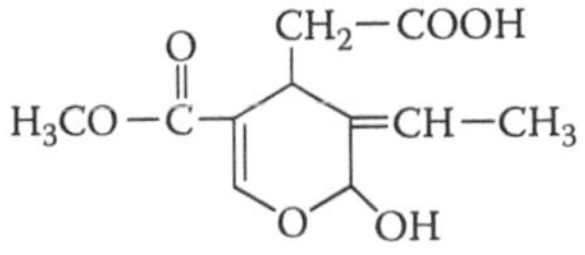

elenolic acid

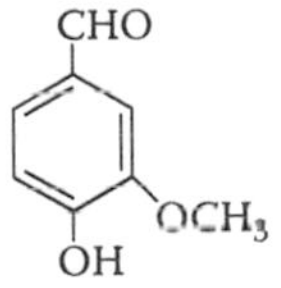

vanillin

cinnamic acid

FIGURE 3.6 Vanillin.

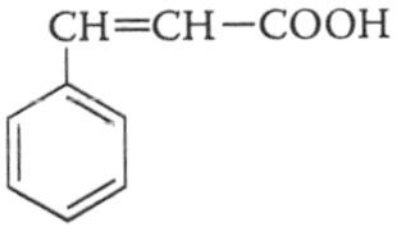

FIGURE 3.7 Nonphenolic compounds.

3.1.2 LEVELS

Wide ranges (50–1000 mg/kg) have been reported for the levels of total polar phenols in olive oils. Usual values range between 100 and 300 mg/kg (Boskou D. et al., 2006). The most abundant phenolic compounds in virgin olive oil are aglycons deriving from secoiridoids present in the fruit. These substances are relatively polar and they are partitioned between the oil and the vegetation water.

The effect of variety, system of extraction, conditions of prossessing, packing, distribution, and storage have been discussed by Aparicio and Luna (2002), Salvador et al. (2003), and Boskou D. et al. (2006). Due to natural variability and strong dependence on so many factors (and especially the index of maturation), it is difficult to establish levels for individual phenols. Servili and Montedoro (2002) gave average values from the analysis of 116 samples of industrial olive oils for hydroxytyrosol, tyrosol, vanillic acid, caffeic acid, 3,4-DHPEA-DEA, p-HPEA-EDA, and 3,4-DHPEA-EA. The prevailing phenols were 3,4-DHPEA-EDA (range 63–840 mg/kg), 3,4-DHPEA-EA (range 85–310 mg/kg), and p-HPEA-EDA (range 15–33 mg/kg). Free hydroxytyrosol and tyrosol were found only in trace amounts (less than 10 mg/kg oil).

In a recent paper Romani and co-corkers (Romani et al., 2007) analyzed samples of bottled extra virgin olive oil from a specific Italian cultivar and provided a graphic representation of the levels of total minor polar compounds, hydroxytyrosol, tyrosol, elenolic acid derivatives, deacetoxy-oleuropein aglycon, oleuropein aglycon, other secoiridoid derivatives, and the flavones luteolin and apigenin. Total minor polar components concentration was 350 mg/kg. This concentration is mainly due to a secoiridoid group of compounds (binding with tyrosol and hydroxytyrosol), deacetoxy-oleuropein aglycone, and elenolic acid. The authors conclude that secoiridoids, particularly deacetoxy-oleuropein-aglycon, should be monitored to evaluate olive oil stability during storage. However, this study ignores the levels of two major components, lignans and hydroxytyrosol acetate (4-acetoxyethyl-1,2-dihydroxybenzene). Lignans were found to range from 112–275 mg/kg in virgin olive oils from Arbequina cv and hydroxytyrosol acetate from 21–131 mg/kg (Tovar et al., 2001). M.P. Romero et al. (2002) gave even higher values for hydroxytyrosol acetate and lignans in virgin olive oils from young olive trees grown under different deficit irrigation strategies. Brenes and co-investigators (Brenes et al., 2001) reported values ranging from 3–67 mg/kg for 1-acetoxypinoresinol and from 19–41 mg/kg for pinoresinol in five Spanish olive oils. The two compounds were identified on the basis of their mass spectra and ^{13}C NMR spectra. 1-Acetoxypinoresinol as determined by combined gas chromatography–mass spectrometry was used by Brenes et al. (2002) as a means to authenticate Picual olive oils. The level of this phenol in this cultivar is much lower in comparison to other Spanish varieties.

Luteolin levels were reported to be around 10 mg/kg in some Spanish olive oils (Brenes et al., 1999). Murkovic et al. (2004) reported values ranging from 0.2–7 mg/kg for Greek olive oils. Usually, the glucosides of flavonoids decrease with maturation, but at the same time the production of free aglycons could increase. Thus, higher concentrations of free flavones may be found. Biochemical routes and changes of the main individual phenols (hydroxytyrosol, tyrosol, vanillic acid, p-coumaric acid, ferulic acid, vanillin, apigenin, luteolin, hydroxytyrosol acetate, and glycoside aglycons) during maturation have also been studied by Brenes (Brenes et al., 1999).

3.1.3 EFFECT ON THE STABILITY

Polar phenols and tocopherols are important for the stability of virgin olive oil. This effect has been discussed extensively (Papadopoulos et al., 1993; Gennaro et al., 1998; Monteleone et al., 1998; Brenes et al., 2001; Cinquanta et al., 2001; Mateos et al., 2003; Boskou, D. et al., 2006; Rahmouni et al., 2006; Tsimidou, 2006). Some important aspects related to the oxidative stability of virgin olive oil during storage as well as at the high temperatures of food preparation have also been discussed by Velasco and Dobarganes (2002). The crucial role of polar phenolic compounds has been well established. Most of the phenols present in olive oil are antioxidant compounds, but the components that are mainly responsible for the remarkable resistance of olive oil to oxidation are the dialdeydic form of elenolic acid linked to hydroxytyrosol (3,4-DHPEA-EDA), decarboxymethyl oleuropein aglycon, and hydroxytyrosol (Baldioli et al., 1996; Fogliano et al., 1999; Briante et al., 2001; Gutierrez-Rosales and Arnaud, 2001; Gomez-Alonso et al., 2003; Mateos et al., 2003; Carrasco-Pancorbo et al., 2006; Romani et al., 2007). Tyrosol, lignans, and ligstroside aglycon are weaker antioxidants. Morello and co-investigators (Morello et al., 2004) studied the changes in the phenolic fraction and the oil during storage. These changes indicate that secoiridoids and hydoxytyrosol acetate contribute most to the stability. Gennaro et al. (1998) evaluated by thermogravimetric analysis the stability of olive oil spiked with different amounts of phenols such as tyrosol, hydroxytyrosol, oleuropein, oleuropein aglycon, caffeic acid, and BHT. Their data showed that the natural antioxidants present in olive oil and especially hydroxytyrosol and its derivatives can extend the olive oil shelf life and protect it from decomposition occurring during thermal treatment.

According to Owen and co-investigators (Owen et al., 2000a,b), lignans constitute an important contribution to the phenolic fraction of olive oil and therefore may contribute to the stability of the oil.

Phenolic compounds can inhibit oxidation in many ways. Three known mechanisms are radical scavenging, hydrogen atom transfer, and metal chelating. Bendini et al. (2006) conducted a study to investigate the protective effect of olive oil phenols on the oxidative stability of the oil in the presence and absence of copper ions. The experimental results of this study also indicate that polar phenols reduce the oxidized forms of alpha-tocopherol and that certain oleuropein aglycons possess a copper-chalating ability. Tocopherols are more quickly consumed in olive oils that have low content of ortho-diphenols.

The antioxidant activity of phenols is enhanced by the presence of tocopherols (Blekas et al., 1995; Pellegrini et al., 2001). This synergism is more evident when the level of phenols is relatively low. The contribution of tocopherols to radical-scavenging activity was 39–61% in virgin olive oil, which suggests that both tocopherols and phenolic compounds contribute to radical-scavenging activity, according to Jiang et al. (2005).

In olive oil models devoid of prooxidants and antioxidants the effect of alpha-tocopherols was antioxidant in the range of polar phenols concentration 100–1000 mg/kg. The best effect was found for the lowest levels of addition (Blekas et al., 1995; Baldioli et al., 1996). This is explained probably by the participation of tocopherols in the autoxidation process after a sufficient amount of hydroxyperoxides is accumulated, although Morello and co-workers (Morello et al., 2004) claimed that alpha-tocopherol is consumed from the beginning. In all cases, although not as strong an antioxidant as polar phenols, alpha-tocopherol contributes significantly to the oil's resistance to autoxidation. Baldioli et al. (1996) observed a synergistic effect of 3,4-DEPEA and its oleosidic forms with tocopherol during autoxidation of an olive oil–purified triacylglycerol mixture.

It has also been suggested that luteolin and apigenin present in olive oil in minute quantities may have a synergistic action (Visioli et al., 2002), but this has to be verified by more experimental work.

3.1.4 Bitter Index, Bitter Phenols, Pungency

Bitterness is a sensorial characteristic related to the presence of phenols. It is more pronounced in certain olive oil varieties and it can be enhanced if this is desirable from nonripe fruits. During ripening bitterness decreases.

The standard method of evaluating the bitter taste is by sensory analysis using a panel of tasters, but instrumental methods have also been proposed. *Bitter index* can be evaluated by the extraction of the bitter substances of an oil sample dissolved in hexane and passed through a C18 cartridge. The cartridge is previously activated with methanol. The cartridge is washed with hexane to remove liposoluble substances and the retained compounds are eluted with a methanol–water mixture 1:1 and diluted to 25 ml. The absorbance is measured at 225 nm in a 1-cm cuvette and the results are expressed as specific UV absorbance (Gutierrez et al., 1992; Garcia et al., 1996; Tovar et al., 2001; Romero, M.P. et al., 2002; Morello et al., 2004). The intensity, measured at 225 nm, is closely related to the intensity of bitter taste estimated by a panel of tasters.

Gutierrez-Rosales et al. (2003) correlated bitter intensity of a large number of virgin olive oil samples with the concentration of individual phenols. Solid phase extraction, preparative high-performance liquid chromatography (HPLC), analytical HPLC, and online liquid chromatography–electrospray ionization mass spectrometry were used to separate, identify, and determine the concentration of individual phenols. The dialdehydic and aldehydic forms of decarboxymethyl oleuropein aglycon and the dialdehydic form of decarboxymethyl-ligstroside aglycon were found to be the components mainly responsible for the bitter taste. These compounds and derivatives or isomers of ligstroside and oleuropein aglycons, which were all bitter, were tentatively identified by Andrewes and his research team (Andrewes et al., 2003), who attempted to establish a relation between sensory properties and level of individual phenols. The fraction containing deacetoxy-ligstroside aglycon produced a strong, burning, pungent sensation at the back of the throat. Oils rich in this compound were oils with a pungent taste. The deacetoxy oleuropein aglycon gave a slightly burning sensation; tyrosol was found to be astringent but not bitter.

Mateos and collaborators (Mateos et al., 2004) identified the main compounds that are responsible for the bitterness. They correlated the intensity of bitterness with the concentration of secoiridoids as determined by HPLC and proposed a method of evaluation of bitterness based on the quantification of secoiridoid derivatives. The compounds mainly responsible for the bitter taste were found to be the dialdehydic forms of decarboxymethyl oleuropein and ligstroside aglycons, and the aldehydic forms of oleuropein and ligstroside aglycons.

Siliani et al. (2006) attempted to define the contribution of each individual phenol to the bitter sensory note. Concentrations of secoiridoids and lignans were processed as a function of bitter intensity by regression analysis. The results of their study confirmed that there is a positive correlation between total phenolic content and bitter intensity. The highest statistical significance was obtained from the exponential relationship between oleuropein aglycon (3,4-DHPEA-EA) and bitter intensity.

In a recent report Beltran et al. (2007) tried to establish a relationship between phenol content and K225. They also obtained a prediction model for the intensity of bitterness based on the phenol content. In order to provide an easy means to estimate bitterness, oils were classified by their phenol content in four categories. Oils with nonbitter taste or with almost imperceptible bitterness correspond to levels lower than 220 mg phenols per kilogram. Slightly bitter oils correspond to 220–340 mg/kg, bitter oils have a total phenol content ranging from 340–410 mg/kg, and very bitter oils have polar phenols content higher than 410 mg/kg. The study was based on the analysis of a big number of oils from the cultivars Frantoio, Holiblanca, Picual, and Arbequina.

Oleocanthal. Freshly pressed extra virgin olive oil contains a compound that has the same pharmacological activity as the nonsteroidal anti-inflammatory drug ibuprofen. A recent paper by Beauchamp and his research team (Beauchamp et al., 2005) pointed out that the dialdehydic form of deacetoxy-ligstroside aglycon is structurally related to the anti-inflammatory drug ibuprofen. This compound was identified in the past as a key factor for pungency (Andrewes et al., 2003). The authors demonstrate that this aglycon shares with ibuprofen the throat-irritating sensation and the ability to inhibit the cyclooxygenase enzymes COX-1 and COX-2. These findings offer a possible explanation for some of the various health benefits attributed to a Mediterranean diet rich in olive oil; the authors, based on a daily consumption of approximately 10 mg of oleocanthal, suggested that the cardiovascular-protective effects of the Mediterranean diet may be expected from the regular intake of this secoiridoid aglycon. The conclusions of this study stimulated the interest of the mass media, especially in countries surrounding the Mediterranean Sea where olive oil is the staple fat. The theory was critically discussed by Vincenzo Fogliano (2006), who examined the levels of possible daily intake in relation to the level of oleocanthal in acceptably bitter olive oils and also intestinal absorption and biotransformation. Fogliano concluded that there is no doubt that olive oil may modify body functions but it should be evaluated using a more general approach that takes into consideration all the compounds present and not just any single one. It is more likely that other structurally related phenols enhance the anti-inflammatory action of oleocanthal.

3.2 STRATEGIES TO PRESERVE NATURAL ANTIOXIDANTS IN OLIVE OIL

Levels of individual phenols in olive oil vary because of the natural variability and the dependence on ripeness, history of production, and age. Free phenols are found at higher levels in stored oils; fresh oils contain more complex forms of secoiridoid aglycons. The biotransformation of phenolic compounds in *Olea europaea* L., the importance of agronomic factors and variety, and the effect of maturation on the fate of phenolics in various cultivars have been discussed by many authors (Amiot, 1989; Esti et al., 1998; Brenes et al., 1999; Ranalli et al., 2000; Briante et al., 2001; Ryan et al., 2002; Briante et al., 2002a,b; Boskou D. et al., 2006; Cipriani et al., 2006; Cerretani et al., 2006).

3.2.1 IRRIGATION

Growing conditions are important for olive oil quality (Patumi et al., 2002). Regulated deficit irrigation strategies applied to olive trees have been found to affect polar phenols content and consequently the bitter index and oxidative stability (Romero et al., 2002; Tovar et al., 2002). The effect of full irrigation and deficit irrigation on the various classes of olive oil polar phenols was investigated also by Servili et al. (2007).

3.2.2 Harvest Time

The evaluation of the influence of olive oil degree of ripeness on its oxidative stability is important for the assessment of overall quality. The decision to produce a pungent olive oil or a mellower product is based on many factors such as cultivar, processing, and time of harvest. The latter is the most important factor. Studies conducted on the level of phenolic substances indicated that during ripening the concentration of phenols increases gradually to a maximum level and decreases rapidly as ripening is progressing. The lowest amount of phenolic compounds is observed at the black stage of maturation. The peak is at the half pigmentation stage; oils produced from olives harvested at such a pigmentation stage may present higher stability and better sensorial profiles. Salvador et al. (2001) conducted a study to correlate fruit ripening with analytical parameters determining oil quality. For the Cornicarba olives they found that the best stage for processing of the olives is the stage when the ripeness is between 3.0 and 4.5 (as determined by the International Olive Oil Council method). However, it is difficult to generalize as to where the optimal point is, and in spite of the number of relative studies, there is much to be learned about each individual olive cultivar (Garcia et al., 1986, 1996; Ranalli et al., 2000; Rotondi et al., 2004; Mailer et al., 2005; Boskou, D. et al., 2006; Cipriani, 2006; Van Hoed et al., 2006).

3.2.3 Processing

Currently, technological improvements in the olive oil industry are oriented to the preservation of minor constituents originally present in the fruits that are related to important nutritional properties, stability, and quality of the oil. By modulating technology it is possible to some extent to optimize the transfer of some polar minor constituents into the oil or reduce their level in the case of extremely pungent oils.

The main systems currently applied for the extraction of olive oil from olives are pressing, centrifugation, and percolation (Petrakis, 2006). (See Figure 3.8.)

Levels of individual phenols in olive oil are different because of the natural variability and the dependence on ripeness, history of production, and age. Free phenols are found in stored oils; fresh oils contain more complex forms of secoiridoid aglycons.

The effect of the processing system on olive oil quality and level of phenols is well documented. Results have been extensively discussed by Monteleone et al. (1998), Schiratti (1999), DiGiovacchino et al. (2001), Servili and Montedoro (2002), Salvador et al. (2003), Petrakis (2006), Poerio et al. (2006), and many others.

3.2.3.1 Pressing and Centrifuging

In the traditional or "classical" system a first extraction by pressure is obtained by primary hydraulic presses, followed by a second extraction with second presses (260–280 kg/cm^2). The olives are crushed by millstones. The resultant mash is spread on round mats that are stacked one upon the other and pressed by a heavy beam. The products — oil, pomace, and water — are then separated in the clarifiers. In the 1950s such systems were replaced by hydraulic super presses, with a service pressure up to 400 atm. These presses work with gradual increase of the pressure and have increased yields. To obtain good quality olive oil in this machinery with a high content of polyphenols, it is necessary to process the fruits as soon as possible and to keep the mats properly clean at all times.

In the 1960s the development of new processes began that were based on centrifuging and that expanded quickly. Currently, two types of centrifugal systems are used, the three-phase and the two-phase systems. In the three-phase system the crushed olives are mixed with water. A horizontal centrifuge separates the mass into pomace, which is further separated into oil and vegetable water.

Press Olive Oil Extraction

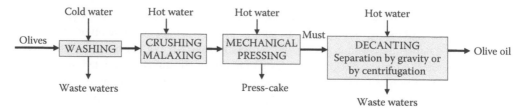

Two-Phase Centrifugal Olive Oil Extraction

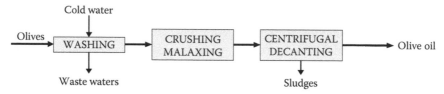

Three-Phase Centrifugal Olive Oil Extraction

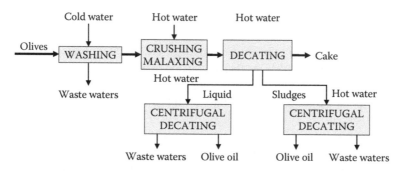

FIGURE 3.8 The main systems currently applied for the extraction of olive oil from olives.

In the two-phase decanters water is not added. Crushed olives are separated into oil and water plus husks. Both systems produce good quality oil, but since in the two-phase system no water is added, the oil usually has higher phenol content and longer induction periods.

3.2.3.2 Percolation

Percolation is a very good system because the operation takes place at room temperature and no process water is added; losses of polar phenolic compounds are smaller. Percolation is based on the difference of the surface tension between the oil and the "vegetable" water. The oil phase is separated when a steel blade is plunged into the paste. The blade coated with oil is then withdrawn and the oil drips off. The system does not allow complete extraction and it is therefore combined with centrifugation.

3.2.3.3 Crushing

To upgrade the quality of olive oil when olives are very rich in phenols, olives can be crushed with a stone mill. In this way bitterness and pungency may decrease. On the contrary, to have an increased level of total polar phenolic compounds, hammer crushers are suitable (Caponio et al., 1999). With hammer crushers even the rotation may be critical (Fogliano et al., 1999). A higher speed causes a better fragmentation of the tissues and a release of some forms of elenolic acid–hydroxytyrosol ester. Servili at al. (2002) reported on the effectiveness of a blade crusher in comparison to a hammer crusher. The level of phenols was not different but the use of the blade crusher influenced favorably the volatile compounds and organoleptic properties of the oil. The temperature of crushing also seems to be critical.

3.2.3.4   Malaxation

Malaxation is important because during this step of processing, hydroxytyrosol is freed by glycosidases and esterases (Boskou D. et al., 2006). The conditions of kneading are generally important factors for the level of total phenol content. Malaxation is not just a mechanical procedure for the separation of olive droplets from the solid phase, but it also involves a series of complex biochemical changes due to various enzymic activities. The biotransformations occurring may be beneficial or negative factors for the quality of the oil (Angerosa et al., 2001; Garcia et al., 2001; DiGiovacchino, 2002; Gomez-Rico, 2006). Non-proper conditions may reduce the level of phenols significantly. Temperature and duration of malaxation are critical (Angerosa et al., 2001; DiGiovacchino, 2002). Kalua et al. (2006) studied virgin olive oils produced at different malaxation temperatures (15, 30, 45, and 60°C) and various periods (30, 60, 90, and 120 min). Variables measured to discriminate malaxation time and temperature were hexanal, 3,4-dihydroxyphenyl ethyl alcohol, decarboxymethyl elenolic acid dialdehyde (3,4-DHPEA-DEDA), free fatty acids content, 1-penten-3-ol, E-2-hexenal, octane, tyrosol, vanillic acid, Z-2-penten-1-ol, and (+)-acetoxypinoresinol. Caponio and Gomes (2001) found that total phenols and levels of hydroxytyrosol, tyrosol, affeic acid, and oleuropein were higher when pastes were obtained from previously refrigerated olives (6°C).

Exposure of the oil paste to air during malaxation results in oxidation of aglycons by oxidizing enzymes (Servili et al., 2003; Migliorini et al., 2006). To protect olive paste against any oxidation during the malaxation state, machines can be designed to work with an inert gas (nitrogen) (Petrakis, 2006). Recently, Parenti and collaborators (Parenti et al., 2006) conducted a study at a laboratory scale to observe the effect of carbon dioxide, naturally evolved from the paste during malaxation, on the quality of the oil and total phenol content. Another approach to solve partially the problem is to remove the stones and extract the oil from the stoned olive paste, as most of the peroxidases are concentrated in the stone.

Addition of pectinases and other enzymes during malaxation has also been suggested for difficult pastes (Petrakis, 2006); the enzymatic action releases more natural antioxidants from the olive pulp, but this practice is not in accordance with the definition of virgin olive oil (the oil obtained from the fruit only by mechanical means).

3.2.3.5   Storage of Olives before Milling

Extra virgin olive oil is obtained from the fruits only by mechanical means (crushing, malaxation, centrifugation) and its production takes place during the period of olive harvest. The work in olive mills should be organized in such a way that the plant can cope with large loads of raw material in a short time. The maximum time of storage for obtaining oil without defects is approximately 48 h. Stocking the raw material for longer periods will result in oils with defects due to hydrolytic and oxidative reactions. Recently some attempts have been made to use freezing storage before crushing olives or to keep the olives at low temperatures under controlled atmospheres such as humidified air or air with 3% oxygen and 5% carbon dioxide (Clodoveo et al., 2007; Poerio et al., in press). Such approaches, however, have to be further evaluated from the point of view of practical applicability and cost, as cost increases significantly.

3.2.3.6   Storage of Oil

There is extensive literature on the changes in the phenol fraction during storage. Various conditions have been studied, even frozen storage (Cerretani et al., 2005b).

3.3   PROPOSALS TO ENRICH VIRGIN OLIVE OIL WITH PHENOLS

The avalanche of publications that indicate a beneficial role of antioxidants, in general, and of olive oil phenols, in particular, has led to many efforts to increase polyphenol content in the oil with the addition of leaves before crushing or obtain pure phenols from waste products and leaves. The latter may be added to refined oils used for cooking or frying, food products subject to oxidation, nutritional supplements, and cosmetics.

Gibriel and collaborators (2006) studied the effect of mixing olive leaves with olives during crushing and also adding fungal pectinases in the malaxation stage. Kachouri and Hamdi (2004) proposed an enhancement of polyphenols in olive oil by contact with olive mill waste water fermented by *Lactobacillus plantarum*. Incubation of olive oil with fermented olive mill waste water caused a reduction of polyphenols in the waste water and an increase in the oil due to depolymerization of the high molecular weight phenolics by the microorganism.

3.4   EXTRACTION OF BIOPHENOLS FROM OLIVES AND OLIVE PROCESSING BY-PRODUCTS

The methodology of obtaining extracts rich in polar phenols is based on the defatting of oil mill waste waters, extraction with organic solvents, and fractionation with various methods. (For a review see Boskou, D. et al. [2006].) Other approaches of valorization of olive oil by-products are based on nanofiltration/reverse osmosis systems of the waste and recovery by extraction. Fernandez-Bolanos et al. (2002, 2006) claimed that production of large quantities of highly purified hydroxytyrosol can be obtained from "alperujo," the liquid-solid waste product of the two-phase olive processing system. The principle of the method applied in a flash hydrolysis laboratory pilot unit is steam treatment, hydrolysis, and purification by a patented simple and inexpensive chromatographic system. According to the authors, after purification, 3 kg of hydroxytyrosol of 90–95% purity can be obtained from 1000 kg of alperujo. The authors have also patented a method (2005) to obtain purified hydroxytyrosol from products and by-products derived from olive milling. The procedure is a two-step chromatographic treatment. The invention uses a nonactivated ion exchange resin chromatographic separation, followed by a second treatment on an XAD-type absorbent nonionic resin that concentrates and completely purifies the hydroxytyrosol by means of elution with a methanol or ethanol/water mixture. The method can also be applied to pomaces from the two- and three-phase extraction systems.

Fki and co-workers (2005) proposed an ethyl acetate extraction of the mill waste water using a counter–counter unit. The antioxidants obtained can be added to refined olive oil and refined husk oil to increase stability.

A patented method (Cuomo et al., 2002) uses as a first step an extraction with a polar aqueous solvent to recover antioxidants from olives, the olive pulp (the cake that remains as a by-product after milling), olive oil, and waste waters. The second step is trapping of the antioxidants in a solid matrix (a resin like amberlite) and the third washing with a polar organic solvent such as methanol, ethanol, propanol, isopropanol, acetone, and others. The efficiency of the procedure may be improved by extracting the starting material in an acidic polar solvent that causes hydrolysis of oleuropein and an enhancement of the antioxidant activity. If waste waters are used as the raw material, these pass directly through a solid matrix. The invention also provides antioxidant compositions and methods to increase the antioxidant activity of a product.

Crea (2005) developed a process without solvents. The raw material is olives from which the pits have been removed prior to milling. The fruit water, rich in polar phenols, contains citric acid which hydrolyses oleuropein and aglycons and acts at the same time as an antioxidant. Another product, an olive pulp extract, rich in hydroxytyrosol and verbascoside, has also been patented (Indena, 2004, http://www.foodnavigator.com.news). The olives are selected from a variety that is rich in polyphenols. The extraction method uses only water and ethanol. The extract has already been formulated in food supplements.

A different approach to recover phenols was proposed recently by Garcia et al. (2006). The idea is to add a washing step before refining in the processing of the residue of two-phase milling, which is used for the recovery of the so-called "second centrifugation oil." This water washing will remove the most polar phenols such as hydroxytyrosol and tyrosol from the oil. A concentration up to 1400 mg hydroxytyrosol per liter can be obtained.

3.4.1 OLIVE LEAVES

Paiva-Martins et al. (2005) proposed the addition of extracts obtained from olive leaves to refined olive oil. The latter is poor in phenolics as these compounds are polar and completely removed during the refining process. According to the authors this unusual practice may increase the nutritional value and stability of refined oil. Salta and co-workers (2007) suggested the addition of extracts from olive leaves to virgin olive oil, sunflower, cotton seed, and palm oil at levels necessary to bring the final concentration to 200 mg polyphenols per kilogram of oil. Calculation of the increase of the antioxidant capacity was based on EC_{50} values, determined by the 1,1-diphenyl-2-picrylhydrazyl radical method. The enrichment resulted in the supplementation of commercial oils mainly with oleuropein, hydroxytyrosol, and quercetin. In a recent report, Rada et al. (2006) tried to optimize a process to extract and isolate hydroxytyrosol from olive leaves, since the compound has a high added value with applications in cosmetics, pharmaceutical products, and food supplements. The technique is based on ethanol extraction and fractionation by Short Path Distillation.

Japon-Lujan et al., in two papers (2006a,b), proposed microwave and ultrasound assistance to accelerate ethanol–water extraction of biophenols from olive leaves. The results were verified by analysis of the target analytes. Oleuropein, verbascoside, apigenin-7-glucoside, and luteolin-7-glucoside were identified and quantified using an HPLC-photodiode array detector assembly. In comparison to conventional extraction with ethanol/water mixtures, the time of extraction was reduced from many hours to minutes. Japon-Lujan and de Castro, in a more recent publication (2007), report extraction conditions for the recovery of biophenols not only from the leaves but also from the small branches (fibrous softwood) of the olive tree. The target analytes oleuropein, verbascoside, tyrosol, alpha-taxifolin, and hydroxytyrosol are practically completely removed. Extraction accelerated by microwave assistance may be implemented in continuous and discontinuous extractors using ultrasound assistance and superheated liquids as auxiliary energies.

Briante et al. (2002a) proposed a method of production of hydroxytyrosol based on the use of nonhomogenous hyperthermophilic beta-glycosidase immobilized on chitosan. According to the authors the method is simple and provided a natural, nontoxic product. Leaves with high oleuropein content have to be selected to obtain a good substrate for biotransformation. The bioreactor eluates were examined as substitutes for synthetic antioxidants commonly used to increase the shelf life of food products and also for their possible effect in human cells.

Such proposals to use leaves, however, have to be considered carefully and examined if they are nutritionally and toxicologically correct. The mode of extraction is critical as the leaf extracts may contain traces of bioactive compounds and contaminants not properly studied.

3.4.2 FUNCTIONALIZATION OF FOOD COMPOSITIONS

Food compositions fortified with antioxidants from olive oil or olives have been proposed by van der Boom and Manon (2004). Their invention is suited for compositions containing water such as spreads, processed tomato products, and dressings. The principle of the method is exposing olive oil under hydrolytic conditions to an aqueous phase, so that lipophilic phenolic compounds will hydrolyze and migrate to this phase. Thus, the nutritional value of the product is enhanced.

A very different approach for the production of a protein-based functional food with antioxidative and antimicrobial properties was proposed by Baycin et al. (2007). The two most abundant polyphenols in olive leaves, oleuopein and rutin, are first extracted from olive leaves with 70% ethanol aqueous solution. The crude extract is then dissolved in a solvent and mixed with silk fibroin. The final product is silk fibroin containing adsorbed polyphenols. This product can be considered as a natural preservative because it has antioxidant and antimicrobial properties.

Other attempts aim at obtaining more lipophilic derivatives that are effective in protecting edible oils or can be used in food preparations with a protective action against oxidative stress. Enzymatic esterification of hydroxytyrosol for the synthesis of lipophilic antioxidant was first suggested by Buisman et al. (1998). The phenol was enzymatically converted into its octanoic acid ester using various lipases. The octanoate ester was tested in refined sunflower oil for its antioxidant activity and compared to BHT. By esterification the phenol was found to become a less effective antioxidant. Gordon et al. (2001) prepared hydroxytyrosol acetate synthetically and assessed its antioxidant activity in relation to hydoxytyrosol, oleuropein, an isomer of oleuropein aglycon and alpha-tocopherol. Hydroxytyrosol acetate had a weaker DPPH radical scavenging activity than hydroxytyrosol and oleuropein but it had a radical scavenging activity similar to that of alpha-tocopherol. In oil and in emulsions the ester had an antioxidant activity that was more or less similar to that of free hydroxytyrosol. Hydroxytyrosol was subjected to a chemoselective lipase acylation that affords 10 derivatives with C_2 to C_{18} acyl chains at C-1 (Grasso et al., 2007). The lipophilic esters showed a good DPPH radical scavenging activity. Some of them were tested with the Comet test on whole blood cells and were found to have a protective effect against H_2O_2-induced oxidative DNA damage.

Lipophilic derivatives such as hydroxytyrosol acetate, palmitate, oleate, and linoleate were tested for their antioxidant activity in lipid matrices and biological systems (Trujillo et al., 2006). Hydroxytyrosol and its esters were found to be more effective as antioxidants compared to alpha-tocopherol and BHT. The compounds tested showed a capacity to protect proteins and lipids against oxidation caused by peroxyradicals when a brain homogenate was used as an *ex vivo* model.

Manna et al. (2005) prepared synthetically di- and triacetyl derivatives of hydroxytyrosol. The chemical antioxidant activity of these compounds was evaluated by measuring the ferric reducing antioxidant potential (FRAP). The data indicated that the hydroxytyrosol analogues modified in the *o*-diphenolic ring were devoid, as expected, of any chemical antioxidant activity. On the contrary, acetyl derivatives, at micromolar concentrations, protect against *tert*-butylhydroperoxide–induced oxidative damages in Caco-2 cells and human erythrocytes. The authors claim that chemically stable hydroxytyrosol acetyl derivatives, although devoid of chemical antioxidant activity, were as effective as the parent compound in protecting human cells from oxidative stress-induced cytotoxicity after metabolization by esterases at the intestinal level. This suggests a possible utilization in either nutritional (functional food), cosmetic, or pharmaceutical preparations.

Hydroxytyrosol esters have been synthesized by reacting natural or synthetic hydroxytyrosol and natural oleuropein and oleuropein aglycons with an acylating agent (Gonzales et al., 2005). The esters can be used as additives in food preparations and supplements.

Recently, Artajo et al. (2006) conducted a study focusing on the enrichment of different olive oil matrices with individual components from the phenolic fraction of virgin olive oil, and aiming at the possible discovery of functional application in food.

3.4.3 SYNTHESIS OF HYDROXYTYROSOL

Hydroxytyrosol can be synthesized enzymatically from tyrosol, a compound that is commercially available, in the presence of tyrosinase and ascorbic acid (Espin et al., 2001). Tyrosinase may be obtained from mushrooms (Saiz, 2000). The synthesized hydroxytyrosol can be used to functionalize foods such as vegetable oil, butter, and tomato juice (Larrosa, 2003). Conversion of tyrosol to hydroxytyrosol has also been proposed by Allouche et al. (2004) and Bouallagui and Savadi (2006), who used the whole cells of a soil bacterium, *Pseudomonas aeruginosa*, which has the ability to grow on tyrosol as a sole source of carbon and energy. Gambacorta et al. (2007) proposed the preparation of a stable precursor of hydroxytyrosol, its acetonide, which is synthesized by a high yield procedure; it is purifiable and stable over a wide range of pH. These properties allow long-term storage. The protection is removed quantitatively, when needed, and pure hydroxytyrosol becomes available for uses in food preparations and cosmetic products.

3.5 TABLE OLIVES AS SOURCES OF BIOPHENOLS

Table olives are well-known sources of compounds with biological properties. They are important from a nutritional point of view for the general population in many Mediterranean countries, especially during the long periods of fasting. They are more important for the Christian Orthodox monks and nuns who consume large quantities of olives. In the northeastern part of Portugal, stoned halved table olives known as "alcaparra" are largely consumed and their production is an important agroeconomic factor for the local producers (Sousa et al., 2006).

The chemistry and levels of polar phenols present in olives and table olives have been discussed by Bianco and Uccella (2000), McDonald et al. (2001), Servili et al. (2002), and Boskou, D. et al. (2005). The phenolic profile by GC/MS and antioxidant capacity of five different varieties of Greek table olives were studied by Boskou, G. et al. (2006).

The major compounds present in olive fruits are anthocyanins (cyanidin and delphinidin glucosides), flavonols (mainly quercetin-3-rutinoside), flavones (luteolin and apigenin glucosides), phenolic acids (hydroxybenzoic, hydroxycinnamic, others), phenolic alcohols (tyrosol and hydroxytyrosol), secoiridoids (olcuropein, demethyloleuropein, ligstroside, nuzhenide), and *verbascoside*, a hydroxycinnamic acid derivative. In the oil of seeds the oleuropein glucoside, nuzhenide, with a strong antioxidant activity, was found to be the phenolic with the highest concentration (Silva et al., 2006).

Table olives have a phenol composition that differs from that of olive oil and nonprocessed olives. This is due to the debittering, which causes diffusion of phenols from the fruit to the water or brine and vice versa. When lye is used sodium hydroxide and constituents with carboxylic and hydroxyl groups react and the hydrophilic derivatives are washed away. Oleuropein and verbascoside are hydrolyzed to a great extent during the lye treatment. Acid hydrolysis of hydroxytyrosol, tyrosol, and luteolin glycosides takes place during the fermentation in brine when naturally black olives are prepared. Thus, the prevailing phenols in table olives are hydroxytyrosol, tyrosol, luteolin, and phenolic acids (Blekas et al., 2002; Boskou, G. et al., 2006).

Table olive samples from the retail market were analyzed for individual phenols by RP-HPLC by Blekas et al. (2002). Higher levels, ranging from 100–760 mg/kg, were found in Greek-style naturally black olives and Spanish-style green olives in brine. Hydroxytyrosol and caffeic acid are eliminated during the preparation of California-type black olives. The diminution of *ortho*-diphenols in the flesh of this type of oil is related to the browning. Iron salts used for color fixation catalyze the oxidation of hydroxytyrosol, which disappears or is reduced significantly.

Pereira and co-workers (2006) measured the levels of some phenolic compounds in four types of table olives from Spanish varieties. The compounds identified and quantified by HPLC in the methanol extract of the olive pulp were hydroxytyrosol, tyrosol, 5-*O*-caffeoyl quinic acid, verbascoside, luteolin, and luteolin 7-*O*-glycoside. High levels of hydroxytyrosol, verbascoside, and luteolin were determined in naturally black olives and olives turning color in the brine method. High levels of hydroxytyrosol and luteolin were found in green olives in brine. Black ripe olives, produced by the Californian method, had lower levels of hydroxytyrosol, verbascoside, and luteolin. Three flavonoids — luteolin 7-*O*-glycoside, apigenin 7-*O*-glycoside, and luteolin — were identified as the main constituents in the Portuguese "alcaparra" table olives by Sousa et al. (2006). These olives are prepared from healthy green or yellow-green fruits by destoning. The pulp is then sliced into two parts and placed in water, which is replaced every day until the bitterness is removed. This mode of preparation may explain the different chemical composition.

3.6 OLIVE OIL PHENOLS IN OTHER PLANT MATERIALS

3.6.1 Hydroxytyrosol and Tyrosol Derivatives

Oleuropein, an ester of 3,4-dihydroxyphenylethanol with elenolic acid glucoside, belongs to a specific group of coumarin-like compounds called secoiridoids. The latter are abundant in *Oleaceas, Cornales,* and other plants. Oleuropein is present in high amounts in the leaves of olive trees and also in unripe olives. Oleuropein occurs not only in the *Olea* genus but also in many other genera belonging to the Oleaceae family and has been described in *Fraximus excelsior, F. angustifolia, F. chinensis, Syringa josikaea, S. vulgaris, Philyrea latifolia, Ligustrum ovalifolium, L. vulgare,* and many others (Soler-Rivas et al., 2000). The methanolic extract of the leaves of the plant *Syringa oblata* Lindl var. alba was examined as a source of oleuropein by Nenadis et al. (2006). The extract had a high total phenol content and a radical scavenging activity similar to that of olive leave extracts. The most abundant phenolic compounds in the extract, as characterized by HPLC and LC-MS, were oleuropein and syringopicroside. The latter was identified by LC-MS and homonuclear two-dimensinal correlated NMR spectroscopy. Other compounds detected were oleuropein aglycon, verbascoside, ligstroside (a tyrosol derivative), luteolin rutinoside, and syringopicroside derivatives.

3.6.2 Phenolic Acids

Phenolic acids are widely distributed in nature. Top sources of hydroxycinnamic and hydroxybenzoic acids are berries, cherries, citrus fruits, plums, prunes, apples, pears, kiwi fruits, aubergine, and many other plant materials. (For a review see Clifford [2000], Manach et al. [2004], and Boskou [2006].)

3.6.3 Flavones

Flavones are encountered in many plant materials. Rich sources of flavones are parsley, potato peels, celery, capsicum peppers, and other plant materials.

3.6.4 Lignans

Sesame seed and flaxseed are rich sources of lignans (Kamal-Eldin et al., 1994; Kato et al., 1998). (+)-Pinoresinol was identified in *Forsynthia suspensa* (Davin et al., 1992). Lignans are also present in the bark of *Olea* plants (Tsukamoto et al., 1984). Important sources in the diet are beverages, vegetables, nuts and seeds, bread, and fruit. Some lignans, including pinoresinol, are considered important precursors of enterolignans (enterolactone and enderodiol) that are formed in the colonic microflora. Enterolignans are biologically important phytoestrogens that can potencially reduce the risk of certain cancers and cardiovascular diseases (see also Chapter 7). Therefore, databases are now developed to estimate lignan intakes from representative samples of the population (Milder et al., 2005a,b).

Pinoresinol and syringaresinol (the lignan identified in olive oil by Professor Photis Dais and his research team; see Chapter 5) are also present in the plants of the Aviceniaceae family (Sharp et al., 2001).

3.7 ANTIOXIDANT ACTIVITY: *IN VITRO* AND ANIMAL STUDIES

The increasing interest in the antioxidant properties of natural compounds and food components is due to their ability to protect fats present in foods and the hypothesis that they prevent the effects of reactive species on the human body. Phenols present in olive oil are investigated more and more actively, as information accumulated indicates a plethora of biological activities suggesting that these compounds may have a favorable effect on health. Oil is among those natural agents that have widely been considered to have antioxidant and free radical scavenging capabilities.

Antioxidant activity measurements may be divided into two categories. One class of determinations aims at evaluating the effect of phenols on the stability of the oil to autoxidation and has a purely technological character. The other class is a series of approaches to evaluate better the possible biological effects.

3.7.1 ANTIOXIDANT PROPERTIES WITH TECHNOLOGICAL IMPORTANCE

Evaluation of antioxidant activity of the total polar phenol fraction or individual phenols is usually based on determinations of the shelf life of the oil or accelerated tests such as Rancimat analysis at 120°C. Methods have been developed to measure the antioxidant activity directly in the oil in addition to methods for the effect of phenolic extracts, pure phenols, or fractions obtained by preparative HPLC. Papadopoulos and Boskou (1991) compared the antioxidant effect of phenolic acids and simple phenols on refined olive oil. Hydroxytyrosol and caffeic acid were found to be more powerful antioxidants in relation to BHT when the stability and keepability of the oil containining these additives were examined. Baldioli et al. (1996) used Rancimat to study the effect of various phenols and secoiridoid derivatives on purified olive oil stability. The concentration of hydroxytyrosol, the dialdehydic form of elenolic acid linked to hydroxytyrosol, and an isomer of oleuropein aglycon were found to correlate well to the oxidative stability of purified oil.

Fogliano et al. (1999) obtained by semipreparative HPLC fractions containing individual phenols and evaluated the relative antioxidant efficiency in relation to BHT by monitoring the peroxidation at 240 nm using the ABAP (2,2-azo-bis-2-amidinopropane hydrochloride) reagent.

Oxygen radical absorbance capacity (ORAC) of olive oil was investigated by Ninfali et al. (2001) using a spectrofluorometric method that measures the protection of the phenolic substances of the oil on the b-phycoerythrin fluorescence decay in comparison with Trolox. This value, which indicates the capacity to trap peroxyl radicals, was proposed as a new parameter to assess the quality and stability against oxidation of extra virgin olive oil.

Quiles et al. (2002) proposed the use of electron spin resonance (ESR) spectroscopy to evaluate antioxidant capacity in virgin olive oil. The method is based on the determination of remaining galvinoxyl (a synthetic radical) by integration of the ESR spectrum after addition of an ethanol solution of the oil. Electron paramagnetic resonance (EPR) was also used by Ottaviani et al. (2001), who identified and quantified free radicals by means of the spin-trapping technique using alpha-phenylnutylnitrone (PBN) as a spin trap. From their study the authors concluded that EPR can be applied to check storage and handling conditions that significantly influence the radical concentration in olive oils.

In general the antioxidant activity of phenols is higher in *ortho*-diphenols or phenols with *o*-methoxy groups. The activity of simple phenols, secoiridoids, and lignans as antioxidants was recently investigated by Carrasco-Pancorbo et al. (2006) by the DPPH radical test and measurement of oxidation stability. The study confirmed previous findings indicating that the presence of a second hydroxyl group at *ortho*-position enhances signigicantly the ability to act as an antioxidant.

A theoretical approach to the radical scavenging potential of phenolic compounds encountered in olives and olive oil and olive leaves was reported by Nenadis et al. (2005). This approach is based on quantum chemical calculations of bond dissociation enthalpy (BDE) of phenolic hydroxyl groups and the ionization potential (P) values and aims at predicting the H-donating and electron-donating abilities. Catechols were found to have the lowest BDE values. Lignans and monophenols had much higher BDE values (a lower potential for radical scavenging). In real systems, however, activity may vary due to differences in lipophility.

Roche et al. (2005) characterized olive oil phenols by the number of radicals trapped per antioxidant molecule and by the rate constants K_1 for the first H-atom abstraction by the radical DPPH.

Oleuropen, hydroxytyrosol, and caffeic acid have the largest K_1 values, whereas dihydrocaffeic acid, an intestinal metabolite of caffeic acid, was found to be the best antioxidant in terms of stoichiometry (number of radicals trapped per molecule). The study indicated that overall, olive phenols are efficient scavengers of hydrophilic peroxyl radicals with a long-lasting antioxidant effect. The latter is due to the residual activity of their oxidation products.

A different approach for evaluation of the antioxidant power of olive oil was proposed by Mannino and co-workers (Mannino et al., 1999). The method is based on a FIA system with an amperometric detector. According to the authors the method is sensitive and offers an alternative to the Rancimat method for direct and reliable monitoring of the total antioxidant power of olive oil. The method is also better correlated to the real keepability than the Rancimat method, in which severe oxidation conditions are used.

The effect of pH and ferric anions on the antioxidant activity of olive oil polyphenols in oil-in-water emulsions was studied by Paiva-Martins and Gordon (2002). Antioxidant behavior is more complex in emulsions than in bulk oil as there are more variables involved in lipid oxidation (pH, emulsifiers). Four olive oil phenols were examined: oleuropein, hydroxytyrosol, 3,4-dihydroxyphenylethanol-elenolic acid, and 3,4-dihydroxyphenylethanol-elenolic acid dialdehyde. The effect of each antioxidant on DPPH radical concentration and the FRAP was also determined. The work has shown that phenolic compounds of olive oil have a high antioxidant capacity at pH range 3.5–7.4, but their activity may be reduced in the presence of ferric anions.

3.7.2 Antioxidant Properties with Biological Importance

3.7.2.1 LDL Oxidation

The protective effect of olive oil phenolic compounds on oxidation of human low-density lipoprotein has been reported in a series of papers published by F. Visioli, C. Galli, G. Galli, D. Caruso, and others from the Department of Pharmacological Sciences, University of Milano; and by M.I. Covas, R. de la Torre, M. Fito, J. Marrugat, and others from the Lipids and Cardiovascular Epidemiology Unit, Institut Municipal d'Investigació Mèdica (IMIM–Hospital del Mar, Barcelona; see Chapter 6). Both hydroxytyrosol and oleuropein potently and dose dependently inhibit copper sulfate-induced oxidation of low-density lipoproteins (LDL) (for reviews see Visioli et al., 2002, 2006).

A group of researchers in the Netherlands (Leenen et al., 2002) conducted a study to indicate the effect of olive oil phenols on the resistance of LDL against oxidation. To better mimic the *in vivo* situation, plasma was incubated with olive oil phenols and LDL was isolated and challenged for its resistance to oxidation. The study supports the hypothesis that extra virgin olive phenols protect LDL in plasma against oxidation.

Masella et al. (1999) studied the effects of 3,4-dihydroxyphenylethanol-elenolic acid and protocatechuic acid on the oxidative modification of copper-stimulated human LDL. Modification was tested by measuring the formation of intermediate and end products of lipid peroxidation (conjugation, hydroperoxide formation, cholesterol oxidation products, and increase in LDL negative charges). The results of this study demonstrated that the two examined phenols show an antioxidant activity that is comparable to that of caffeic acid, hydroxytyrosol, and oleuropein. (For an in-depth discussion of LDL oxidation see Chapter 6.)

3.7.2.2 Radicals and Reactive Species

There is a plethora of studies with respect to the potential of olive oil phenols to scavenge synthetic radicals, superoxide radicals, and peroxyradicals or neutralize reactive species and reduce damages caused by hydrogen peroxide and peroxynitrate ion. The existing literature has been reviewed by Visioli et al. (2002), Boskou et al. (2005), Boskou, D. et al. (2006), and Visioli et al. (2006).

Pellegrini et al. (2001) evaluated the total antioxidant activity of extra virgin olive oil and individual phenols with the long-living ABTS [2,2′-azinobis (3-ethylbenz-thiazoline-6-sulfonic) diammonium salt] radical cation decolorization assay. The results were expressed in millimole Trolox per kilogram oil. Silva et al. (2006) used the ABTS$^+$ method to evaluate the antioxidant activity of extracts obtained from olive fruits, olive seeds, and olive leaves.

A number of investigators have used the DPPH (2,2-diphenyl-1-picrylhydrazyl) radical to characterize total free radical scavenging capacity of olive oil or its fractions (methanolic, lipidic) and individual phenols. The disappearance of the radical is measured at 515 or 517 nm (Mosca et al., 2000). The results are usually expressed in EC_{50} or Trolox equivalents (Carlos-Espin, 2000) or the reciprocal of EC_{50}, which corresponds to the phenolic extract concentration able to reduce 50% of the DPPH· radical content (Rotondi et al., 2004). Free radical scavenging activity of the polar fraction of olive oil or hydroxytyrosol and its derivatives was also measured by Saija et al. (1998), Gordon et al. (2001), Tuck et al. (2002), Lavelli (2002), Gomez-Alonso et al. (2003), Valavanidis et al. (2004), Romani et al. (2007), and many others.

Gorinstein and co-investigators (Gorinstein et al., 2003) used four different methods to measure antioxidant activity in samples of Spanish olive oils. Among the four methods — DPPH radical test, antioxidant potential by ABAP, total antioxidant status by ABTS, and beta-carotene-linoleate system — the best correlation between total phenols and antioxidant capacity was found for the beta-carotene/linoleate conjugated oxidation.

The radical hydrogen donor ability of antioxidants was measured colorimetrically using the stable red radical cation DMPD$^+$ (Briante et al., 2003) and also the xanthine oxidase/xanthine system (Lavelli, 2002).

The methanolic fraction of olive oil containing the polar olive oil phenols was used by Valavanidis et al. (2004) for measurements of the radical scavenging capacity toward the most important oxygen-free radicals, superoxide ion ($O_2^{·}$) and hydroxyl OH· radicals. Superoxide radical was generated by potassium superoxide in DMSO. The antioxidant activity measurement was based on the spin trapping of $O_2^{·}$ in DMSO with the addition of 18-crown-6 ether to complex K$^+$ and the EPR spectra of superoxide anion spin-trapped by DMPO (spin adduct DMPO-OOH). To measure the antioxidant activity of methanolic extracts toward hydroxyl radicals, a Fenton system ($H_2O_2/F = 2$/EDTA-Na$_2$) was used. The radicals were again spin-trapped by DMPO.

Deiana and others (Deiana et al., 1999) studied peroxynitrite-dependent nitration of tyrosine and DNA damage and found a protective role of hydroxytyrosol. The same phenol, oleuropein, and caffeic acid were also found to reduce the amount of nitric oxide (formed by nitroprusside) and also to reduce chemically generated peroxinitrate. According to De la Puerta et al. (2001), however, oleuropein may have both the ability to scavenge nitric oxide and to cause an increase in the inducible nitric oxide synthase (INOS) expression in the cell.

A scavenging effect of hydroxytyrosol and oleuropein was demonstrated with respect to hypochlorous acid (HOCL) (Visioli et al., 2002). HOCL is an oxidative substance produced *in vivo* by neutrophil myeloperoxidase at the site of inflammation and can cause damage to proteins including enzymes. Very dilute preparations of the substance may also be used in the food industry to prevent prespoilage proliferation of bacteria on fresh meat.

Antioxidant, anti-inflammatory, and hypolipidemic properties of olive oil minor compontents and their effects on vascular dysfunction and the mechanisms by which they modulate enthothelial activity (involving the release of nitric oxide, eicosanoids, and adhesion molecules) are discussed in Chapters 6 and 8. (See also Perona et al., 2006.)

3.7.2.3 Hydroxy-Isochromans

Lorenz et al. (2005) conducted a study to investigate the scavenging activity of polyphenolic isochromans and assess the relation between structure and scavenging. 1-(3′-Ethoxy-4′-hydroxy-phenyl)-6,7-dihydroxy-isochroman, the natural hydoxy-isochroman, was found to have a radical scavenging capacity when tested with the DPPH radical, a scavenging capacity for enzymatically generated superoxide in a hypoxanthin-xanthinoxidase reaction. The compound also scavenged peroxynitrate anion (ONOO⁻) and in all tests it superseded the scavenging effect of troloc (the hydrophilic analogue of alpha-tocopherol). The authors suggest that the excellent radical and reactive species (reactive oxygen and nitrogen species, ROS/RNS) scavenging species make hydroxyl-1-aryl-isochromans candidates for pharmaceutical applications.

3.7.2.4 Other Studies

Saija et al. (1998) conducted measurements to obtain more information for the scavenging activity against peroxyl radicals near the membrane surface and within the membranes. For their studies they used a model consisting of phospholipid/linoleic acid unilamellar vesicles and an azo compound as a free radical generator.

3.7.2.5 Other Mechanisms of Antioxidant Activity

The antioxidant effect of certain olive oil phenols, as indicated by a series of experiments (Visioli et al., 2002; Briante et al., 2003; Bendini et al., 2006), may be partly due to a metal chelation. The presence of metals in virgin olive oil is due to plant metabolism (endogenous factors), contamination by agricultural practices, and contamination during processing of oils or storage (exogenous factors). Traces of metals such as iron and copper, dissolved in the oil as metal salts with fatty acids, act as prooxidants yielding radicals that initiate radical chain oxidation.

3.7.3 EXPERIMENTS WITH ANIMALS

Dietary nontocopherol antioxidants present in extra virgin olive oil were found to increase the resistance of low-density lipoproteins to oxidation in rabbits (Wiseman et al., 1996).

Tuck et al. (2002) studied the scavenging activity not only of hydroxytyrosol but also of its metabolites in rats (homovanillic acid, homovanillic alcohol, glucuronide conjugate, sulfate conjugate) on human low-density lipoprotein and on cell cultures. Based on the results of *in vitro* and cell culture investigations indicating the ability of certain olive oil phenols to inhibit the oxidative process, Coni and his research team (Coni et al., 2000) conducted a study with laboratory rabbits fed special diets that contained olive oil and oleuropein. The results indicated that the addition of oleuropein increased the ability of LDL to resist oxidation and at the same time reduced the plasmatic levels of total, free, and esterified cholesterol.

Gorinstein and collaborators (Gorinstein et al., 2002) indicated that olive oil can improve lipid metabolism and increase antioxidant potentials in rats fed diets containing cholesterol. The effect of olive oils on lipid metabolism and antioxidant activity was investigated on 60 male Wistar rats adapted to cholesterol-free or 1% cholesterol diets. The results of the study demonstrated that virgin olive oil possesses antioxidant properties that should be attributed mostly to the phenolic compounds present in the oil. Krzeminski et al. (2003) studied the mechanism of the hypocholesterolemic effect of olive oils in rats adapted to cholesterol-containing and cholesterol-free diets. The antioxidants present in olive oil, evaluated by plasma total radical-trapping antioxidant potential (TRAP), were found to play a leading role in the mechanism of the hypocholesterolemic effect.

The potential protective effects of oleuropein have been investigated in the isolated rat heart by Manna et al. (2004). The organs were subjected to 30 min of no-flow global ischemia and then reperfused. At different intervals, the coronary heart effluent was collected and assayed for creatine kinase activity and reduced and oxidized glutathione. The extent of lipid peroxidation was evaluated by measuring thiobarbituric acid–reactive substance concentration in the muscle. The findings of the study, according to the authors, strengthten the hypothesis that the health benefits of olive oil are related to the oleuropein derivatives present in olive oil.

One-month administration of hydroxytyrosol to hyperlipemic rabbits may improve blood lipid profile and antioxidant status and reduce atherosclerosis development, according to Gonzalez-Santiago et al. (2006). Hydroxytyrosol supplementation improved the antioxidant status in rabbit groups and reduced the size of atherosclerotic lesions measured as initial layer areas of the aortic arch when compared with control animals. The authors, based on the results of their study, conclude that hydroxytyrosol may have a cardioprotective effect *in vivo* (see also Chapters 6 and 8). In a more recent work, Fki and co-workers (Fki et al., 2007) studied the hypocholesteremic effects of hydroxytyrosol purified from olive mill waste water in rats fed cholesterol-rich diets. Administration of low doses of hydroxytyrosol significantly lowered the serum levels of total cholesterol and low-density lipoprotein cholesterol and increased the serum levels of high-density lipoprotein cholesterol. The thiobarbituric acid reactive substances (TBARS) content in liver, heart, kidney, and aorta decreased significantly after oral administration of hydroxytyrosol. The olive mill wastewater phenolics increased catalase and superoxide dismutase activities. The results suggest that the hypocholesterolemic effect of hydroxytyrosol might be due to the ability to lower total cholesterol and low-density lipoprotein cholesterol levels, to a retardation of the lipid peroxidation process, and to enhancement of antioxidant enzyme activities.

3.7.4 Experiments with Cells

The effect of hydroxytyrosol on hydrogen peroxide (H_2O_2)–induced oxidative alterations was investigated in human erythrocytes (Manna et al., 1999). The data collected indicated that hydroxytyrosol prevents oxidative alterations and provides protection against peroxide-induced cytotoxicity in erythrocytes.

Experimental and clinical evidence suggesting that oxidative stress causes cellular damages and functional alterations of the tissue, and the implication of radicals in the pathogenesis of a number of human diseases, prompted many attempts to obtain results with cells. Giovannini et al. (1999), in an effort to analyze the oxidative damage induced by oxidized LDL to intestinal mucosa, examined the effect of tyrosol by evaluating morphological and functional changes induced by oxidized LDL in the human colon adenocarcinoma cell line, Caco-2 cells. The authors conclude that some biophenols present in olive oil may counteract the reactive oxygen metabolite–mediated cellular damage and related diseases, by improving *in vivo* antioxidant defense.

De la Puerta et al. (1999) determined the anti-eicosanoid and antioxidant effects in leukocytes of the principal phenolic compounds from the polar fraction of olive oil (oleuropein, tyrosol, hydroxytyrosoland, caffeic acid). In intact rat peritoneal leukocytes stimulated with calcium ionophore, all the phenols tested inhibited leukotriene B_4 generation at the 5-lipogygenase level. They also quenched the chemiluminescence signal due to reactive oxygen species generated by phorbol myristate acetate–stimulated rat leukocytes.

Kohyama et al. (1997) investigated the effects of olive fruit extracts on arachidonic acid lipoxygenase activities using rat platelets and rat polymorphonuclear leukocytes. Hydroxytyrosol was one of the compounds responsible for the inhibition of lipoxygenase (12-LO and 5-LO) activity.

Recently, Paiva-Martins et al. (2006) assayed the capacity of olive oil phenolic compounds to protect erythrocytes from oxidative injury induced by hydrogen peroxide and the azo compound AAPH (a radical generator).

There is generally a rapidly growing interest in cheap and abundant sources of phenolics such as olive oil, as there are indications that plant foods rich in antioxidants modulate positively surrogate markers of many human pathological changes. The studies now are extended to the effect of olive oil phenols to deleterious effects of oxidative stress on brain cell survival. In a very recent publication Schaffer et al. (2007) report on the efficacy of hydroxytyrosol-rich extracts to attenuate Fe^{++} and nitric oxide (NO)–induced cytotoxicity in murine-dissociated brain cells.

3.8 ANTIMICROBIAL PROPERTIES

3.8.1 Olive Oil Phenols

The antimicrobial effect of olive polar phenols has been discussed by Soler-Rivas et al. (2000), Saija and Uccella (2001), and Tripoli et al. (2005). There are many publications related to the *in vitro* antimicrobial properties of oleuropein and its hydrolysis products as well as ligstroside aglycon (Walter et al., 1973; Tassou and Nychas, 1994; Bisignano et al., 1999; Keceli and Robinson, 2002; Furneri et al., 2004; Pereira et al., 2006; Romero et al., 2007). Olive oil phenols have generally been demonstrated to inhibit *in vivo* or delay the growth of bacteria such as salmonella, cholera, pseudomonas, staphylococcus, fungi, viruses, and parasites. Such findings suggest a possible beneficial role of olive oil and its polar phenolic compounds in promoting intestinal and respiratory wellness in humans.

Hydroxytyrosol was highly toxic to *Pseudomonas syringae* pv *savastanoi* and *Corynebacterium michiganense* (Capasso et al., 1995). Aziz et al. (1998) indicated that oleuropein can completely inhibit the growth of *Escherichia coli, Klebsiella pneuomoniae,* and *Bacillus cereus.* Bisignano et al. (1999) studied the *in vitro* antimicrobial activity of pure oleuropein provided by Exra Synthese and pure hydroxytyrosol chemically synthesized. Five bacterial strains (*Haemophilus influenza* ATCC 9006, *Moraxela catarrhalis* ATCC 8176, *Salmonella typhi* ATCC 6539, *Vibrio parahaemolyticus* ATCC 17802, *Staphylococcus aureus* ATCC 25923) and 44 fresh clinical isolates, causal agents of infections of the intestinal or respiratory tract, were tested for *in vitro* susceptibility to the two above phenols. Results were compared to ampicilin activity. According to the authors the olive tree can be a source of antimicrobial agents for the treatment of infections of the intestinal and respiratory tract.

Hydroxytyrosol, chemically synthesized, was studied by Furneri et al. (2004) for its *in vitro* antimycoplasmal activity. Twenty strains of *Mycoplasma hominis*, three strains of *M. fermentance,* and one strain of *M. pneumoniae* were used in the study. The results indicated that hydroxytyrosol can be considered as an agent for the treatment of infection. According to the authors, "one might speculate that dietary intake of the oil that contains the phenol could reduce the risk of mycoplasmal infections."

Rubia-Soria et al. (2006) studied the production of bacterial isolates from retail table olives. Brenes et al. (2006) and also Medina et al. (2006, 2007) conducted studies to indicate that olive oil is a potential biopreservative for foods. They investigated the antimicrobial activity of individual phenols after separation and isolation with HPLC. The dialdeydic form of decarboxymethyl oleuropein and ligstroside aglycons, hydroxytyrosol and tyrosol, were the phenols that are statistically correlated to bacterial survival. The bactericidic action measured was against a broad spectrum of microorganisms. The effect was higher against Gram-positive than Gram-negative bacteria. The antimicrobial effect of virgin olive oil was also confirmed on mayonnaise inocculated with *S. enterica* and *L. monocytogenes.* It is also worth mentioning that the bactericidal activity shown was not only against harmful bacteria of the intestinal microbiota (*E. coli, C. perfingens*) but also against beneficial *Lactobacillus acidophilus* and *Bifidobacterium bifidum.*

In a recent report C. Romero and collaborators (Romero et al., 2007) found that the phenolics present in olive oil exert *in vitro* a strong bactericidal activity against eight strains of *Helicobacter pylori*, which are linked to a majority of peptic ulcers and certain types of gastric cancer. Some strains are resistant to a number of antibiotics. The authors used simulated conditions to indicate that polar phenols diffuse from the oil into the gastric juice. Among the various phenolics studied the dialdeydic form of decarboxymethyl ligstroside aglycon demonstrated the strongest activity. According to the author a chemopreventive role of olive oil in relation to peptic ulcer or gastric cancer could be suggested, but this has to be confirmed by *in vivo* studies.

Phenolic acids *p*-hydroxybenzoic, vanillic, and *p*-coumaric acids were found to completely inhibit the growth of *E. coli, K. peneumoneae,* and *B. cereus* (Aziz, 1998).

3.8.2 GREEN OLIVES AND TABLE OLIVES

Antimicrobial compounds were isolated from green olives by Walter et al. (1973) and Fleming et al. (1973). Oleuropein was isolated from the fruits using solvent extraction and countercurrent distribution. The dried extract of oleuropein (molecular weight 540) was further purified and hydrolyzed to give three hydrolysis products, 3,4-dihydroxy-phenylethyl alcohol (hydroxytyrosol, molecular weight 154), oleuropein aglycon (molecular weight 378), and elenolic acid (molecular weight 378).

Recently, Pereira et al. (2006) and collaborators as well as Sousa and investigators (2006) evaluated extracts from Portuguese table olives for their *in vitro* activity against microorganisms that can be the cause of intestinal and respiratory tract infections. The microorganisms tested were Gram-positive bacteria *(B. cereus, B. substilis, S. aureus),* Gram-negative bacteria *(P. aeruginosa, E. coli, K. pneumoniae),* and fungi *(Candida albicans and Cryptococcus neoformans).* Three flavonoid compounds — luteolin, apigenin, and 7-*O*-glucosides — were identified by HPLC and their levels correlated to antimicrobial activity. All the extracts tested were found to inhibit most of the bacteria. *B. cereus* and *K. pneumoniae* were the most sensitive. The fungal species investigated (*C. albicans* and *C. neoformans*) were resistant to the extracts (Sousa et al., 2006).

Verbascoside (see Figure 3.9). Verbacoside, the caffeic acid ester of hydroxytyrosol rhamnoglycoside present in olives, shows antibacterial activity against *S. aureus, E. coli,* and other clinical bacteria (Soler-Rivas, 2000; Pardo et al.,1993).

3.8.3 OLIVE LEAVE EXTRACTS

Markin et al. (2003) investigated the antimicrobial effect of olive leaf water extracts against bacteria and fungi. *E. coli* cells exposed to a small concentration of the water extract showed complete destruction, as indicated by scanning electron microscopy. *C. albicans* exposed to 40% olive leaf extract showed invaginated and amorphous cells.

Antiviral activity. The olive leaf extracts were also investigated for their antiviral activity against viral hemorrhagic septicemia virus (VHSV) (Micol et al., 2005) and against HIV-1 infection and replication. Cell-to-cell transmission of HIV was inhibited in a dose-dependent manner, and HIV replication was inhibited in an *in vitro* experiment (Lee-Huang et al., 2003). Oleuropein has been patented for antiviral activity against viral disease, including herpes, mononucleosis, and hepatitis (Fredrickson, 2000).

Claims for pills and tinctures prepared from olive leaf extracts — capsules, tinctures, and teas prepared mainly in the United States, Australia, and Italy from olive leaves — have been advertised for years for their content of oleuropein and their "vast healing powers and ability to eliminate viruses, fungi, bacteria and parasites" (olive leaf extract, http://www.altcancer.com/oliveleaf.htm; organic herbal olive leaf tea, http://www.alibaba.com/catalog/11499524/Organic Olive Leaf Tea html).

Advertisements usually contain the statement that these extracts have not been evaluated by the U.S. Food and Drug Administration. They also contain instructions for use and some warnings to avoid abuse, or interference, with medicines such as antibiotics or blood pressure or blood sugar–lowering drugs, how or if they can be used by pregnant women, the effect on probiotics, and others.

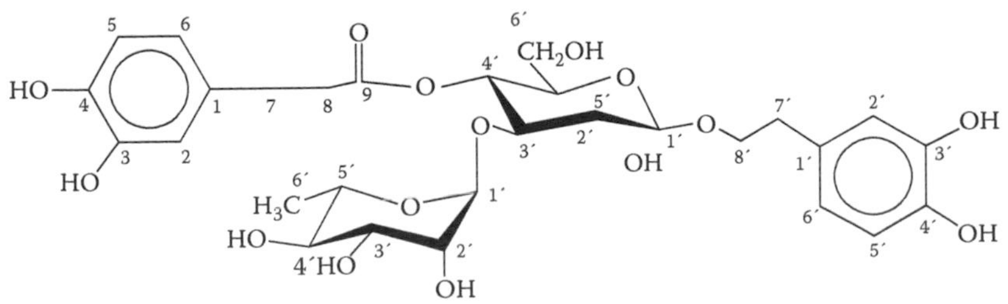

FIGURE 3.9 Verbascoside.

Olive leaf extracts are also sold as strong antioxidants with the claim that they fight free radicals and help maintain a healthy cardiovascular system. The ORAC expressed in µmol of Trolox equivalents per gram of such supplements has been reported to be very high, much higher than that of grape seed and green tea extract (http://www.EnvirOlea.com).

3.8.4 Mechanism of Antimicrobial Activity

The precise mechanisms of antimicrobial action of olive oil phenols are not fully described (Soler-Rivas et al., 2000; Tripoli et al., 2005).

Olive oil biophenols have been shown to be able to penetrate structurally different cell membranes of Gram-negative and Gram-positive bacteria and inhibit irreversibly microbial replication. An example of a structural characteristic is that the glycoside group may modify the ability to penetrate the cell membrane and attain the target site (Saija and Uccella, 2001). An effective interference with the production procedures of certain amino acids necessary for the growth of specific microorganisms has also been suggested. Another mechanism proposed is the direct stimulation of phagocytosis as a response of the immune system to microbes of all types.

3.8.5 Safety Assessment of Olive Extracts

Olive oil and olive fruit have a rich history of nutritional and medicinal use. This may explain why the available safety–toxicity literature on olive oil polyphenols such as hydroxytyrosol is not extensive. The toxicity profile of a patented hydrolyzed aqueous olive pulp extract was characterized in a series of toxicological studies described by Christian et al. (2004). In a recent report Soni et al. (2006) examined the literature related to studies on oral bioavailability of hydroxytyrosol, urinary excretion, and acute and subchronic toxicity in rats. In the oral bioavailability studies urinary excretion of hydroxytyrosol and its glucoronide was found to be directly associated with the intake. Oral bioavailability of hydroxytyrosol in olive oil and in aqueous solution was reported as 99 and 75%, respectively. The LD_{50} of the extract and hydroxytyrosol was reported to be higher than 2000 mg/kg. The NOAEL (no observed adverse effect level) of the water extract obtained from olive pulp, in a subchronic study in rats, was found to be 2000 mg/kg/day. Soni and collaborators (Soni et al., 2006) also conducted developmental and reproductive toxicity studies with olive pulp extract rich in hydroxytyrosol. The extract did not cause toxicity at levels up to 2000 mg/kg/day. In an *in vivo* micronucleus assay oral exposure of rats to the extract, in doses up to 5000 mg/kg/day for 29 days, did not induce any increase in polychromatic erythrocytes in bone marrow. According to the authors the consumption of the patented water olive pulp extract containing hydroxytyrosol should be considered safe at levels not exceeding 20 mg/kg/day.

REFERENCES

Allouche, N., Damak, M., Ellouz, R., and Sayadi, S., 2004, Use of whole cells of *Pseudomonas aeruginosa* for synthesis of antioxidant hydroxytyrosol via conversion of tyrosol, *Appl. Environ. Microb.*, 70, 2105–2109.

Amiot, M.J., Fleuriet, A., and Macheich, J.J., 1989, Accumulation of oleuropein derivatives during olive maturation, *Phytochemistry*, 28, 67–69.

Andrewes, P., Busch, J., De Joode, T., Groenewegen, A., and Alexander, H., 2003, Sensory properties of virgin olive oil polyphenols: identification of deacetoxy-ligstroside aglycon as a key contributor to pungency, *J. Agric. Food Chem.*, 51, 1415–1420.

Angerosa, F., Mostallino, R., Basti, C., and Voto, R., 2001, Influence of malaxation temperature and time on the quality of virgin olive oils, *Food Chemistry*, 72, 19–28.

Aparicio, M. and Luna, G., 2002, Characterization of monovarietal virgin olive oils, *Eur. J. Lipid Sci. Technol.*, 104, 614–637.

Artajo, L.S., Romero, M.P., and Moltiva, M.J., 2006, Enrichment of olive oil: antioxidant capacity functionalized with phenolic compounds, *4th EuroFed Lipid Congress, Madrid,* Book of Abstracts, p. 471.

Aziz, N.H., Farag, S.E., Mousa, L.A., and Abo-Zaid, M.A., 1998, Comparative antibacterial and antimicrobial effects of some phenolics comounds, *Microbios.*, 93, 43–54.

Baldioli, M., Servilli, M., Perretti, G., and Montedoro, G., 1996, Antioxidant activity of tocopherols and phenolic compounds of virgin olive oil, *J. Amer. Oil Chem. Soc.*, 73, 1589–1593.

Baycin, D., Altiok, A., Ulku, S., and Bayractar, O., 2007, Adsorption of olive leaf (*Olea europaea* L.) antioxidants on silk fibroin, *J. Agric. Food Chem.*, 55, 1227–1236.

Beauchamp, G., Keast, R., Morel, D., Lin, J., Pika, J., Han, Q., et al., 2005, Ibuprofen-like activity in extra virgin olive oil, *Nature*, 437, 45–46.

Beltran, G., Ruano, M.T., Jimenez, A., Uceda, M., and Aguilera, M.P., 2007, Evaluation of virgin olive oil bitterness by total phenol content analysis, *Eur. J. Lipid Sci. Technol.*, 108, 193–197.

Bendini, A., Cerretani, L., Vecchi, S., Carrassco-Pancorbo, A., and Lercker, G., 2006, Protective effects of extra virgin olive oil phenolics on oxidative stability in the presence or absence of copper ions, *J. Agric. Food Chem.*, 54, 4880–4887.

Bendini, A., Cerretani, L., Carrasco-Pancorbo, A., Gomez-Caravaco, A.M., Segura-Cerretano, A., Fernandez-Gutierrez, A., et al., 2007, Phenolic molecules in virgin olive oils; a survey of their sensory properties, health effects, antioxidant activity and analytical methods. An overview of the last decade, *Molecules*, 12, 1679–1719.

Bianco, A. and Uccella, N., 2000, Biophenolic components of olives, *Food Res. Int.*, 33, 475–485.

Bianco, A., Chiachio, M., Guiso, M., et al., 2001, Presence in olive oil of a new class of phenolic compounds hydroxyl-isochromans, *Food Chem.*, 77, 405–411.

Bianco, A., Chiacchio, M., Grassi, G., Iannazzo, D., Piperno, A., and Romeo, R., 2006, Phenolic components of *Olea europaea*: isolation of new tyrosol and hydroxytyrosol derivatives, *Food Chem.*, 95, 562–565.

Bisignano, G., Tomaino, A., LoCascio, R., Crisafi, G., Uccele, N., and Saija, A., 1999, On the in-vitro antimicrobial activity of oleuropein and hydroxytyrosol, *J. Pharm. Pharmacol.*, 51, 971–974.

Bitler, C.M., Crea, R., Viale, T.M., and Damai, B., 2005, Hydrolyzed olive vegetation water in mice has anti-inflammatory activity, *J. Nutr.*, 135, 1475–1479.

Blekas, G., Tsimidou, M., and Boskou, D., 1995, Contribution of alpha-tocopherol to olive oil stability, *Food Chem.*, 52, 289–294.

Blekas, G., Vassilakis, C., Harizanis, C., Tsimidou, M., and Boskou, D., 2002, Biophenols in table olives, *J. Agric. Food Chem.*, 50, 3688–3692.

Boskou, D., 2006, Sources of natural antioxidant phenols, in *Natural Antioxidant Phenols: Sources, Structure-Activity Relationship, Current Trends in Analysis and Characterization*, Boskou, D., Gerothnassis, I., and Kefalas, P., Eds., Research Signpost, Trivandrum, Kerala, 1–14.

Boskou, D., Blekas, G., and Tsimidou, M., 2005, Phenolic compounds in olive oil and olives, *Curr. Top. Neutraceut. Res.*, 3, 125–136.

Boskou, G., Salta, F.N., Chrysostomou, S., Mylona, A., Chiou, A., and Andikopoulos, K., 2006, Antioxidant capacity and phenolic profile of table olives from the Greek market, *Food Chem.*, 94, 558–564.

Boskou, D., Tsimidou, M., and Blekas, D., 2006, Polar phenolic compounds, in *Olive Oil, Chemistry and Technology*, Boskou, D., Ed., AOCS Press, Champaign, IL, 73–92.

Bouallagui, Z. and Savadi, S., 2006, Production of high hydroxytyrosol yields via tyrosol conversion by *Pseudomonas aeruginosa* immobilized resting cells, *J. Agric. Food Chem.*, 54, 9906–9911.

Brenes, M., Garcia, A., Garcia, P., Rios, J.J., and Garrido, A., 1999, Phenolic compounds in Spanish olive oils, *J. Agric. Food Chem.*, 47, 3535–3540.

Brenes, M., Garcia, A., Garcia, P., and Garrido, A., 2001, Acid hydrolysis of secoiridoid aglycons during storage of virgin olive oil, *J. Agric. Food Chem.*, 49, 5609–5614.

Brenes, M., Garcia, A., Rios, J.J., Garcia, P., and Garrido, A., 2002, Use of 1-acetoxypinoresinol to authenticate Picual olive oils, *Int. J. Food Sci. Technol.*, 37, 615–623.

Brenes, M., Romero, C., and Garcia, A., 2004, Phenolic compounds in olive oil intended for refining: formation of 4-ethylphenol during olive paste storage, *J. Agric. Food Chem.*, 52, 8177–8181.

Brenes, M., Medina, E., De Castro, A., and Romero, C., 2006, Antimicrobial activity of olive oil, *4th EuroFed Lipid Congress, Madrid*, Book of Abstracts, p. 68.

Briante, R., La Cara, F., Tonziello, M.P., Febbrio, F., and Nucci, R., 2001, Antioxidant activity of the main bioactive derivatives from oleuropein hydrolysis by hyperthermophilic beta-glycosidase, *J. Agric. Food Chem.*, 49, 3198–3203.

Briante, R., La Cara, F., Febbraio, F., Patumi, M., and Nucci, R., 2002a, Bioactive derivatives from oleuropein by a biotransformation on *Olea europaea* leaf extracts, *J. Biotechnol.*, 93, 109–119.

Briante, R., Patumi, M., Limongelli, S., Febbraio, F., Vaccaro, C., DiSalle, A., et al., 2002b, Changes in phenolic and enzymic activities content during fruit ripening in two Italian cultivars of *Olea europaea* L., *Plant Sci.*, 162, 791–798.

Briante, R., Febbraio, F., and Nucci, R., 2003, antioxidant properties of low molecular weight phenols present in the Mediterranean diet, *J. Agric. Food Chem.*, 51, 6975–6981.

Buisman, G.J.H., van Helteren, C.T.W., Kramer, G.F.H., Veldsink, J.W., Derksen, J.W., and Cuperus, F.P., 1998, Enzymatic esterifications of functionalized phenols for the synthesis of lipophilic antioxidants, *Biotechnol. Lett.*, 20, 131–136.

Capasso, R., Evidente, A., Shivo, L., Orru, M., Marcialis, M.A., and Cristinzio, G., 1995, Antibacterial polyphenols from olive oil mill waste waters, *J. Appl. Bacteriol.*, 79, 393–398.

Caponio, F. and Gomes, T., 2001, Influence of olive crushing temperature on phenols in olive oil, *Eur. Food Res. Technol.*, 212, 156–159.

Caponio, F., Aloggio, V., and Gomes, T., 1999, Phenolic compounds in virgin olive oil: influence of paste preparation techniques, *Food Chem.*, 64, 203–209.

Carrasco-Pancorbo, A., Cerretani, L., Segura-Carretero, A., Gallina-Toschi, T., Lercker, G., and Fernandez-Gutierrez, A., 2006, Evaluation of individul antioxidant activity of single phenolic compounds on virgin olive oil, *Prog. Nutr.*, 8, 28–39.

Caruso, D., Colombo, R., Patelli, R., Giavarini, F., and Galli, G., 2000, Rapid evaluation of phenolic profile and analyis of oleuropein aglycon in olive oil by atmospheric pressure chemical ionization–mass spectrometry (APCI–MS), *J. Agric. Food Chem.*, 48, 1182–1185.

Cerretani, L., Bendini, A., Rotondi, A., Lercker, G., and Toschi, T.G., 2005a, Analytical comparison of monovarietal virgin olive oils obtained by both a continuous industrial plant and a low-scale mill, *Eur. J. Lipid Sci. Technol.*, 107, 93–100.

Cerretani, L., Bendini, A., Biguzzi, B., Lercker, G., and Toschi, T.G., 2005b, Freezing storage can affect the oxidative stability of not filtered extra-virgin olive oils, *J. Commod. Sci.*, 44, 3–16.

Cerretani, L., Bendini, A., Del Caro, A., Piga, A., Vacca, M., Caboni, T., et al., 2006, Preliminary characterization of virgin olive oils obtained from different cultivars in Sardinia, *Eur. Food Res. Technol.*, 222, 354–361.

Christian, M., Sharper, V.A., Hoberman, A.M., Seng, J.E, Covell, D., Diemer, R.B., et al., 2004, The toxicity profile of hydrolyzed aqueous olive pulp extract, *Pharmacol. Toxicol.*, 27, 309–330.

Christophoridou, S., Dais, P., Tseng, L.H., and Spraul, M., 2005, Separation and identification of phenolic compounds in olive oil by coupling high-performance liquid chromatography with post column solid-phase extraction to nuclear magnetic resonance spectroscopy (LC-SPE-NMR), *J. Agric. Food Chem.*, 53, 4667–4679.

Cinquanta, L., Esti, M., and Matteo, M., 2001, Oxidative stability of virgin olive oils, *J. Amer. Oil Chem. Soc.*, 78, 1197–1202.

Cipriani, M., Cerretani, L., Bendini, A., Fontanazza, G., and Lercker, A., 2006, Study of phenolic compounds in *Olea europeae* L. fruits of cv. Frantoio, FS 17 and Don Carlo during olives growth, *4th EuroFed Lipid Congress, Madrid*, Book of Abstracts, p. 449.

Clifford, M.N., 2000, Chlorogenic acids and other cinamates — nature, occurrence, dietary burden, absorption and metabolism, *J. Sci. Food Agric.*, 80, 1033–1043.

Clodoveo, M.L., Delcuratoro, D., Gomes, T., and Celelli, G., 2007, Effect of different temperatures and storage atmospheres on Coratina olive oil quality, *Food Chem.*, 102, 571–576.

Coni, E., Benedetto, R., Pasquale, M., Masella, R., Modesti, D., Mattei, R., et al., 2000, Protective effect of oleuropein, an olive oil biophenol, on low density lipoprotein oxidizability in rabbits, *Lipids*, 35, 45–54.

Crea, R., HIDROX, 2005, Proprieatary Hydroxytyrosol, Creagri Inc., http://www.creagri.com/hidrox/5.

Cuomo, J. and Rabovski, A.B., Usan Inc., 2002, Antioxidant Compositions Extracted from a Waste Water from Olive Oil Production, U.S. Patent 6,361,803.

Davin, B.D., Bedgar, D.L., Katayama, T., and Lewis, N.G., 1992, On the stereoselective synthesis of (+)-pinoresinol in *Forsynthia suspensa* from its achiral precursor, coniferyl alcohol, *Phytochemistry*, 31, 3869–3874.

Deiana, M., Aruoma, O.I., Bianchi, M., Sencer, J.P.E., Kaur, H., Haalliwell, B., et al., 1999, Inhibition of peroxynitrate dependent DNA base modification and tyrosine nitration by extra virgin olive oil–derived antioxidant hydroxytyrosol, *Free Radical Biol. Med.*, 26, 762–769.

De la Puerta, R., Guttierrez, V.R., and Hoult, J.R.S., 1999, Inhibition of leukocyte 5-lipoxygenase by phenolics from virgin olive oil, *Biochem. Pharmacol.*, 57, 445–449.

De la Puerta, R., Dominguez, M.E.M., Ruiz-Guttierrez, V., Flavill, J.A., and Hoult, J.R.S., 2001, Effects of olive oil phenolics on scavenging of reactive nitrogen species and upon nitrergic neurotransmission, *Life Sci.*, 69, 1213–1222.

DiGiovacchino, L., Constantini, N., Serraiocco, A., Surrichio, G., and Basti, C., 2001, Natural antioxidants and volatile compounds of virgin olive obtained by two or three-phase centrifugal decanters, *Eur. J. Lipid Sci. Technol.*, 103, 279–285.

DiGiovacchino, L., Sestili, S., and DiVicenzo, D., 2002, Influence of olive processing on virgin olive oil quality, *Eur. J. Lipid Sci. Technol.*, 104, 587–601.

Espin, J.C., Soler-Rivas, C., and Wichers, H., 2000, Characterization of the total free radical scavenger capacity of vegetable oil and oil fractions using 2,2-diphenyl-1-picrylhydrazyl radical, *J. Agric. Food Chem.*, 48, 648–656.

Espin, J.C., Soler-Rivas, C., Cantos, E., Tomas-Barberan, F.A., and Wichers, H., 2001, Synthesis of the antioxidant hydroxytyrose using tyrosinase biocatalyst, *J. Agric. Food Chem.* 49, 1187–1193.

Esti, M., Cinquanta, L., and La Notte, E., 1998, Phenolic compounds in different olive varieties, *J. Agric. Food Chem.*, 46, 32–35.

Fernandez-Bolanos, J., Rodriguez, G., Rodriguez, R., Heredia, A., Guillen, R., and Jimenez, A., 2002, Production in large quantities of highly purified hydroxytyrosol from liquid-solid waste of two-phase olive oil processing or "alperujo," *J. Agric. Food Chem.*, 50, 6804–6811.

Fernandez-Bolanos, J., Heredia, A., Rodriguez, G, Rodriguez, R., Jimenez, A., and Guillen, R., 2005, Method for Obtaining Purified Hydroxytyrosol from Products and By-Products Derived from the Olive Tree, U.S. Patent 6,849,770.

Fernandez-Bolanos, J., Rodriguez, G., Guillen, R., Rodriguez, R., and Rodriguez, R., 2006, Valorisation of olive oil by-products, *4th EuroFed Lipid Congress, Madrid*, Book of Abstracts, p. 288.

Fki, I., Allouche, N., and Sayadi, S., 2005, The use of polyphenolic extract, purified hydroxytyrosol and 3,4-dihydroxyphenyl acetic acid from olive oil waste water for the stabilization of refined oils: a potential alternative to synthetic antioxidants, *Food Chem.*, 93, 197–204.

Fki, I., Sahoun, Z., and Sayadi, S., 2007, Hypocholesteremic effects of phenolic extracts and purified hydroxytyrosol recovered from olive mill wastewater in rats fed a cholesterol diet, *J. Agric. Food Chem.*, 55, 624–631.

Fleming, H.P., Walter, W.M., and Ethchels, J.L., 1969, Isolation of a bacterial inhibitor from green olives, *Appl. Microb.*, 18, 856–860.

Fogliano, V., 2006, Oleocanthal in olive oil: between myth and reality, *Mol. Nutr. Food Res.*, 50, 5–6.

Fogliano, V., Ritieni, S., Monti, S., Gallo, M., Madaglia, D.D., Ambrosino, M.L., and Sacchi, R., 1999, Antioxidant activity of virgin olive oil phenolic compounds in a micellar system, *J. Sci. Food Agric.*, 79, 1803–1808.

Fredrickson, W.R., F and S Group, Inc., 2000, Method and Composition for Antiviral Therapy with Olive Leaves, U.S. Patent 6,117,884.

Fregapane, G., Lavelli, V., Leon, S., Kapuralin, J., and Desamparados Salvador, M., 2006, Effect of filtration on virgin olive oil stability during storage, *Eur. J. Lipid Sci. Technol.*, 108, 134–142.

Furneri, P.M., Piperno, A., Saija, A., and Bisignano, G., 2004, Antimicrobial activity of hydroxytyrosol, *Antimicrob. Agents Chemother.*, 48, 4892–4894.

Gambacorta, A., Tofani, D., Bernini, R., and Migliorini, A., 2007, High-yielding preparation of a stable precursor of hydroxytyrosol by total synthesis and from the natural glycoside oleuropein, *J. Agric. Food Chem.*, 55, 3386–3391.

Garcia, A., Brenes, M., Romero, C., Alba, J., Garcia, P., and Garrido, A., 2001, HPLC evaluation of phenols in virgin olive oil during extraction at laboratory and industrial scale, *J. Amer. Oil Chem. Soc.*, 78, 625–629.

Garcia, A., Ruiz-Mendez, M.V., Romero, C., and Brenes, M., 2006, Effect of refining on the phenolic composition of crude olive oil, *J. Amer. Oil Chem. Soc.*, 83, 159–164.

Garcia, J.M., Seler, S., and Perez Camino, M.C., 1986, Influence of fruit ripening on olive oil quality, *J. Agric. Food Chem.*, 44, 3516–3520.

Garcia, J.M., Seller, S., and Perez Camino, M.C., 1996, Influence of fruit ripening on olive oil quality, *J. Agric. Food Chem.*, 44, 3516–3520.

Gennaro, l., Bocca, A.P., Modesti, D., Masela, R., and Coni, E., 1998, Effect of biophenols on olive oil stability evaluated by thermogravimetric analysis, *J. Agric. Food Chem.*, 46, 4465–4469.

Gibriel, A.Y., EL-Razik, A., Abb El Razik, F.A.A., and Abou-Zaid, F.O.F., 2006, *4th EuroFed Lipid Congress, Madrid*, Book of Abstracts, p. 414.

Giovannini, G., Straface, E., Modesti, D., Coni, D., Cantafora, A., De Vincenci, M., et al., 1999, Tyrosol, the major olive oil biophenol, protects against oxidized-LDL induced injury in Caco-2-cells, *J. Nutr.*, 129, 1269–1272.

Gomez-Alonso, S., Fregapane, G., Salvador Desamparados, M., and Gordon, M.H., 2003, Changes in phenolic composition and antioxidant activity of virgin olive oil during frying, *J. Agric. Food Chem.*, 57, 667–672.

Gomez-Rico, A., Inarejos-Garcia, A.M., Fregapane, G., and Salvador, M.D., 2006, Study of malaxation on volatile and phenolic compounds in virgin olive oil processing technology, *4th EuroFed Lipid Congress, Madrid*, Book of Abstracts, p. 71.

Gonzales, F.A., Ventula, A.C., Sanchez, J.L.E., Briz, R.M., and Perez-Lanzac, M.T., 2005, Method of Preparing Hydroxytyrosol Esters, Patent Intern. Applic. No. PCT/ES2003/000.327.

Gonzalez-Santiago, M., MartinBatista, E., Carrero, J.J., Fonolla, J., Baro, L., Bartolome, M.V., et al., 2006, One-month administration of hyroxytyrosol, a phenolic antioxidant present in olive oil, to hyperlipemic rabbits improves blood lipid profile, antioxidant status and reduces atherosclerosis development, *Atherosclerosis*, 188, 35–42.

Gordon, M.H., Paiva-Martins, F., and Almeida, M., 2001, Antioxidant activity of hydroxytyrosol acetate compared with that of other olive oil polyphenols, *J. Agric. Food Chem.*, 49, 2480–2485.

Gorinstein, S., Leontowitcz, H., Loiek, A., Leontowicz, M., Ciz, M., Krzemiski, R., et al., 2002, Olive oil improves lipid metabolism and increases antioxidant potential in rats fed diets containing cholesterol, *J. Agric. Food Chem.*, 50, 6102–6108.

Gorinstein, S., Martin Belloso, O., Katrich, E., Lojek, A., Czek, M., and Gligelmo-Miguel, N., 2003, Comparison of the contents of the main biochemical compounds and the antioxidant activity of some Spanish olive oils as determined by four different radical scavenging tests, *J. Nutr. Biochem.*, 14, 154–159.

Grasso, S., Siracusa, L., Spatafora, C., Renis, M., and Tringali, C., 2007, Hydroxytyrosol lipophilic analogues: enzymatic synthesis, radical scavenging activity and DNA oxidative damage protection, *Biorg. Chem.*, 35, 137–152.

Gutierrez, F., Perdiguero, S., Gutierrez, R., and Olias, J.M., 1992, Evaluation of the bitter taste in virgin olive oil, *J. Amer. Oil Chem. Soc.*, 69, 394–395.

Gutierrez-Rosales, F.T. and Arnaud, T., 2001, Contribution of polyphenols on the oxidative stability of virgin olive oil, *24th World Congress ISF, Berlin, Proceedings*, pp. 61–62.

Gutierrez-Rosales, F., Rios, J.J., and Gomez-Rey, M.L., 2003, Main polyphenols in the bitter taste of virgin olive oil. Structural confirmation by on-line high-performance liquid chromatography electrospray ionization mass spectrometry, *J. Agric. Food Chem.*, 51, 6021–6025.

Japon-Lujan, R. and Luque de Castro, M.D., 2007, Small branches of olive tree: a source of biophenols complementary to olive leaves, *J. Agric. Food Chem.*, 55, 4584–4588.

Japon-Lujan, R., Luque-Rondriguez, J.M., and Luque de Castro, M.D., 2006a, Multivariate optimization of the microwave-assisted extraction of oleuropein and related biophenols from olive oil leaves, *Anal. Bioanal. Chem.*, 385, 753–759.

Japon-Lujan, R., Luque-Rondrigez, J.M., and Luque de Castro, M.D., 2006b, Dynamic ultrasound-assisted extraction of oleuropein and related biophenols from olive leaves, *J. Chromatogr. A*, 1108, 76–82.

Jiang, L., Tomoko Yamaguchi, T., Hitoshi Takamura, H., and Teruyoshi Matoba, T., 2005, Characteristics of Shodo Island olive oils in Japan: fatty acid composition and antioxidative compounds, *Food Sci. Technol. Res.*, 11, 254–260.

Kachouri, F. and Hamdi, M., 2004, Enhancement of polyphenols in olive oil by contact with fermented olive mill wastewater by *Lactobacillus plantarum*, *Process Biochem.*, 39, 841–845.

Kalua, C.M., Bedgood, D.R., Bishop, A.G., and Prenzer, P.D., 2006, Changes in volatile and phenolic compounds with malaxation and temperature during virgin olive oil production, *J. Agric. Food. Chem.*, 54, 7641–7651.

Kamal-Eldin, A., Appelquist, L.A., and Yousif, G., 1994, Lignan analysis in seed oils from four sesamum species: comparison of different chromatographic methods, *J. Amer. Oil Chem. Soc.*, 71, 141–145.

Kato, M.J., Chu, A., Davin, L.B., and Lewis, N.G., 1998, Biosynthesis of antioxidant lignans in *Sesamum indicum* seeds, *Phytochemistry*, 47, 583–591.

Keceli, T. and Robinson, R.K., 2002, Antimicrobial activity of phenolic extracts from virgin olive oil, *Milchwissenschaft*, 57, 436–440.

Kohyama, N., Nagata, T., Fujimoto, S., and Sekiya, K., 1997, Inhibition of arachidonate lipoxygenase activities by 2-(3,4-dihydrophenyl)ethanol, a phenolic compound from olives, *Biosci. Biotech. Biochem.*, 61, 347–350.

Krzeminski, R., Gorinstein, S., Leontowicz, H., Leontowcz, M., Gralak, M., Czerwinski, J., et al., 2003, Effect of different olive oils on bile excretion in rats fed cholesterol-containing and cholesterol-free diets, *J. Agric. Food Chem.*, 51, 5774–5779.

Larrosa, M., Carlos-Espin, J., and Tomas-Barberan, A.F., 2003, Antioxidant capacity of tomato juice functionalized with enzymatically synthesized hydroxytyrosol, *J. Sci. Food Agric.*, 83, 658–666.

Lavelli, V., 2002, Comparion of the antioxidant activities of extra virgin olive oils, *J. Agric. Food Chem.*, 50, 7704–7708.

Lee-Huang, S., Zhang, L., Chang, Y.Y., and Huang, P.L., 2003, Anti-HIV activity of olive leaf extract (OLE) and modulation of host cell gene expression by HIV-1 infection and OLE treatment, *Biochem. Biophys. Res. Commun.*, 307, 1029–1037.

Leenen, R., Roodenberg, A.J.C., Vissers, M.N., Schuurbiers, J.A.E., van Putte, K.P.A.M., Wiseman, S.A, et al., 2002, Supplementation of plasma with olive oil phenols and extracts: influence on LDL oxidation, *J. Agric. Food Chem.*, 50, 1290–1297.

Litridou, M., Linssen, H., Schols, H., Bergmans, M., Tsimidou, M., and Boskou, D., 1997, Phenolic compounds of virgin olive oils: fractionation by solid phase extraction and antioxidant activity assessment, *J. Sci. Food Agric.*, 74, 169–174.

Lorenz, P., Zeh, M., Lobenhoffer-Martens, J., Schmidt, H., Wolf, G., and Horn, T.F., 2005, Natural and newly hydroxyl-aryl-isochromans: a class of potential antioxidants and radical scavengers, *Free Radic. Res.*, 39, 535–545.

Mailer, R., Conlan, D., and Ayton, J., 2005, Olive Harvest, Rural Industries Research and Development Corporation, Wagga Wagga, Australia, Publication 05/013.

Manach, C., Scalbert, A., Morand, C., Remesy, C., and Jimenez, L., 2004, Polyphenols: food sources and bioavailability, *Am. J. Clin. Nutr.*, 79, 727–747.

Manna, C., Galletti, P., Cuciolla, V., Montedoro, G., and Zappia, V., 1999, Olive oil hydroxytyrosol protects human erythrocytes against oxidative damages, *J. Nutr. Biochem.*, 10, 159–165.

Manna, C., Migliardi, V., Golino, P., Scognmiglio, A., Galetti, P., Chiariello, M., et al., 2004, Oleuropein prevents oxidative myocardial injury by ischemia and reperfusion, *J. Nutr. Biochem.*, 15, 461–468.

Manna, C., Migliardi, V., Sannino, F., De Martino, A., and Capasso, R., 2005, Protective effects of synthetic hydroxytyrosol acetyl derivatives against oxidative stress in human cells, *J. Agric. Food Chem.*, 53, 9602–9607.

Mannino, S., Buratti, S., Cosio, M.S., and Pellegrini, M., 1999, Evaluation of the "antioxidant power" of olive oils based on a FIA system with amperometric detection, *Analyst*, 124, 1115–1118.

Markin, D., Duek, L., and Berdicevsky, I., 2003, *In vitro* antimicrobial activity of olive leaves, *Mycoses*, 46, 132–136.

Masella, R., Cantafora, A., Modesti, D., Cardilli, A., Gennaro, L., Bocca, A., et al., 1999, Antioxidant activity of 3,4-DHPEA-EA and protocatechuic acid: a comparative assessment with other olive oil biophenols, *Redox Rep.*, 4, 113–121.

Mateos, R., Dominguez, M.M., Espartero, J.L., and Cert, A., 2003, Antioxidant effect of phenolic compounds, alpha-tocopherol and other minor components in virgin olive oil, *J. Agric. Food Chem.*, 51, 7170–7175.

Mateos, R., Cert, A., Perez-Camino, M.C., and Garcia, J.M., 2004, Evaluation of virgin olive oil bitterness by quantification of secoiridoid derivatives, *J. Amer. Oil Chem. Soc.*, 81, 71–76.

McDonald, S., Prenler, P.D., Antolovich, M., and Robards, K., 2001, Phenolic content and antioxidant activity of olive extracts, *Food Chem.*, 73, 73–84.

Medina, E., De Castro, A., Romero, C., and Brenes, M., 2006, Phenolic compounds in olive oil and other plant oils: correlation with antimicrobial activity, *J. Agric. Food Chem.*, 54, 4954–4961.

Medina, E., Romero, C., Brenes, M., and de Castro, A., 2007, Antimicrobial activity of olive oil, vinegar and various beverages against foodborne pathogens, *J. Food Protection*, 70, 1194–1199.

Micol, V., Caturla, N., Perenz-Fons, L., Mas, L., Perez, L., and Estepa, A., 2005, The olive leaf extract exhibits antiviral activity against viral haemorrhagic septicaemia rhabdovirus (VHSV), *Antivir. Res.*, 66, 129–136.

Migliorini, M., Mugelli, M., Cherubini, C., Viti, P., and Zaroni, B., 2006, Influence of O_2 on the quality of virgin olive oil during malaxation, *J. Sci. Food Agric.*, 86, 2140–2146.

Milder, I.E.J., Arts, I.C.W., van de Putte, B., Dini, V.P., and Hollman, P.C.H., 2005a, Lignan contents of Dutch plant foods: a database including lariciresinol, pinoresinol, secoisolariciresinol and matairesinol, *Br. J. Nutr.*, 93, 393–402.

Milder, I.E.J., Feskens, E.J.M., Arts, I.C.W., Bas Bueno de Mesquita, H., Hollman, P.C.H., et al., 2005b, Intake of the plant lignans secoisolareciresinol, matairesinol, lariciresinol and pinoresinol in Dutch men and women, *J. Nutr.*, 135, 1202–1207.

Monteleone, E., Caporale, G., Carlucci, A., and Pagliarini, E., 1998, Optimisation of extra virgin olive oil quality, *J. Sci. Food Agric.*, 77, 31–37.

Morello, J.R., Motilva, M.J., Tovar, M.J., and Romero, M.P., 2004, Changes in commercial virgin olive oil (cv Arbequina) during storage, with special emphasis on the phenolic fraction, *Food Chem.*, 65, 357–364.

Mosca, L., De Marco, C., Visioli, F., and Canella, C., 2000, Enzymatic assay for the determination of olive oil polyphenol content: assay conditions and validation of the method, *J. Agric. Food Chem.*, 48, 297–301.

Murkovic, M., Lechner, S., Pietzka, A., Bratakos, M., and Katzogiannos, M., 2004, Analysis of minor constituents in olive oil, *J. Biochem. Methods*, 61, 155–160.

Nenadis, N., Wang, L.F., Tsimidou, M.Z., and Zhang, H.Y., 2005, Radical scavenging potential of phenolic compounds encountered in *O. europaea*. Products as indicated by calculation of bond dissociation enthalpy and ionization potential values, *J. Agric. Food Chem.*, 53, 295–299.

Nenadis, N., Vervoort, J., Boeren, S., and Tsimidou, M., 2006, *Syringa oblate* Lindl var. alba as a source of oleuropein and related compounds, *J. Sci. Food Agric.*, 87, 160–166.

Ninfali, P., Aluigi, G., Bacchiocca, M., and Magnani, M., 2001, Antioxidant capacity of extra-virgin olive oil, *J. Amer. Oil Chem. Soc.*, 78, 243–247.

Ottaviani, M.F., Spallaci, M., Cangiotti, M., Bacchiocca, M., and Niffali, P., 2001, Electron paramagnetic resonance investigations of free radicals in extra virgin olive oil, *J. Agric. Food Chem.*, 49, 3691–3696.

Owen, R.W., Mier, W., Giacosa, A., Hull, W.E., Spiegelhalder, B., and Bartsch, H., 2000a, Identification of lignans as major components in the phenolic fraction of olive oil, *Clin. Chem.*, 46, 976–988.

Owen, R.W., Mier, W., Giacosa, A., Hull, W.E., Spiegelhalder, B., and Bartsch, H., 2000b, Phenolic compounds and squalene in olive oils: the concentration and antioxidant potential of total phenols, simple phenols, secoiridoids, lignans and squalene, *Food Chem. Toxicol.*, 38, 647–659.

Paiva-Martins, F. and Gordon, M.H., 2002, Effects of pH and ferric ions on the antioxidant activity of olive oil polyphenols on oil-in-water emulsions, *J. Amer. Oil Chem. Soc.*, 79, 571–576.

Paiva-Martins, F., Felix, S., Correia, R., Ferreira, P., and Gordon, M., 2005, Enriched refined olive oil with olive tree phenolic copounds, *Int. Soc. Fat Research, 26th World Congress, Prague,* Book of Abstracts, pp. 96–97.

Paiva-Martins, F., Fernandes, J., Santos, V., Borges, F., Belo, L., and Santos-Silva, A., 2006, Effect of olive oil polyphenols on erythrocytes oxidative damage, *4th EuroFed Lipid Congress, Madrid,* Book of Abstracts, p. 455.

Papadopoulos, G. and Boskou, D., 1991, Antioxidant effect of natural phenols on olive oil, *J. Amer. Oil Chem. Soc.*, 68, 669–671.

Papadopoulos, G., Tsimidou, M., and Boskou, D., 1993, Stability of virgin olive oil: assessment of natural antioxidants and other related factors, in *Food Flavours, Ingredients and Composition*, Charalambous, G., Ed., Elsevier, Amsterdam, pp. 321–326.

Pardo, F., Perich, F., Villaroel, L., and Torres, R., 1993, Isolation of verbascoside, an antimicrobial constituent of *Buddleja globosa* leaves, *J. Ethnopharmacol.*, 39, 221–222.

Parenti, A., Spugnoli, P., Massela, P., Calamai, L., and Pantani, O.L., 2006, Improving olive oil quality using carbon dioxide evolved from pastes during processing, *Eur. J. Lipid Sci. Technol.*, 108, 904–912.

Patumi, M., d'Adria, R., Marsilio, V., Fontanazza, G., Morelli, G., and Lanza, B., 2002, Olive and olive oil quality after intensive monocone olive growing (*Olea europaea* L., cv. Lalamata) in different irrigation regimes, *Food Chem.*, 77, 27–34.

Pellegrini, N., Visioli, F., Buratti, S., and Brighenti, F., 2001, Direct analysis of total antioxidant activity of olive oil and studies on the influence of heating, *J. Agric. Food Chem.*, 49, 2532–2538.

Pereira, J.A., Pereira, A.P.G., Ferreira, I.C.F.R., Valentao, P., Andrade, B.P., Seabra, R., et al., 2006, Table olives from Portugal: phenolic compounds, antioxidant potential and antimicrobial activity, *J. Agric. Food Chem.*, 54, 8425–8431.

Perona, J.S., Cabello-Moruno, R., and Ruiz-Gutierrez, V., 2006, The role of virgin olive oil consumption in the modulation of endothelial function, *J. Nutr. Biochem.*, 17, 429–445.

Petrakis, C., 2006, Olive oil extraction, in *Olive Oil, Chemistry and Technology*, Boskou, D., Ed., AOCS Press, Champaign, IL, pp. 191–225.

Poerio, A., Cerretani, L., Bendini, A., Lercker, G., and Gallina Toschi, T., 2006, Evaluation of phenolic fraction in edible olive oils obtained by different technological systems, *4th EuroFed Lipid Congress, Madrid,* Book of Abstracts, p. 454.

Poerio, A., Bendini, A., Cerretani, L., Bonoli, M., and Lercker, G., in press, Effect of olive fruit freezing on oxidative stability of virgin olive oil, *Eur. J. Lipid Sci. Technol.*

Quiles, J.L., Ramirez-Tortoza, M.C., Gomez, J.A., Huertas, J.R., and Mataix, J., 2002, Role of vitamin E and phenolic compounds in the antioxidant capacity, measured by ESR, of virgin olive oil, olive and sunflower oils after frying, *Food Chem.*, 76, 461–468.

Rada, M., Albi, T., Guinda, A., and Cayuela, J.A., 2006, Extraction of hydroxytyrosol from the olive leaves and isolation by molecular distillation, *4th EuroFed Lipid Congress, Madrid*, Book of Abstracts, p. 425.

Rahmouni, K., Bouhafa, H., Labidi, A., Nafti, A., and Hamdi, S., 2006, Olive oil oxidation: relation between alpha-tocopherol and peroxide value, *Olivae*, 106, 24–31.

Ranalli, A., Modesti, G., Patumi, M., and Fontanazza, G., 2000, The compositional quality and sensory properties of virgin olive oil from a new olive cultivar I-77, *Food Chem.*, 69, 37–46.

Roche, M., Dufour, C., Mora, N., and Dangles, O., 2005, Antioxidant activity of olive phenols: mechanistic investigation and characterization of oxidation products by mass spectrometry, *Org. Biomol. Chem.*, 3, 423–430.

Romani A., Lapucci, C., Cantini, C., Ieri, F., Mulinaci, N., and Visioli, F., 2007, Evolution of minor polar compounds and antioxidant capacity during storage of bottled extra virgin olive oil, *J. Agric. Food Chem.*, 55, 1315–1320.

Romero, C., Brenes, M., Garcia, P., and Garrido, A., 2002, Hydroxytyrosol 4-β-D-glucoside, an important compound in olive oil fruits and derived products, *J. Agric. Food Chem.*, 50, 3835–3839.

Romero, C., Medina, E., Vargas, J., Brenes, M., and DeCastro, A., 2007, *In vitro* activity of olive polyphenols against *Helicobacter pylori*, *J. Agric. Food Chem.*, 55, 680–686.

Romero, M.P., Tovar, M.J., Girona, J., and Motilva, M.J., 2002, Changes in the HPLC phenolic profile of virgin olive oil from young trees (*Olea europaea* L. cv Arbequina) grown under different deficit irrigation strategies, *J. Agric. Food Chem.*, 50, 5349–5354.

Rotondi, A., Bendini, A., Cerretani, L., et al., 2004, Effect of ripening degree on the oxidative stability and organoleptic properties of cv Nostrana di Brisighella extra virgin olive oil, *J. Agric. Food Chem.*, 52, 3649–3654.

Rubia-Soria, A., Abriouel, H., Lucas, R., Omar, N.B., Martinez-Canamero, M., and Galvez, A., 2006, Production of antimicrobial substances by bacteria isolated from fermented table olives, *World J. Microb. Biotechnol.*, 22, 765–768.

Ryan, D., Antonovitch, M., Prenzel, P., and Lavee, S., 2002, Biotransformation of phenolic compounds in *Olea europea* L., *Sintia Hort.*, 92, 147–176.

Saija, A. and Uccella, N., 2001, Olive oil biophenols: functional effects on human well-being, *Trends Food Sci. Technol.*, 11, 357–363.

Saija, A., Trombetta, A., Tomaino, A., Lo Cascio, R., Princi, P., Ucella, N., et al., 1998, *In vitro* evaluation of the antioxidant activity and biomembranes interaction of the plant phenols oleuropein and hydroxytyrosol, *Int. J. Pharmacol.*, 166, 123–133.

Saiz, Y.H., 2000, Enzymatic Synthesis of Antioxidant Hydroxytyrosol, Patent 20000207373, Food Additive, Concejo Superior de Investigaciones Cientificas (CSIC) Spain, AGRO013.

Salta, F.N., Mylona, A., Chiou, A., Boskou, G., and Andrikopoulos, N., 2007, Oxidative stability of edible vegetable oils enriched in polyphenols with olive leaf extract, *Food Sci. Technol. Intern.* 13, 413–417.

Salvador, M.D., Aranda, F., and Fregapane, G., 2001, Influence of fruit ripening on "Cornicabra" virgin olive oil quality. A study of four successive crop seasons, *Food Chem.*, 73, 45–53.

Salvador, M.D., Aranda, F., Gomez-Alonso, S., et al., 2003, Influence of extraction system, production year and area on Cornicabra virgin olive oil; a study of five crop seasons, *Food Chem.*, 80, 359–366.

Schaffer, S., Podstava, M., Visioli, F., Bogani, P., Muller, W.E., and Eckert, P., 2007, Hydroxytyrosol-rich olive mill wastewater extract protects brain cells *in vitro* and *ex vivo*, *J. Agric. Food Chem.*, 55, 5043–5049.

Schiratti, G., 1999, Presentation of the study on the influence of environmental, agronomic and processing variables on the characteristics and levels of minor components in extra virgin olive oil, *Olivae*, 79, 38–40.

Servili, M. and Montedoro, G., 2002, Contribution of phenolic compounds to virgin olive oil quality, *Eur. J. Lipid Sci. Technol.*, 104, 602–613.

Servili, M., Piackuadio, P., De Stefano, G., Taticchi, A., and Sciancalepore, V., 2002, Influence of a new crushing technique on the composition of the volatile compounds and related sensory quality of virgin olive oil, *Eur. J. Lipid Sci. Technol.*, 104, 483–489.

Servili, M., Salvaggini, R., Taticchi, A., Esposto, S., and Montedoro, G., 2003, Air exposure of olive pastes during the extraction process and phenolic and volatile composition of virgin olive oil, *J. Amer. Oil Chem. Soc.*, 80, 685–690.

Servili, M., Esposito, S., Lodonini, E., Selvagini, R., Taticchi, A., Urbani, S., et al., 2007, Irrigation effects on quality, phenolic composition and selected volatiles of virgin olive oils cv Leccino, *J. Agric. Food Chem.*, 55, 6609–6618.

Sharp, H., Thomas, D., Currie, F., Bright, C., Latif, Z., Satyajit, D., et al., 2001, Pinoresinol and syringaresinol: two lignans from *Avicennia germinans* (Avicenniaceae), *Biochem. System Ecol.*, 29, 325–327.

Siliani, S., Mattei, A., Innocent, L.B., and Zanono, B., 2006, Bitter taste and phenolic compounds in extra virgin olive oil: an empirical relationship, *J. Food Qual.*, 29, 431–441.

Silva, S., Gomez, L., Leitao, F., Coelho, A.V., and Vilas Boas, L., 2006, Phenolic compounds and antioxidant activity of *Olea europea* L. fruits and leaves, *Food Sci. Technol. Int.*, 12, 385–395.

Soler-Rivas, C., Carlos-Espin, J., and Wichers, H.J., 2000, Oleuropein and related compounds, *J. Sci. Food Agric.*, 80, 1013–1023.

Soni, M.G., Burdock, G.A., Christian, M.S., and Botler, C.M., 2006, Safety assessment of aqueous olive pulp extract as an antioxidant or antimicrobial agent in foods, *Food Chem. Toxicol.*, 44, 903–915.

Sousa, A., Ferreira, I., Calhelha, R., Andrade, P.B., Valenta, P., Seabra, R., et al., 2006, Phenolics and antimicrobial activity of traditional stoned table olives "alaparra," *Biorgan. Med. Chem.*, 14, 8533–8538.

Tassou, C.C. and Nychas, G., 1994, Inhibition of *Staphylococcus aureus* by olive phenolics in broth and in model system, *J. Food Prot.*, 57, 120–124.

Tovar, M.J., Motilva, M.J., and Romero, M.P., 2001, Changes in the phenolic composition of virgin olive oil from young trees (*Olea europaea* L. cv Arbequina) grown under linear irrigation strategies, *J. Agric. Food. Chem.*, 49, 5502–5508.

Tovar, M.J., Romero, M.P., Alegre, S., Girona, J., and Motilva, M.J., 2002, Composition and organoleptic characteristics of oil from Arbequina olive (*Olea europaea* L.) trees under deficit irrigation, *J. Sci. Food Agric.*, 82, 1755–1763.

Tripoli, E., Giammanco, M., Tabacchi, G., DiMajo, D., Giammanco, S., and LaGuardia, M., 2005, The phenolic composition of olive oil: structure, biological activity, and beneficial effects on human health, *Nutr. Res. Rev.*, 18, 98–112.

Trujillo, M., Mateos, R., Collantes de Teran, L., Espartero, J., Cert, R., Jove, M., et al., 2006, Lipophilic hydroxytyrosol esters. Antioxidant activity in lipid matrices and biological systems, *J. Agric. Food Chem.*, 54, 3779–3785.

Tsimidou, M., 2006, Olive oil quality, in *Olive Oil, Chemistry and Technology*, Boskou, D., Ed., AOCS Press, Champaign, IL, pp. 93–112.

Tsukamoto, H., Hisada, S., and Nishibe, S., 1984, Lignans from the bark of the *Olea* plants, *Chem. Pharm. Bull.*, 32, 2730–2735.

Tuck, K.L., Hayball, P., and Stupans, I., 2002, Structural characterization of metabolites of hydroxytyrosol, the principal phenolic component of olive oil, *J. Agric. Food Chem.*, 50, 2404–2409.

Valavanidis, A., Nisiotou, C., Papageorgiou, Y., Kremli, I., Satravelas, N., Zinieris, N., et al., 2004, Comparison of the radical scavenging potential of polar and lipidic fractions of olive oil and other vegetable oils under normal conditions and after thermal treatment, *J. Agric. Food Chem.*, 52, 2358–2365.

Van der Boom, S. and Manon, J., 2004, Food Compositions Fortified with Anti-Oxidants, U.S. Patent 6,746,706.

Van Hoed, V., Andjekivic, M., Verhe, R., Berti, L., Maestri, E., and Marmiroli, N., 2006, Influence of harvest date on the chemical composition of olive oil of the three main Corsican olive cultivars, *4th EuroFed Lipid Congress, Madrid*, Book of Abstracts, p. 447.

Velasco, J. and Dobarganes, C., 2002, Oxidative stability of virgin olive oil, *Eur. J. Lipid Sci. Technol.*, 104, 661–676.

Visioli, F., Galli, C., Galli, G., and Caruso, D., 2002, Biological activities and metabolic fate of olive oil phenols, *Eur. J. Lipid Sci. Technol.*, 104, 677–684.

Visioli, F., Bogani, P., and Galli, C., 2006, Healthful properties of olive oil minor components, in *Olive Oil, Chemistry and Technology*, Boskou, D., Ed., AOCS Press, Champaign, IL, pp. 173–190.

Walter, W.M., Fleming, H.P., and Etchells, J.L., 1973, Preparation of antimicrobial compounds by hydrolysis of oleuropein from green olives, *Appl. Microb.*, 26, 773–776.

Wiseman, S.A., Mathot, J., Fouw, N.J., and Tijburg, L., 1996, Dietary non-tocopherol antioxidants present in extra virgin olive oil increase the resistance of low density lipoproteins to oxidation in rabbits, *Atherosclerosis*, 120, 15–23.

4 Other Important Minor Constituents

Dimitrios Boskou

CONTENTS

4.1 SQUALENE

Squalene (2,6,10,15,19,23-hexamehyl-2,6,10,14,18,22-tetracosanehexaene) is an unsaturated terpene widely distributed in nature. Chemically it is an all-*trans* isoprenoid containing six isoprene units. Squalene is an intermediate in the biosynthesis of sterols in plants and animals, a precursor of phytosterols in plants, and a precursor of cholesterol in humans. It occurs in high concentrations in the liver oil of certain sharks and in smaller amounts in olive oil, rice bran oil, and yeast. It is also found in palm oil and the palm fatty acid distillate (Gapor Md Top and Abd Rahman, 2000). Squalene is widely distributed in human tissues, most prominently in human sebum, the oily lubricant secreted by the skin's tiny sebaceous glands.

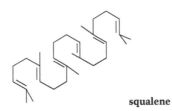

squalene

Squalene accounts for more than 50% of the unsaponifiable matter of olive oil and its level in the oil may range from 200–7500 mg/kg, although much higher levels (up to 12,000 mg/kg) have been reported (Manzi et al., 1998; Boskou et al., 2006). Murkovic et al. (2004) reported a concentration of squalene ranging from 5.1–9.6 g/l in seven samples of Greek olive oils. When the oil is refined the squalene level is reduced dramatically.

Squalene supplements are considered a promising anticancer agent, although human trials have yet to be performed that could verify its usefulness in cancer therapy. Researchers believe that squalene is a constituent of olive oil that has a significant contribution to the health effects and the

45

chemopreventive action against certain cancers (Rao et al., 1998; Smith et al., 1998; Newmark, 1999). Squalene inhibits 3-hydroxy-3-methylglutaryl coenzyme A reductase activity. This reduces farnesyl pyrophosphate availability for prenylation of the ras oncoproteins. This activity may account for the observed antiproliferative effects of squalene in some animal cancer models.

In a study conducted by Smith and others (1998) it was found that mice fed diets rich in olive oil and squalene had significantly fewer lung tumors than those fed a vegetable oil control diet. Tumorogenesis was induced by selected doses of 4-(methylnitrosamino)-1-(3-pyridyl)-1-butanone (NNK). The squalene diet decreased lung hyperplasia by 70%. Another animal study determined that squalene helps to protect against colon cancer (Rao et al., 1998). These findings support the hypothesis that squalene posseses a chemopreventive activity, further suggesting that frequent olive oil consumption may be a protective factor against lung or colon cancer (Bartoli, 2000). The abstract of a patent published in 1999 indicates that a functional food can be produced by mechanical extraction of grain germs (rich sources of tocopherols) and olive oil (a rich source of squalene and bioactive phenols) (Eyres, 1999). Squalene's chemopreventive activity was questioned by Scolastici et al. (2004), who conducted a hepatocarcinogenesis model study with Wistar rats.

As an ingredient in body care products squalene is an effective moisturizer, wrinkle remover, and wound healer (for a review of the clinical use of squalene see Kelly [1999]). The hydrocarbon appears to function on the surface of the skin as an antioxidant, capable of quenching singlet oxygen and protecting the skin from damage due to exposure to ultraviolet and other sources of ionizing radiation (Kelly, 1999; Kohno, 1995).

Pharmacokinetics. After ingestion, more than 60% of squalene is absorbed from the small intestine. It is then carried from there in the lymph in the form of chylomicrons into the systemic circulation. In the blood it is carried mainly in the very-low-density lipoprotein (VLDL) fraction to be distributed to the tissues of the body. Squalene is metabolized to cholesterol but the increase in cholesterol synthesis is not associated with a consistent increase in serum cholesterol level.

4.1.1 Role of Squalene in Olive Oil Stability

Psomiadou and Tsimidou (1999) studied the role of squalene in the stability of olive oil for various levels and experimental conditions. No effect was found in induction periods at elevated temperatures used in the Rancimat apparatus. A concentration-dependent weak antioxidant activity was shown when samples were stored at 40°C in the dark. In the presence of other antioxidants such as alpha-tocopherol and phenolic acids the contribution of squalene was insignificant. Mateos et al. (2003) also found a negligible antioxidant effect when purified olive oil was spiked with the hydrocarbon and subjected to an accelerated oxidation in a Rancimat apparatus. According to Psomiadou and Tsimidou (1999), the weak antioxidant activity could be explained by the competitive oxidation of the different lipids leading to a reduction of the oxidation rate. Dessi et al. (2002) suggested that squalene acts as a peroxyl radical scavenger and provides protection to polyunsaturated fatty acids against autoxidation.

In a recent report Malecka (2006) reported that the addition of 0.1–1% squalene to rapeseed oil reduced significantly changes due to heating at 170°C. The addition of about 0.5% squalene was proposed as a practically applicable concentration to retard degradation of unsaturated fatty acids and oxidative polymerization in heated rapeseed oil.

4.1.2 Recovery of Squalene from Olive Oil Residues

Bondioli et al. (1993) proposed a process for the recovery of squalene by supercritical carbon dioxide extraction from the deodorization distillates. The latter may contain squalene in a concentration ranging from 10–30% (see also FAIR-CT95-1075). Recently, a countercurrent supercritical carbon dioxide extraction for the recovery of squalene from residues was studied (Vazquez et al., 2007). The raw material used for the recovery was obtained by distillation and ethylation of olive oil deodorization distillates, which contained mainly squalene and fatty acid esters.

4.1.3 Determination of Squalene

The official method for the determination of squalene is the one proposed by the Association of Official Analytical Chemists (1999) that is based on saponification, repeated extractions with solvents, and fractionation through column chromatography. For the determination of squalene in olive oil, fractional crystallization for sample preparation and reversed-phase high-performance liquid chromatography (RP-HPLC) with detection at 208 nm was proposed by Nenadis and Tsimidou (2002). Grigoriadou et al. (2007) optimized a solid-phase extraction procedure for the subsequent extraction of squalene and alpha-tocopherol prior to HPLC analysis of triacylglycerols. The extraction of squalene from a silica cartridge is obtained with n-hexane, while alpha-tocopherol is isolated with a mixture of hexane/diethylether 99:1 v/v. According to the authors the procedure is useful in the official control of virgin olive oil, since silica cartridges are marginally used for the purification of samples before HPLC analysis of triacylglycerols or gas chromatographic (GC) analysis of methylesters.

Methods for HPLC and GC analysis of squalene in vegetable oils have been reviewed by Moreda et al. (2001).

4.2 TOCOPHEROLS

Vitamin E is the generic name for a group of lipid-soluble compounds encountered in plants that includes four tocopherols (alpha-, beta-, gamma-, and delta-) and four tocotrienols (alpha-, beta-, gamma-, and delta-). The different forms of vitamin E differ in their biological activities; alpha-tocopherol is the most common form of vitamin E occurring in human blood and tissues and it has the highest biological activity among the tocopherols and tocotrienols.

alpha-tocopherol

According to Kamal-Eldin and Appelquist (1996), tocopherols can act as antioxidants by two mechanisms. The first is a chain-breaking electron donor mechanism in which the tocopherol donates its phenolic hydrogen atom to lipid radicals. The second is a chain-breaking acceptor mechanism that includes singlet oxygen scavenging or quenching and inhibits oxidation induced by excited singlet oxygen. There is extensive literature on the role of alpha-tocopherol *in vivo* and its activity in relation to chronic inflammatory conditions, cardiovascular, cancer, and other diseases and cell aging.

The level and importance of tocopherols present in olive oil have been discussed by Boskou et al. (2006). From the eight known E-vitamers (four tocopherols, four tocotrienols) the alpha-homologue in the free form comprises 90% of the total tocopherol content. The rest is beta-tocopherol, gamma-tocopherol, and delta-tocopherol (levels ranging from 10–20 mg/kg oil). Wide ranges for alpha-tocopherol have been reported in Italian, Spanish, and Greek oils. Usual values are from 100–250 mg/kg oil. Lo Curto et al. (2001) investigated the variation in tocopherol content in Italian virgin olive oils. Alpha-tocopherol was found to range from 36–314 mg/kg oil. Values of beta-tocopherol and gamma-tocopherol ranged from 1–17 and 0.5–22 mg/kg, respectively.

Although, in general, the tocopherols decrease during olive ripening, gamma-tocopherol levels increase. Differences between crop years show a higher content in low-rainfall-year oils (Beltran et al., 2005). The level of tocopherols is also influenced by nitrogen fertilization (Fernandez-Escobar et al., 2006). In a recent report, Grigoriadou et al. (2005) reported levels of alpha-tocopherol content in 120 virgin olive oil samples sold in 16-l containers throughout Greece. Alpha-tocopherol levels higher than 200 mg/kg were found mainly in extra virgin oil quality. The authors stress that reducing the packing capacity to 5 l and improvement of handling and storage may contribute to an increase of alpha-tocopherol and polyphenol levels and consequently to an improvement of the nutritional quality of the oils that finally reach the consumer's table.

Alpha-tocopherol acts as an antioxidant in many ways and its presence is related to the quality of the oil (Tsimidou, 2006). Its antioxidant activity depends on its concentration in relation to polar phenols (Mateos et al., 2003; Blekas et al., 1995; see also Chapter 3). When olive oil is heated, hydroxytyrosol derivatives are lost but alpha-tocopherol and tyrosol are more stable and they are fully destroyed when a high accumulation of hydroperoxides occurs (Nissiotis and Tasioula-Margari, 2002; Morello et al., 2004). Jiang et al. (2005) determined radical-scavenging activity of olive oils spectrophotometrically by measuring the disappearance of DPPH radical. The contribution of tocopherols to radical-scavenging activity was 39–61% in virgin olive oil, which suggests that both tocopherols and phenolic compounds contribute to radical-scavenging activity. According to Pellegrini et al. (2001) polyphenols act as stabilizers of alpha-tocopherol during olive oil heating. This stabilizing effect was also reported by Valavanidis et al. (2004).

Determination of alpha-tocopherol. Tocopherols in oils are usually determined by direct normal-phase HPLC or RP-HPLC after saponification. Fluorescence or UV detection is employed for identification and quantification. The International Union of Pure and Applied Chemistry (IUPAC method 2.432, 1988) method for the determination of tocopherols in virgin olive oil employs direct analysis of the oil sample with normal phase separation and fluorescence or UV detection. In the American Oil Chemists' Society method a Lichrosorb Si-60 column is used (250 mm × 4.6 mm, particle size 5 μm). The oil is diluted in hexane and elution is performed with hexane/propanol. A fluorescence detector with excitation and emission wavelength set at 290 and 330 nm may be used (Salvador et al., 2001). Grigoriadou et al. (2005) determined alpha-tocopherol in olive oils using normal-phase HPLC, a Lichrospher 100Si 5-μm column (250 × 4 mm), and an elution system consisting of n-hexane/2-propanol 98:2. Nissiotis and Tasioula-Margari (2002) proposed a method for the simultaneous determination of alpha-tocopherol, tyrosol, and hydroxytyrosol based on the use of an octadecyl 104 C18 25-cm column, a gradient elution (acetic acid in water, methanol, acetonitrile, and isopropanol).

4.3 TRITERPENIC ACIDS

Triterpene acids such as *oleanolic acid* (3β-hydroxyolean-12-en-28-oic acid), *maslinic acid* (2α,3β-dihydroxyolean-12-en-28-oic acid), *ursolic acid* (3β-hydroxyurs-12-en-28 oic acid), and *betulinic acid* (3β-hydroxylup-20(29)-en-28 oic acid) are present in small amounts in olive oil (Boskou et al., 2006). They occur mainly in the olive husk and a small quantity is extracted during processing. Total triterpene acid content of extra virgin oils was found to range from 40–185 mg/kg. Oils with high acidity and crude solvent–extracted olive oils may have levels as high as 580 and 10,000 mg, respectively (Perez-Camino and Cert, 1999). When the oil is refined significant losses occur. Severge (1983) reported that the presence of oleanolic acid may cause turbidity in physically refined oil. This is due to the omission of caustic soda in the refining process and removal with the soap.

oleanolic acid

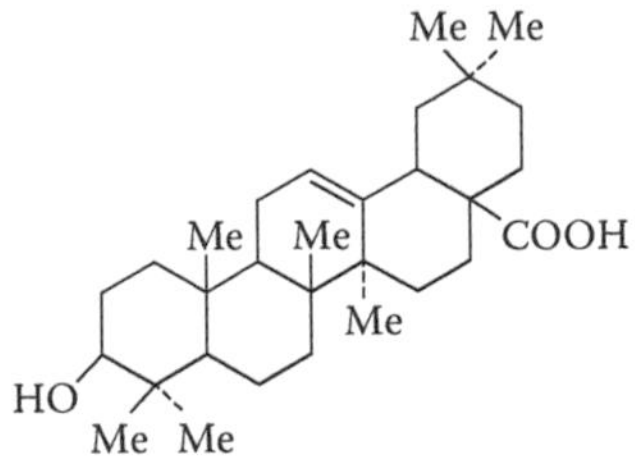

maslinic acid

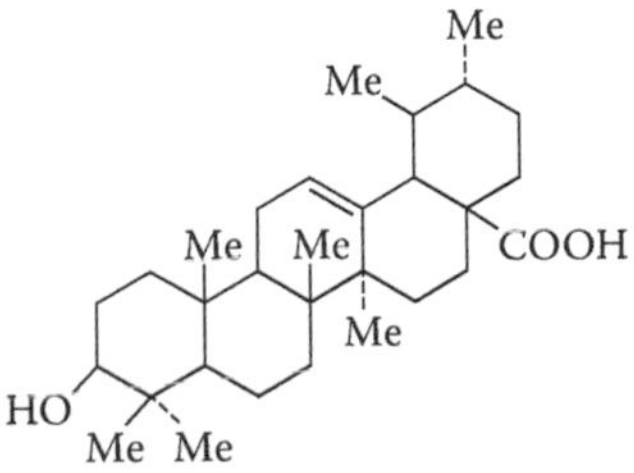

ursolic acid

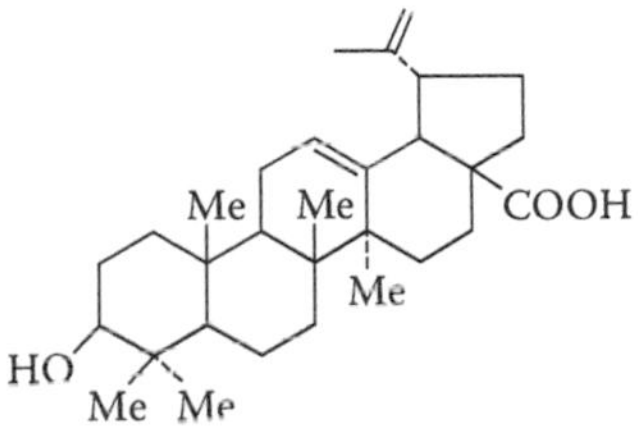

betulinic acid

Triterpenic acids are compounds with important biological properties. They are widespread in plants in the form of free acids or derivatives. They are used in the pharmaceuticals industry, among others, for their antitumoral, anti-inflammatory, and germicide activities (see also Chapters 7 and 8). For the triterpenic acids present in olive pomace oil, the oil obtained from the milling residue by solvent extraction or specific centrifugation, there is a plethora of publications suggesting a biological role. Claims exist that these acids may even become part of the fight against human immunodeficiency virus (HIV), the cause of AIDS (*Medical Research News*, July 9, 1998). Marquez-Martin et al. (2006a) tested the effect of maslinic acid upon oxidative stress and cytokine production using peritoneal murine macrophages. Maslinic acid significantly inhibited the enhanced production of nitric oxide (NO) induced by lyposaccharide (LPS) when it was measured by nitrite production. According to the authors such properties suggest a possible biopharmaceutical use of hydroxyl-pentacyclic triterpenes present in olive pomace oil for the prevention of oxidative stress and pro-inflammatory cytokine generation.

Rodriguez-Rodriguez et al. (2006) conducted an *in vitro* study to analyze the vasorelaxation induced in isolated aorta from spontaneously hypertensive rats by the triterpenes present in olive pomace oil. The triterpenes examined (erythrodiol, uvaol, maslinic acid, oleanolic acid) induced concentration-dependent vasorelaxation, involving mostly endothelial NO.

Also, in a very recent report Rodriguez-Rodriguez and her research team (Rodriguez-Rodriguez et al., 2007) examined the effect of dietary pomace olive oil on animal models of hypertension.

Pomace olive oil (olive residue oil) has the same fatty acid composition but a higher proportion of oleanolic acid than olive oil. During 12 weeks, hypertensive rats were fed with a control diet and a diet containing refined olive oil, pomace olive oil, and pomace oil supplemented in oleanolic acid (up to 800 mg/kg). Then vascular reactivity and endothelial nitric oxide synthase expression were studied in aortic rings. The authors conclude, based on the experimental evidence, that the effects of pomace oil on endothelial function in hypertensive animals is related to the presence of oleanolic acid.

Juan et al. (2006) also recently investigated the effect on cell proliferation and apoptosis in HT-29 human colon cancer cells of an extract obtained from the skin of olives. This extract was rich in pentacyclic triterpenes, mainly maslinic and oleanolic acids. The results of this study indicated inhibition of cell proliferation without cytotoxicity and the restoration of apoptosis in colon cancer cells by maslinic and oleanolic acids present in olive fruit.

Garcia-Granados and De Herro (1998) from the University of Granada patented a method for obtaining oleanolic and maslinic acid from milled olives or from oil cakes produced in oil mill expellers, mainly from the oil foot refuse taken from the two-phase extraction system.

The summary of a patented process for producing oleanolic acid and/or maslinic acid was reported in 2003 (Kuno Noriyasu and Shinohara Gou, 2003). The proposed process involves extraction of olives or olive plant products with water and an organic solvent followed by fractionation. In another patent it is claimed that an olive oil fortified with oleanolic acid can be produced by subjecting harvested olives to a malaxation treatment, where the malaxation mash contains olive leaves. The collected oil after the separation of the phases may contain at least 300 mg/kg oleanolic acid (van Putte, 1999).

Albi et al. (2001) proposed a process to obtain oleanolic acid from olive leaves, which is based on solid/liquid extraction with ethanol. The raw material is a by-product from the pruning of olive groves. The same authors proposed a method for quantification of the terpenic acids in the ethanol extract with three steps: addition of betulinic acid as an internal standard, fractionation by preparative thin layer chromatography (TLC), and GC analysis.

For the quantitative determination of hydroxyl pentacyclic triterpene acids in vegetable oils Perez-Camino and Cert (1999) described a method based on solid-phase extraction. The acids were isolated using bonded aminopropyl cartridges. The extract was silylated and analyzed by gas chromatography.

Ruiz-Mendez and Dobarganes (2005) analyzed for tritepenic acids samples of the "second centrifugation olive oil" and crude pomace olive oils, produced from the pomace of a two-phase decanter. The authors discuss the possibility for the recovery of triterpenic acids. Taking into consideration the biological properties of oleanolic acid, Guinda et al. (2004) conducted a study aimed at isolating oleanolic acid from olive leaves and supplementing various oils at concentrations from 200–1000 mg/kg.

Betulinic acid. Betulinic acid has several sources but it can also be chemically derived from betulin, a substance found in abundance in the outer bark of birch trees. In olive oil it occurs in ppm quantities. Betulinic acid has been found to have an antiangiogenic effect (Mukherjee et al., 2004) and its compositions are used for inhibiting angiogenesis (for the anticancer activity of triterpenic acids see Chapter 7). It has also been reported to be an effective anti-inflammatory agent (Banno et al., 2005).

4.4 TRITERPENE DIALCOHOLS

Erythrodiol (homo-olestranol,5-olean-12-ene-3β,28-diol) and uvaol (Δ12-ursen-3β,28-diol) are pentacyclic triterpenes found mainly in the nonglyceride fraction of olive oil and beta-residue oil (orujo oil, olive pomace oil) (Boskou et al., 2006). Erythrodiol occurs in the free and esterified form.

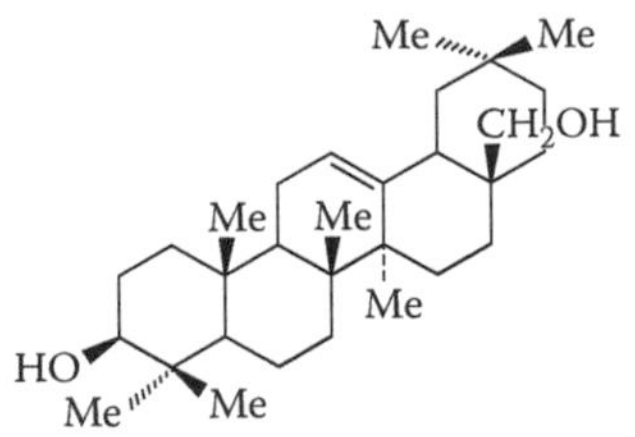

erythrodiol

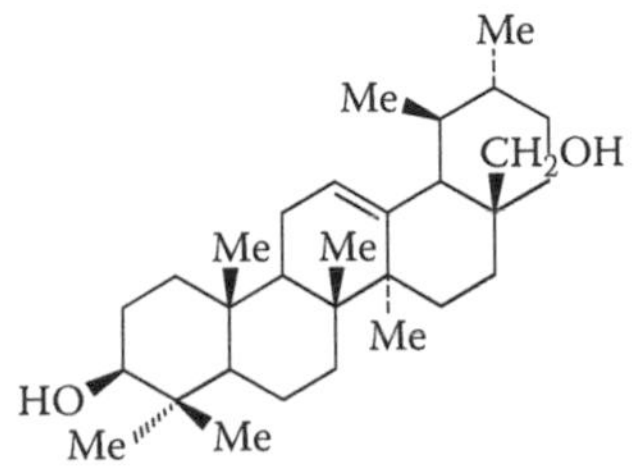

uvaol

The levels of these compounds in virgin olive oil are strongly affected by cultivar. The range of total erythrodiol was found between 19 and 69 mg/kg (Aparicio and Luna, 2002). The levels of triterpene alcohols are much higher in olive pomace oil; these compounds are accumulated in the flesh and skin of olive fruits. Thus, the oil obtained by solvent from the solid residue after the mechanical extraction of olive pastes is particularly rich in these compounds. Percentages of erythrodiol and uvaol in relation to sterols provide a good means for the differentiation between mechanically and solvent extracted oils. In virgin olive oil the percentage of dialcohols is not more than 4.5 of the total sterol fraction. For refined residue (pomace) oil the limit is 12% of the total sterol fraction.

For the analysis of triterpene dialcohols the same methodology applied to sterols is used (separation of unsaponifiables, preparative TLC or HPLC, silylation, and GC (Angerosa, 2006).

Triterpene dialcohols and triterpenic acids have been studied for their effect on pro-inflammatory cytokine production by human peripheral blood mononuclear cells (Marquez-Martin et al., 2006b). (For modulation of the immune response see also Chapter 7). Vasorelaxant effects of erythrodiol in rat aorta were studied by Rodriguez-Rodriguez et al. (2004). (See also Chapter 8.)

4.5 STEROLS

Phytosterols are very important for human nutrition. Various studies indicate that these compounds decrease serum total and LDL cholesterol levels. Still, the level of sterols in olive oil, usually 0.1–0.2%, is rather low compared to that (8%) of the commercial hypocholesteremic spreads. In a recent report for oils obtained in a laboratory scale from many olive varieties the levels of total sitosterol were found to change between 1.03 and 2.01 g/kg, followed by avenasterol ranging from 0.07–0.44 g/kg (Gul and Seker, 2006).

The major common (4a-desmethyl) sterol is beta-sitosterol, followed by delta-5-avenasterol and campesterol. Other sterols present in smaller quantities or in trace amounts are stigmasterol, cholesterol, brassicasterol, chlerosterol, ergosterol, sitostanol, campestanol, delta-7-avenasterol, delta-7-cholesterol, delta-7-campesterol, delta-7-stigmastenol, delta-5,23-stigmastadienol, delta-5,24-stigmastadienol, delta-7,22-ergastadienol, delta-7,24-ergostadienol,24-methylene-cholesterol, and 22,23-dihydrobrassicasterol (for a review see Boskou et al., 2006).

Olive oil sterols are analyzed by gas chromatography (Angerosa, 2006). To predict the chromatographic retention times for a group of natural sterols found in olive oil, a new approach was proposed by Hueso-Urena et al. (2003). By a quantitative structure property relationship treatment of an initial set of a very large number of molecular descriptors, models were obtained that permit the calculation of retention indices on two different columns (SE-54 and SE-52) for sterols naturally occurring in olive oil and their trimethyl-silyl ethers.

Phytosterols may also have other important biological properties related to the reduction of reactive oxygen species produced by regulating enzymes and inflammatory effects (see Chapter 8).

There are several reports on antitumor effects of phytosterols, especially β-sitosterol, that have been discussed by Assmann and Wahrburg (2006). When cholesterol-treated controls were compared with human prostate cancer cells treated with β-sitosterol, β-sitosterol was found to decrease growth and induce apoptosis (apoptosis is the so-called programmed cell death, a prophylactic mechanism by which cells commit suicide, e.g., when they have converted into cancer cells, in order to avert damage to the body). β-Sitosterol also had a favorable effect in the treatment of benign prostatic hyperplasia. There are also other reports on the *in vitro* effects of β-sitosterol on colon cancer cells and breast cancer cells.

4.6 CAROTENOIDS

The main carotenoids present in olive oil are lutein and beta-carotene (Su et al., 2002; Boskou et al., 2006). Total carotenoid content usually ranges between 1 and 20 mg/kg. Antioxidant and pro-oxidant properties have been assigned to carotenoids, which depend on the substrate, concentration, and levels. The low amount of beta-carotene and lutein present in olive oil, however, limits their importance in autoxidation mechanisms (Tsimidou, 2006).

4.7 ELENOLIC ACID

Elenolic acid (see also Chapter 3) is not a phenol but it is present in the methanol extract containing the polar phenols, deriving from the hydrolysis of ligstroside and oleuropein. Elenolic acid was found to have a very weak antioxidant capacity (Carrasco-Pancorbo et al., 2006). It is a medically potent chemical compound and has antibacterial, antiviral, and other properties.

REFERENCES

Albi, T., Guinda, A., and Lanzon, A., 2001, Obtaining procedure and determination of terpenic acids of olive leaf (*Olea europaea*), *Grasas Aceites*, 52, 275–278.

Angerosa, F., 2006, Analysis and authentication, in *Olive Oil, Chemistry and Technology*, Boskou, D., Ed., AOCS Press, Champaign, IL, pp. 113–172.

AOAC (Association of Official Analytical Chemists), 1999, Squalene in oils and fats. Titrimetric method, *Official Method* AOAC 943.04.

Aparicio, R. and Luna, G., 2002, Characterization of monovarietal virgin olive oils, *Eur. J. Lipid Sci. Technol.*, 104, 614–627.

Assmann, G. and Wahrburg, U., 2006, Health Effects of the Minor Components of Olive Oil, http://www.food-info.net/uk/products/olive/olive06.htm.

Banno, N., Akihisa, T., Tokuda, H., Yasukawa, K., Taguchi, Y., Akazawa, H., et al., 2005, Anti-inflammatory and antitumor-promoting effects of the triterpene acids from the leaves of *Eriobotrya japonica*, *Biol. Pharmac. Bull.*, 28, 1995–1999.

Bartoli, R., Fernandez-Balares, F., Navarro, E., Castella, E., Mane, J., Alvarez, M., et al., 2000, Effect of olive oil on early and late events of colon carcinogenesis in rats: modulation of arachidonic acid metabolism and local prostaglandin E_2 synthesis, *Gut*, 46, 91–199.

Beltran, G., Aguillera, M.P., Del Rio, C., Sanchez, S., and Martinez, L., 2005, Influence of fruit ripening process on the natural antioxidant content of Hojiblanca virgin olive oils, *Food Chem.*, 89, 207–215.

Blekas, G., Tsimidou, M., and Boskou, D., 1995, Contribution of alpha-tocopherol to olive oil stability, *Food Chem.*, 52, 289–294.

Bondioli, P., Mariani, C., Lanzani, A., Fedeli, E., and Muller, A., 1993, Squalene recovery from olive oil deodorization distillates, *J. Amer. Oil Chem. Soc.*, 70, 763–766.

Boskou, D., Tsimidou, M., and Blekas, D., 2006, *Olive Oil, Chemistry and Technology*, Boskou, D., Ed., AOCS Press, Champaign, IL, pp. 41–92.

Carrasco-Pancorbo, A., Cerretani, L., Segura-Carretero, A., Gallina-Toschi, T., Lercker, G., and Fernandez-Gutierrez, A., 2006, Evaluation of individul antioxidant activity of single phenolic compounds on virgin olive oil, *Prog. Nutr.*, 8, 28–39.

Dessi, M.A., Deiana, M., Day, B.W., Rosa, A., Banni, S, and Corongiu, F.P., 2002, Oxidative stability of poly-unsaturated fatty acids: effect of squalene, *Eur. J. Lipid Sci. Technol.*, 104, 506–512.

Eyres, L., 1999, Functional food from olive oil and grain germ, Patent abstract, *Lipid Technol.*,11, 22.

FAIR-CT95-1075 programme, FAIR-CT95-1075, Ultrahydrophytosqualene, http://www.biomatnet.org/secure/Fair.

Fernandez-Escobar, R., Beltran, G., Sanchez-Zamora, M.A., Garcia-Novelo, J., and Aguilera, P., 2006, Olive oil quality decreases with nitrogen over-fertilization, *HortScience*, 41, 215–219.

Gapor Md Top, A. and Abd Rahman, H., 2000, Squalene in oils and fats, *Palm Oil Dev.*, 32, 36–39.

Garcia-Granados, A. and De Herro, L., 1998, Process for the Industrial Recovery of Oleanolic and Maslinic Acids Contained in the Olive Milling Sub-Products, U.S. Patent 6,037,492, Application No. 43,318, 1998.

Grigoriadou, D., Androulaki, A., and Tsimidou, M.Z., 2005, Levels of phenolic antioxidants in virgin olive oil purchased in bulk, *Ital. J. Food Sci.*, 17, 195–202.

Grigoriadou, D., Androulaki, A., Psomiadou, E., and Tsimidou, M.Z., 2007, Solid phase extraction in the analysis of squalene and tocopherols in olive oil, *Food Chem.*, 105, 675–680.

Guinda, A., Perez-Camino, M.C., and Lanzon, A., 2004, Supplementation of oils with oleanolic acid from the olive leaf (*Olea europaea*), *Eur. J. Lipid Sci. Technol.*, 106, 22–26.

Gul, M.K. and Seker, M., 2006, Comparative analysis of phytosterol components from rapeseed (*Brassica napus* L.) and olive (*Olea europaea* L.) varieties, *Eur. J. Lipid Technol.*, 108, 759–765.

Hueso-Urena, F., Cabeza, N.I., Jimenez-Pulido, S.B., Morreno-Catretero, M.N., and Martinez-Martos, J.M., 2003, A recalculation of quantitative structure chromatographic retention time relationships of natural phenols and sterols found in olive oil, *Internet Electronic J. Mol. Design*, 2, 000–000, http://www.biochempress.com.

Jiang, L., Yamaguchi, T., Takamura, H., and Matoba, T., 2005, Characteristics of Shodo Island olive oils in Japan: fatty acids composition and antioxidative compounds, *Food Sci.Technol. Res.*, 11, 254–260.

Juan, M.E., Wenzel, U., Ruiz-Guttierrez, V., Daniel, H., and Planas, M., 2006, Olive fruit extracts inhibit proliferation and induce apoptosis in HT-29 human colon cancer cells, *J. Nutr.*, 136, 2553–2557.

Kamal-Eldin, A. and Appelquist, L.A., 1996, The chemistry and antioxidant properties of tocopherols and tocotrienols, *Lipids*, 31, 671–701.

Kelly, G.S., 1999, Squalene and its potential clinical uses, *Altern. Med. Rev.*, 4, 29–36.

Kohno, Y., Egawa, Y., Itoh, S., Nagaoka, S., Takahashi, M., and Mukai, K., 1995, Kinetic study of quenching reaction of singlet oxygen and scavenging reaction of free radical by squalene in n-butanol, *Biochim. Biophys. Acta*, 1256, 52–56.

Kuno Noriyasu and Shinohara Gou, Nisshin Oil Mills, Ltd., 2003, Process for Producing Oleanolic Acid and/or Maslinic Acid, Patent No. EP 1310478, Intern. Application No. PCT/JP/2002/010101.

Lo Curto, S., Dugo, G., Mondello, L., Errante, G., and Russo, M.T., 2001, Variation in tocopherol content in Italian virgin olive oils, *Ital. J. Food Sci.*, 13, 221–225.

Malecka, M., 2006, The effect of squalene on the thermostability of rape seed oil, *Food/Nahrung*, 38, 135–140.

Manzi, P., Panfili, G., Esti, M., and Pizzoferrato, L., 1998, Natural antioxidants in the unsaponifiable fraction of virgin olive oils from different cultivars, *J. Sci. Food Agric.*, 77, 115–120.

Marquez-Martin, A., De la Puerta Vazquez, R., Fernandez-Arche, A., and Ruiz-Gutierrez, V., 2006a, Supressive effect of maslinic acid from pomace olive oil on oxidative stress and cytokine production in stimulated murine macrophages, *Free Rad. Res.*, 40, 295–302.

Marquez-Martin, A., De la Puerta, R., Fernandez-Arche, A., Ruiz-Guttierrez, V., and Yaqoob, P., 2006b, Modulation of cytokine secretion by pentacyclic triterpenes from olive pomace oil in human mononuclear cells, *Cytockine*, 36, 211–217.

Mateos, R., Dominguez, M.M., Espartero, J.L., and Cert, A., 2003, Antioxidant effect of phenolic compounds, alpha-tocopherol and other minor constituents in virgin olive oil, *J. Agric. Food Chem.*, 51, 7170–7175.

Moreda, W., Perez-Camino, M.C., and Cert, A., 2001, Gas and liquid chromatography of hydrocarbons in edible oils, *J. Chromatogr.*, 936, 159–171.

Morello, J.-R., Motilva, M.-J., Tovar, M.-J., and Romero, M.-P., 2004, Changes in commercial virgin olive oil (cv Arbequina) during storage, with special emphasis on the phenolic fraction, *Food Chem.*, 85, 357–364.

Mukherjee, R., Jaggi, M., Rajendram, P., Siddiqui, J.A., Strivastava, S.K., Vardham, A., et al., 2004, Butilinic acid and its derivatives as anti-angiogenic agents, *Biorg. Med. Chem. Lett.*, 14, 2181–2184.

Murkoviz, M., Lechner, S., Pietzka, A., Bratakos, M., and Katzogiannos, M., 2004, Analysis of minor constituents in olive oil, *J. Biochem. Methods*, 61, 155–160.

Nenadis, N. and Tsimidou, M., 2002, Determination of squalene in olive oil using fractional crystallization for sample preparation, *J. Amer. Oil Chem. Soc.*, 79, 257–259.

Newmark, H.L., 1999, Squalene, olive oil and cancer risk: a review and hypothesis, *Ann. N.Y. Acad. Sci.*, 889, 193–203.

Nissiotis, M. and Tasioula-Margari, M., 2002, Changes in antioxidant concentration of virgin olive oil during thermal oxidation, *Food Chem.*, 77, 371–376.

Pellegrini, N., Visioli, F., Burrati, S., and Brigetti, F., 2001, Direct analysis of total antioxidant activity of olive oil and studies on the influence of heating, *J. Agric. Food Chem.*, 49, 2532–2538.

Perez-Camino, M.C. and Cert, A., 1999, Quantitative determination of hydroxyl pentacyclic triterpene acids in vegetable oils, *J. Agric. Food Chem.*, 47, 1558–1562.

Psomiadou, E. and Tsimidou, M., 1999, On the role of squalene in olive oil stability, *J. Agric. Food Chem.*, 47, 4025–4032.

Rao, C.V., Newmark, H.L., and Reddy, B.S., 1998, Chemopreventive effect of squalene on colon cancer, *Carcinogenesis*, 19, 287–290.

Rodriguez-Rodriguez, R., Herrera, M.D., Perona, J., Gutierrez, V., 2004, Potential vasorelaxant effects of oleanolic acid and erythrodiol, two triterpenoids contained in "orujo" olive oil, in aorta, *Brit. J. Nutr.*, 42, 635–642.

Rodriguez-Rodriguez, R., Perona, J.S., Herrera, M.D., and Ruiz-Gutierrez, V., 2006, Triterpenic compounds from "orujo" olive oil elicit vasorelaxation in aorta from spontaneously hypertensive rats, *J. Agric. Food Chem.*, 54, 2096–2102.

Rodriguez-Rodriguez, R., Herrera, M.D., de Sotomayor, M.A., and Guttierrez, V., 2007, Pomace olive oil improves endothelial function in spontaneously hypertensive rats by increasing endothelial nitric oxide synthase expression, *Am. J. Hypertens.*, 20, 728–734.

Ruiz-Mendez, M.V. and Dobarganes, C., 2005, Triterpenic acids from olive pomace, *26th World Congress, Int. Soc. Fat Research, Modern Aspects of Fats and Oils, Prague,* Book of Abstracts, p. 92.

Salvador, M.D., Aranda, F., and Fregapane, G., 2001, Influence of fruit ripening on Cornicabra virgin olive oil quality. A study of four successive crop seasons, *Food Chem.*, 73, 45–53.

Severge, A., 1983, Difficulties in physical refining of olive oil, due to presence of triterpene "oleanolic acid," *J. Amer. Oil Chem. Soc.*, 60, 584–587.

Scolastici, C., Ong, T.P., and Moreno, F.S., 2004, Squalene does not exhibit a chemopreventive activity and increases plasma cholesterol in a Wistar rat hepatocarcinogenesis, *Nutr. Cancer*, 50, 11–109.

Smith, T.J., Yang, G.Y., Seril, D.N., Liao, J., and Sunkbin, K., 1998, Inhibition of 4-(methylnitrosamino)-1-(3-pyridyl)-1-butanone–induced lung tumorigenesis by dietary olive oil squalene, *Carcinogenesis*, 19, 703–706.

Su, Q., Rowley, K.G., Itsiopoulos, C., and O'Dea, K., 2002, Identification and quantitation of major carotenoids in delected components of the Mediterranean diet: green leafy vegetables, figs and olive oil, *Eur. J. Clin. Nutr.*, 56, 1149–1154.

Tsimidou, M., 2006, Olive oil quality, in *Olive Oil, Chemistry and Technology*, Boskou, D., Ed., AOCS Press, Champaign, IL, pp. 93–112.

Valavanidis, A.C., Nisiotou, C., Papageorgiou, Y., Kremli, I., Satravelas, N., Zinieris, N., et al., 2004, Comparison of the radical scavenging potential of polar and lipidic fractions of olive oil and other vegetable oils under normal conditions and after thermal treatment, *J. Agric. Food Chem.*, 52, 2358–2365.

Van Putte, K., 1999, http://www.patentstorm.us/patents/6338865–claims.html.

Vazquez, L., Torres, C.F., Formuri, T., Senorans, F.J., and Reglero, G., 2007, Recovery of squalene from vegetable oil sources using countercurrent supercritical carbon dioxide extraction, *J. Supercrit. Fluids*, 40, 59–62.

5 Detection and Quantification of Phenolic Compounds in Olive Oil, Olives, and Biological Fluids

Photis Dais and Dimitrios Boskou

CONTENTS

5.1 OVERVIEW

Polar phenolic compounds, very often termed "polyphenols," constitute an important class of minor compounds detected in olive fruits and olive oils with strong antioxidant capacities. These compounds not only act as natural antioxidants, protecting the products of olive trees from oxidation caused by atmospheric oxygen, but they are also considered as alternative potent agents to combat chronic degenerative diseases, cardiovascular diseases, and cancer (see Chapters 2 and 6–9).

Due to the wealth of positive effects on human health and the hard work involved in the cultivation of olive trees (*Olea europaea* L.), the collection and processing of olive fruits, and/or the extraction of olive oil, olive oil products have a high commercial price. Therefore, mixing of olive oil of fine quality (extra virgin olive oil, EVOO) with cheaper refined seed oils (e.g., corn oil, sunflower oil, and especially hazelnut oil) and/or olive oils of inferior quality (e.g., refined olive oil) is a constant temptation. Fraud in EVOO will certainly diminish its phenolic content, thus reducing its oxidative stability, and more importantly will deprive EVOO of the associated beneficial effects on human health. For this reason, it is of crucial importance to detect and quantify these bioactive substances from *O. europaea* L. Characterization and quantification of polar phenols can ensure consistency in the selection of cultivars in olive tree breeding and raw material specification, since the distribution of phenols is related to quality attributes such as flavor and antioxidant properties. A good knowledge of polar phenols composition is also needed to:

* Develop technology for antioxidant content optimization in virgin olive oil
* Evaluate table olives as sources of biophenols
* Prepare complete compositional data necessary for calculations of antioxidant intake
* Set out biochemical and other laboratory studies

In recent years, there have been a large number of analytical methods developed for the isolation, separation, structural determination, and quantification of polyphenols in olives and oils. This review describes the various analytical methods currently used for this purpose.

Methods for sample preparation constitute an important step in the determination of phenolic compounds. Extraction of phenolics depends on the nature of the sample. Liquid-liquid extraction and/or solid-phase extraction are generally used for the isolation of phenolic compounds from olive oil. Extraction of phenolics from olive fruits is more demanding due to reduced homogeneity of olives and the increased enzyme content that may cause modification to the phenolic content. It is worth noting that the various extraction procedures have not been subjected yet to rigorous quality tests in order to eliminate the possibility of qualitative and quantitative changes induced by the recovery procedure.

Separation and quantification of phenolic compounds from the complex matrices of olives and oils have been achieved mainly by well-recognized chromatographic methods. Gas chromatography (GC) finds limited application to the separation of phenolic compounds. The high polarity and the limited volatility of phenolics demand a derivatization step, thus lengthening the duration of the analysis. Moreover, thermal decomposition may occur at elevated temperatures of the experiment, hindering further analysis of the higher molecular mass phenolics. Nevertheless, the excellent resolving power and detection capabilities of GC, especially when it is combined with mass spectrometry (GC-MS), has established this technique as a valuable analytical tool.

The most preferred method for the analysis of the phenolic fraction of olives and olive oils is reversed-phase high-performance liquid chromatography (RP-HPLC) with gradient elution. There is a plethora of papers dealing with the various conditions (column, mobile phase, detector, etc.) adopted for the separation of phenolics. A usual problem associated with this methodology may be the use of standards for calibration that may not be available in the market.

Detection in RP-HPLC is typically based on measurements of UV absorption. This type of detection creates problems in quantification, since different phenolic compounds show different absorption maxima and molar absorptivities, and therefore no single wavelength is ideal for all classes of phenolics. Usually, measurements are performed at two to three different wavelengths depending on the chosen class of phenolics to be investigated. Several other detection methods have been adopted in the past (e.g., diode array, amperometry with or without cyclic voltametry). The online coupling of the liquid chromatograph with a mass spectrometer (LC-MS) was a huge step in the analysis of phenolics in olives and oils. This combination, along with the use of pertinent ionization techniques, and invention of various mass spectrometry detection modes allowed the detection of polar nonvolatile and thermolabile phenolics at very low concentrations. Furthermore, the presence of substantial fragmentation from collisionally induced dissociation gave structural information about these molecules.

Multinuclear and multidimensional nuclear magnetic resonance (NMR) spectroscopy represents an alternative effective analytical technique to detect polyphenols in olives and oils and elucidate indisputably their chemical structure. Recently, derivatization of hydroxyl and carboxyl groups with a phosphorus reagent allowed the quantification of several phenolic compounds in olive oil in a single ^{31}P NMR spectrum without previous calibration. The potential of NMR spectroscopy was especially demonstrated when it was coupled with HPLC (LC-NMR). The combined selectivity of LC with the structural information at a molecular level offered by NMR leads to the detection and identification of new phenols in olive oil.

As an alternative to HPLC, capillary electrophoresis (coupled to different detectors such as UV, electrochemical, mass spectrometry) has been proposed recently. Capillary electrophoresis is a new technique in food analysis and when applied to olive oil it provides certain advantages, most important of which are small quantities of sample, short time, separation efficiency, and satisfactory characterization of the individual phenols.

There are a few review articles, including a very recent one (Bendini et al., 2007) dealing with different aspects of phenolic compounds, the analytical methods that have been developed for identification and quantification of these compounds in olive fruits and olive oils, as well as of their metabolites in human biofluids after olive oil ingestion. These articles are mentioned in proper places of the subsequent paragraphs.

Biological fluids. HPLC and the hyphenated analogues GC-MS and LC-MS with minor modifications, and specific isolation procedures have been used with success for the detection and quantification of phenolic metabolites in biological fluids. Bioavailability studies in urine and plasma of humans and/or laboratory animals contributed significantly to a complete clarification of the fate of these compounds after ingestion. Investigation of the bioavailability and metabolism of olive and oil phenolic compounds is of vital importance for assessing their role in human health.

5.2 SPECTROPHOTOMETRY AND CHROMATOGRAPHY

Many different approaches for the spectrophotometric and chromatographic analysis of the olive oil polar phenolics fraction have been reported. These different approaches have led to results that are often difficult to compare. Controversial data reported, the difficulties encountered in the selection of reference compounds, and the expression of results have been discussed by Blekas et al. (2002), Hrncirik and Fritsche (2004), and Angerosa (2006).

5.2.1 SAMPLE PREPARATION

The isolation of phenolic compounds from oil for the spectrophotometric determination of total phenols or the characterization and quantitation of individual compounds by HPLC or GC is very important; some differences encountered in the literature are definitely due to different methods of isolation. The traditional method of isolation is liquid-liquid partition of the oil solution in hexane with portions of water–methanol mixtures. There are many variations of the method.

5.2.1.1 Liquid-Liquid Extraction Techniques

The solvent is usually a mixture of methanol–water and the oil is first diluted in hexane. The ratios of the two solvents of the mixture (methanol/water) may vary. Some researchers have found that a 80:20 v/v methanol/water mixture gives better results (Montedoro et al., 1992; Pirisi et al., 2000; Rotondi et al., 2004). Pirisi et al. used a triple extraction with a 60:40 mixture. The hydroalcoholic fractions are combined, washed with hexane to remove residual oil, and the extract is concentrated by evaporation of the solvent *in vacuo*. Angerosa (2006) suggests the use of absolute methanol, while Cortesi et al. (1995) proposed tetrahydrofuran, which increases the recovery of phenols in comparison to methanol–water extraction. Another solvent, *N,N*-dimethylformamide, has been suggested (Brenes et al., 2002).

5.2.1.2 Solid-Phase Extraction

The extraction procedures are rather laborious and some alterations of the phenolic compounds may occur in the process of isolation. Therefore, attempts have been made to isolate the polar fraction by solid-phase extraction techniques using cartridges (Romani et al., 1999; Servili et al., 1999a; Tsimidou, 1999; Liberatore et al., 2001; Mateos et al., 2001; Pellegrini et al., 2001; Gutierrez-Rosales et al., 2003; Rios et al., 2005; Vinha et al., 2005; Del Carlo et al., 2006). Still, incomplete extraction and partial separation have been reported (Cert et al., 2000; Bendini et al., 2003; Angerosa, 2006). A selectivity of SFE toward individual phenolics, particularly the aglycone-type ones, was found by Hrncirik and Fritsche (2004).

Liberatore et al. (2001) used commercially available C18 cartridges according to the following protocol: 1 g oil is dissolved in 10 ml hexane and put onto a column previously conditioned with 2 × 10 ml methanol and 2 × 10 ml hexane. The column is eluted with 4 × 10 ml hexane to eliminate the lipophile constituents and the retained polar compounds are recovered by eluting with 4 × 10 ml methanol. According to the authors the results do not completely agree with those of liquid-liquid extraction.

To simplify the whole procedure for the preparation of the sample before injection to the liquid chromatograph column or to measure the antioxidant activity, Gomez-Alonso et al. (2003) used a diol-bonded phase cartridge. The latter was conditioned and then the oil solution was applied to the SPE column. The less polar compounds were removed by washing with hexane and hexane/ethyl acetate mixtures and the phenols were recovered by eluting with methanol. Bendini and co-workers (2003) compared many solid-phase extraction techniques (C8-SPE, C18-SPE, Diol-SPE) with liquid-liquid extraction. They concluded that the latter gives better results in terms of recovery of total phenols, *ortho*-diphenols, tyrosol, hydroxytyrosol, and their secoiridoid derivatives.

Solid-phase extraction has also been used in the analysis of other minor constituents such as triterpene acids (Perez-Camino and Cert, 1999; Ruiz-Mendez and Dobarganes, 2005), squalene (Grigoriadou et al., 2007) as well as the isolation of phenolics from biological fluids.

In a very recent report (Armaforte et al., 2007), the two commonly employed extraction methods for the recovery of phenolics, liquid-liquid chromatography and solid-phase extraction, were compared in a number of samples of fresh virgin olive oil that were stored at different temperatures in the presence of oxygen to promote the formation of oxidation products. This work revealed that there is a selective retention of the naturally occurring phenols and polar oxidation products. The latter interfere with the retention of phenols in SPE columns when there is a significant level of oxidation. Thus, SPE seems to be effective only in fresh oil samples. The authors suggest that this difference in the concentration of phenols obtained by liquid-liquid extraction and solid-phase extraction may be used to evaluate the oil freshness.

5.2.1.3 Preparative High-Performance Liquid Chromatography

Preparative HPLC has been used by many investigators to purify polar phenol extracts and isolate the specific fractions for the analysis of individual phenols or for the enrichment of lipid matrices with antioxidants (Artajo et al., 2006). Angerosa et al. (1996) used a Spherisorb semi-prep S5 ODS2 column of 250 × 10 mm i.d. Fogliano et al. (1999) obtained, by semipreparative HPLC, fractions containing individual phenols and evaluated the relative antioxidant efficiency. Semipreparative HPLC analyses were performed by Ryan et al. (1999c) with a ODS-AQ column (10 mm × 250 mm, 5 µm) to isolate phenolic compound fractions before electrospray mass spectrometric analysis. Monti et al. (2001) used preparative HPLC on a Spherisorb S5 ODS-2 reversed-phase column (250 cm, 4.6 mm, particle size 5 µm) to separate virgin olive oil phenolic compounds and collect peaks for further analysis by LC-MS. Gutierrez-Rosales and co-authors (2003) isolated the major peaks found in the phenolic profile using preparative HPLC. The molecules purified were tested for the intensity of bitterness.

Carrasco-Pancorbo et al. (2006b) used semipreparative HPLC to isolate individual phenols and test antioxidant activity with the DPPH radical test. The column was Pheomenex Luna (C_{18}), 10 mm i.d., 25 cm × 10 mm, and the flow rate was 3 ml/min.

5.2.2 High-Performance Liquid Chromatography

The most frequently applied technique to analyze the polar phenol fraction of olive oil is RP-HPLC, using isocratic or gradient elution. The system is equipped with a UV detector operating at 225, 240, or 280 nm. Due to different absorption maxima of the various phenols, the use of a simultaneous multiple UV detector (photodiode array) is recommended, especially when some identification is necessary (Vinha et al., 2002). An improved technique is based on the use of two detection systems, diode array and fluorescence detector. Other detection systems have also been proposed such as amperometric methods, coulometric electrode, and mass spectrometry detector (Tsimidou, 1999; Cert et al., 2000; Angerosa, 2006; Silva, 2006). (For new developments in hyphenated methods see Sections 5.3 and 5.4.)

The columns (C18) have a 5-µm particle size and dimensions 25 cm × 3 mm i.d. or 25 cm x 4.6 mm i.d. For isocratic elution an aqueous solution of sulfuric acid-acetonitrile or methanol-aqueous acetic acid may be used (Cert et al., 2000). Gradient elutions vary from laboratory to laboratory (Cert et al., 2000). Brenes et al. (1999) used an initial composition of 90% water adjusted to pH 3.1 with acetic acid and 10% methanol. Gradually the methanol percentage was raised to 40, 50, and finally to 60, 70, and 100%. Rotondi et al. (2004) separated the phenols with a mobile phase of a water/formic acid 99.5:0.5 mixture and acetonitrile as the mobile phase. Romero et al. (2002) used a 15 cm × 4.6 mm, 5 µm, Intersil ODS-3 column equipped with a 1 cm × 4.6 mm i.d., 5 µm, Spherisorb S5 ODS-2 precolumn. The eluents were 0.2% acetic acid and methanol. Identification was based on the analysis of standards. Quantification of individual phenols was obtained with four-point regression curves. Ferulic acid and flavones were quantified at 339 nm and elenolic at 240 nm. For the rest of the compounds the wavelength 240 nm was used. Vinha et al. (2005) and also Bendini et al. (2003) quantified hydroxytyrosol and oleuropein aglycons at 280 nm. Rotondi et al. (2004) set the wavelengths at 280 nm for phenolic acids, alcohols, and secoiridoids and at 350 nm for flavonoids. Pereira et al. (2006) used the same wavelengths for phenolic alcohols and flavonoids and 350 nm for verbascoside present in olives.

Recently, Selvaggini et al. (2006) proposed a new method for the evaluation of phenolic compounds in virgin olive oil, which is based on direct injection in HPLC with fluorometric detection.

The oil is first diluted with acetone and filtered through a syringe filter 0.2 μm. As compared to the liquid-liquid extraction and HPLC analysis, the new method is more efficient for the quantification of simple alcohols, lignans, and 3,4-DHPEA but the efficiency is lower for the evaluation of 3,4-DHPEA-EDA and p-HPEA-EDA.

HPLC analysis of olive oil phenols finds many applications including detection of olive oil authenticity (Zabaras and Gordon, 2004). Conditions for HPLC analysis of olive oil phenols have been summarized by Bendini et al. (2007). Gikas et al. (2006) used HPLC for a kinetic study of acidic hydrolysis of oleuropein.

5.2.3 Gas Chromatography

Gas chromatography was used mainly by Angerosa (2006), who combined capillary GC with mass spectrometry to identify simple and linked phenols present in olive oil. Quantitative determination of hydroxytyrosol in olive oils was performed by GC-MS (Visioli et al., 2002) using deuterated hydroxytyrosol as an internal standard (see also Section 5.4).

5.2.4 Capillary Zone Electrophoresis

According to Carrasco-Pancorbo et al. (2004), this method is a reliable, sensitive, and rapid one, applicable to phenolic acids present in olive oil. The separation is performed on a fused silica capillary of total length 57 cm (effective length 50 cm), 75 μm i.d., 375 μm o.d., using a 25-mM sodium borate buffer (pH 9.6) at 25 KV. Good repeatability is obtained by rinsing the capillary with 0.1 M sodium hydroxide for 5 min followed by 2 min with Milli-Q-water at the beginning of each experimental run. The optimized running buffer is prepared by dissolving an appropriate amount of solid salt in Milli-Q-water and adding a proper amount of 1.0 M NaOH. Detection is performed at 210 and 215 nm, simultaneously. To obtain spectral data diode array detection can be used over the range 190–600 nm.

Bonoli and co-investigators (2003) optimized the conditions of capillary zone electrophoresis for the analysis of important phenols such as tyrosol, hydroxytyrosol, and oleuropein derivatives. The separation according to the method proposed is obtained in 10 min, using a 40-cm × 50-μm capillary, with a running buffer of 45 mM sodium tetraborate (pH 9.6) at 27 KV and 30°C. As the method has a smaller operative cost than HPLC and a positive correlation with the colorimetric Folin-Ciovalteu determination of total phenols, its use is also proposed as a means to quantify the antioxidant profile of olive oil.

Recently, Carrasco-Pancorbo and collaboratotors (2006a) described the conditions of solid-phase extraction (SPE) and capillary zone electrophoresis (CZE) for coupling to electrospray ion source mass spectrometry. The optimized SPE and CZE parameters increased the number of phenolic compounds that could be detected. Electrophoretic separation was carried out with an aqueous buffer system consisting of 60 mM ammonium acetate with 5% 2-propanol. According to the authors the technique is suitable for the study of compounds present in olive oil such as tyrosol, hydroxytyrosol, hydroxytyrosol acetate, lignans ligstroside, and oleuropein algycons; various forms of aldehydic, dialdehydic, and decarboxylated aglycons; and 10-hydroxy-oleuropein aglycon.

5.2.5 Determination of Total Phenols Content

The colorimetric Folin-Ciocalteu method is broadly used to determine the level of phenols. The results are usually expressed in gallic or caffeic acid. The method is conventional since any reducing substance may interfere; besides, the response of each phenol to the oxidizing agent is different. However, it is very useful, as the values obtained are well correlated to the stability. Blekas et al. (2002) proposed the addition of the measurement to the existing quality criteria of the oil.

An alternative to the spectrophotometric method is HPLC. This technique also has many drawbacks, as many standards are needed for the preparation of standard curves, the whole chromatographic profile is not quite clear, and possibly some minor compounds are not yet fully characterized. Pirisi et al. (2000) indicated that the chromatographic features, the standards used, and the expression of the concentration affect greatly the final values. The authors propose a gradient separation with an eluent mixture of acetonitrile–sulfuric acid, detection at 225 nm, and expression of the results in tyrosol equivalents.

Mosca et al. (2000) proposed a new spectrophotometric assay for the content of polar phenols of olive oil that employs tyrosinase in the presence of excess NADH. The reaction of phenols with the enzyme produces an *o*-quinone, which is detected by recycling between reactions with enzyme and NADH. The quinone products are estimated in the range 380–420 nm. According to the authors the method gives a better estimation of the phenol content in relation to the Folin-Ciocalteu method.

For the rapid determination of certain phenolic classes biosensors have been proposed (Busch et al., 2006; Georgiou et al., 2007). Busch et al. proposed two amperometric enzyme–based biosensors employing tyrosinase or peroxidase for the rapid measurement of polar phenolics of olive oil. The methods have different specificity toward different groups of phenolics and can be used in the evaluation of bitterness and pungency. For the quantification of phenolic compounds in olive oil mill wastewater a laccase biosensor was proposed by Torrecilla et al. (2007). The data collected from amperometric detection of the laccase biosensor are transferred into an artificial neural network (ANN) trained computer for modeling and prediction of output.

Another approach to determine directly the bitterness and total phenolic content, avoiding sensorial analysis, which requires highly specialized experts, was proposed by Garcia-Mesa and Mateos (2007). The method uses a flow injection analysis system based on the spectral shift undergone by phenolic compounds when the pH changes (variation of absorbance at 274 nm).

Determination of o-diphenols. Ortho-diphenols can be determined separately with a solution of sodium molybdate in ethanol/water. The absorbance is measured at 370 nm using gallic acid or caffeic acid for the calibration curve (Blekas et al., 2002; Rotondi et al., 2004). The method is conventional and it is not correlated to stability as total phenol content (Blekas et al., 2002).

5.3 NUCLEAR MAGNETIC RESONANCE SPECTROSCOPY

5.3.1 INTRODUCTION

NMR spectroscopy is a powerful analytical technique suitable for qualitative and quantitative measurements. Nuclei of atoms with magnetic properties (endowed with a magnetic moment) can be excited by a magnetic field emitting radiation at the radiofrequency range. Energy absorption by nuclei occurs whenever the Larmor frequency of the spinning nuclei is in resonance with the radiofrequency of the magnetic field. The excited nuclei at a higher energy state interact with their environment, remove or exchange their energy, and finally return to a lower energy state. This process is detected by the receiver coil of the NMR spectrometer. The thus obtained weak signals are amplified and recorded as a function of frequency. The position of the signals (chemical shift) in the NMR spectrum depends on the chemical environment of the respective nuclei, whereas interaction of the magnetic moments of neighboring magnetically nonequivalent nuclei through bonding electrons results in splitting (spin-spin or scalar coupling) of their signals in the spectrum. The spectroscopic parameters, chemical shifts, and coupling constants (distances between the components of a multiple signal) derived either directly from the spectrum or by spin simulation are the basis for qualitative analysis. The NMR spectrum of a substance is unique and represents its fingerprints for an unambiguous identification at a molecular level. On the other hand, the measured intensity of the signals by digital integration constitutes the basis for quantitative analysis. The signal intensity is proportional to the number of magnetically equivalent nuclei giving rise to that signal. NMR signals integration in combination with (or without) an internal standard is a rapid and accurate process for quantitative analysis, since it does not require calibration with standards as in other analytical techniques. Moreover, NMR spectroscopy is a noninvasive, nondestructive analytical technique, and thus very useful for sensitive samples, and/or for samples that are available in very small quantities.

The advent of the revolutionary pulsed Fourier transform NMR at the beginning of the 1970s and the manufacturing of strong magnetic fields produced by superconducting solenoids and properly designed cryogenic probes shortened considerably the duration of the analysis and increased dramatically the sensitivity and resolution of the NMR experiment. These advances forwarded the recording of NMR spectra for insensitive and less abundant nuclei, such as carbon-13, nitrogen-15, and others. In addition, the pulsed Fourier transform NMR technique made feasible the expansion of the NMR experiment in more than one dimension. Multidimensional NMR spectroscopy based on carefully designed and executed pulse sequences extended the spectroscopic information in two, three, and sometimes four dimensions disclosing hidden information from the crowded spectrum of a complex substance or from that of a multicomponent system, such as food or biological fluids.

Three more NMR spectroscopic parameters can be measured by conducting appropriate experiments: the spin-lattice (T_1) and spin-spin (T_2) relaxation times, and the nuclear Overhauser enhancement (nOe), the latter being originated from the interaction of the nuclear magnetic moments through space. The first two parameters allow the study of molecular dynamics, whereas the third parameter is a valuable aid for the determination of the three-dimensional structure of a molecular system in solution. As can be seen in the following paragraphs, multinuclear multidimensional NMR spectroscopy represents an effective analytical technique in detecting polyphenols in olive fruits and oils and elucidating indisputably their chemical structure. Furthermore, NMR spectroscopy coupled with HPLC allowed the detection and identification of new polyphenols in olive oil.

5.3.2   Identification of Polyphenols by ^{1}H and ^{13}C NMR Spectroscopy

The most important classes of polyphenols in the olive fruit comprise phenolic acids, phenyl alcohols, flavonoids, and secoiridoids. The main phenyl alcohols of olives are hydroxytyrosol and tyrosol, which were found mostly as glucosides. The flavonoids include mostly the flavone luteolin-7-*O*-glucoside and the flavonols rutin or quercetin-3-*O*-rutinoside. Oleuropein glucoside and demethyoleuropein are the predominant secoiridoids of olive fruit, which in addition contain small quantities of ligstroside and verbascoside (Servili et al., 1999a). The composition of the phenolic fraction of olive fruit is very complex depending on several factors, such as the variety and degree of ripeness of the olive fruit, geographical origin, climatic conditions, harvesting period, and agricultural practices. The polar phenol content in olive oil depends on that in olive fruits from which it was extracted, and is influenced by the extraction procedure used. Phenolic acids and phenyl alcohols are encountered in olive oil, but the phenols with a higher level found in olive oil are the secoiridoid derivatives. It is known (Gariboldi et al., 1986; Montedoro et al., 1993; Limiroli et al., 1995; Bianco and Uccella, 2000) that oleuropein and ligstroside undergo enzymatic hydrolysis during olive oil extraction and/or storage, resulting first in oleuropein aglycon and ligstroside aglycon by removal of the attached glucose moiety, and then in a number of metabolites upon further molecular transformations via ring opening and rearranged re-closure (Figure 5.1). The structures of these metabolites and their proportion in the mixture depend heavily on the nature of the solvent and the pH of the hydrolysis medium (Montedoro et al., 1993; Limiroli et al., 1995). Moreover, olive oil contains small quantities of the lignans (+)-pinoresinol, (+)-1-acetoxypinoresinol, and the free forms of phenolic alcohols and flavonoid classes (see Chapter 3).

^{1}H NMR spectroscopy has provided valuable information about lipid classes, fatty acid composition, unsaturation levels, and several minor compounds (sterols, squalene, terpenes, volatile compounds, etc.), whereas ^{13}C NMR gave unique information about the positional distribution of fatty acids on glycerol moiety and the stereochemistry of unsaturation, among other information. However, these spectroscopic techniques have not yet found broad application in the *in situ* determination of polyphenols of olive fruit and olive oils. Strong signal overlap in ^{1}H NMR spectra, dynamic range problems, diversity of intensities due to various concentrations of the food constitu-

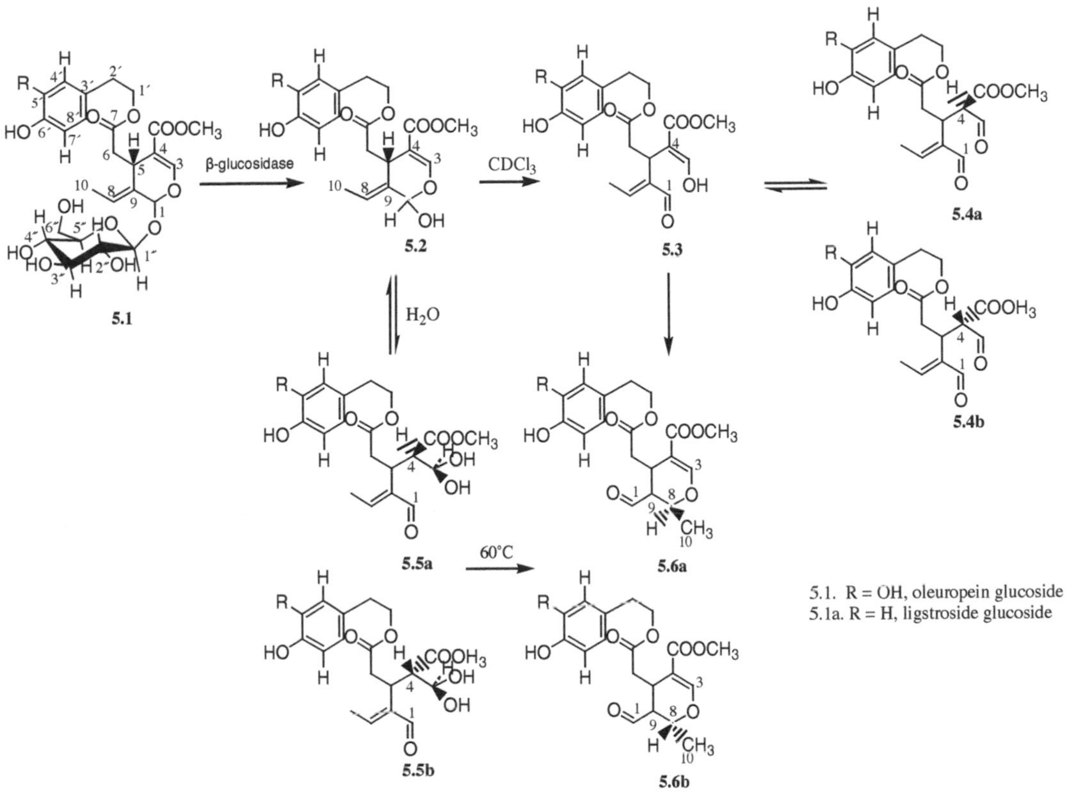

FIGURE 5.1 Enzymatic hydrolysis of oleuropein glucoside and ligstroside in chloroform and water.

ents, and inherent lack of scalar coupling information between different moieties lead to ambiguous or incomplete assignments, thus making their detection and quantification a difficult task even with the use of multidimensional NMR. On the other hand, the low sensitivity and low natural abundance of the ^{13}C nucleus do not allow measurements of polar phenols, which were found at low levels in olive fruit and oil extracts. Therefore, most studies in the literature perform characterization of polyphenols by ^1H and ^{13}C NMR spectroscopy after their separation from the polar part of olive fruit and/or olive oil by preparative or semipreparative chromatography. The isolation procedure is time-consuming, although it has the advantage that the isolated phenols can be used as standards in subsequent experimental work. Thus, Owen and co-workers reported (Owen et al., 2000a) the isolation of the two lignans (+)-pinoresinol and (+)-1-acetoxypinoresinol from methanol extracts of olive oil with preparative thin-layer chromatography, further purification with preparative HPLC, and then chemical structure elucidation by using ^1H and ^{13}C NMR spectroscopy. At the same time, Brenes and co-workers (Brenes et al., 2000), working independently and using mass spectrometry and ^1H NMR spectroscopy, succeeded in characterizing the molecular structure of the same lignans extracted from olive oil and purified by preparative HPLC.

In a subsequent publication Owen et al. (2003), by using the same isolation procedure and NMR spectroscopic techniques, succeeded in elucidating the structure of major phenolic compounds obtained from olive fruits, and from two types (black and green) of brined olive drupes. The data showed that tyrosol, hydroxytyrosol, dihydrocaffeic acid, dihydro-*p*-coumaric acid, verbascoside, and isoverbacoside, along with the flavones apigenin and luteolin, were the major compounds in the phenolic fraction of the black brined olives. Brined green olives contained only hydroxytyrosol and traces of other minor polyphenols. Also, they assessed the antioxidant potential of the purified polyphenols, and that of the commercial olives through their effect on the xanthine oxidase activity monitored by UV spectrometry. Finally, based on these results and those obtained for olive oils (Owen et al., 2000a,b), they concluded that brined olives contain higher concentrations of polyphenols than olive oil.

Characterization of principle components of polyphenols contained in olive fruit and oil (and olive leaf) by ¹H and ³¹C NMR spectroscopy was made by several authors. Oleuropein glucoside (compound 1 in Figure 5.1) (Gariboldi et al., 1986; Montedoro et al., 1993; Servili et al., 1999a), demethyloleuropein (Servili et al., 1999a), verbascoside (Andary et al., 1982; Servili et al., 1999a), and ligstroside (Owen et al., 2000a) were extracted by liquid-liquid or solid-phase extraction, purified, and separated by preparative HPLC, and finally their chemical structure was determined by NMR spectroscopy. Figure 5.2 shows the 500-MHz ¹H NMR spectrum of a commercial sample of oleuropein glucoside in DMSO-d₆ recorded in the NMR Laboratory, Department of Chemistry, University of Crete. The assignment of the various resonances was performed with the aid of homonuclear and heteronuclear two-dimensional NMR experiments.

Evaluation of the metabolic process of oleuropein and the molecular characterization of the various epimeric phenolic metabolites by NMR spectroscopy were reported by Gariboldi and co-workers as early as 1986 (Gariboldi et al., 1986). They examined the extracts obtained from olive leaves. The two isomers 5*S*, 8*S*, 9*S* and 5*S*, 8*R*, 9*S* of the aldehydic form of oleuropein (**6a** and **6b** in Figure 5.1) were separated by column chromatography, purified by HPLC, and finally characterized by ¹H and ¹³C NMR spectroscopy. The stereochemistry and conformation of these two isomers were elucidated by running 2D-NOE (NOESY) experiments. On the basis of the NMR spectroscopic data (chemical shifts and coupling constants) obtained for compound **6a**, elenolic acid (**7**) and its methyl ester (**8**) (Scheme 5.1) were identified as the final products of the biotransformation of oleuropein. Oleuropein glucoside (**1**), the aldehydic form of oleuropein (**6**), elenolic acid (**7**), and the hemiacetal form (**9**) of the latter compound were detected and characterized by NMR in the phenolic extract of virgin olive oil after separation by preparative HPLC (Montedoro et al.,

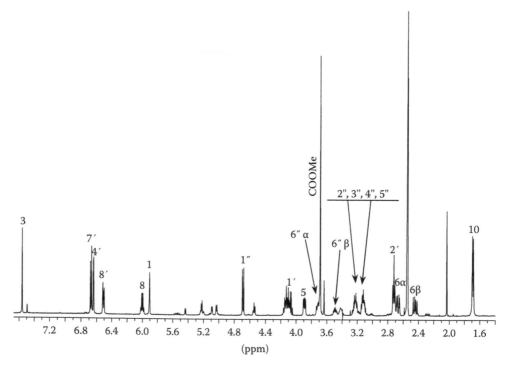

FIGURE 5.2 500-MHz 1H NMR spectrum of oleuropein glucoside in DMSO-d6 solution. Protons were numbered as in compound 1 in Figure 5.1.

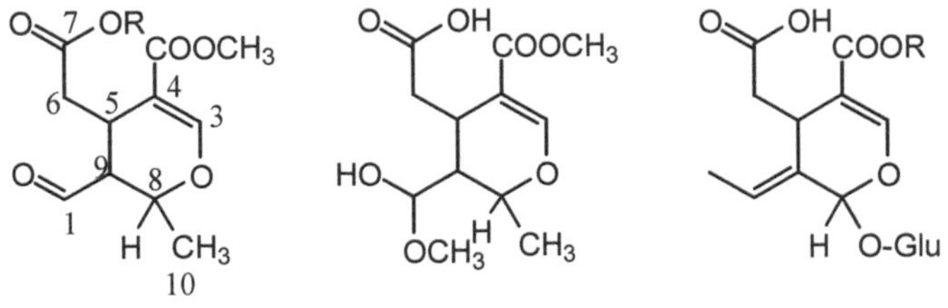

O 7 OR
COOCH$_3$
6 5 4
3
O 9 8 O
1
H CH$_3$
10

7. R = H
8. R = CH$_3$

O OH
COOCH$_3$
HO
H
OCH$_3$ CH$_3$

9

O OH
COOR
O
H O-Glu

10. R = CH$_3$
11. R = H

SCHEME 5.1

1993). In addition, four new phenolic compounds were identified and their chemical structures were confirmed by ^{1}H and ^{13}C NMR spectroscopy in chloroform-d solutions. These compounds were metabolites of oleuropein and ligstroside, namely, their aglycons (compound **2** in Figure 5.1) and their dialdehydic forms (**4** in Figure 5.1), but lacked the carboxymethyl group at C-4. No isomers of compound **4** were detected in this study. The NMR spectra of the dialdehydic forms of oleuropein and ligstroside lacking a carboxymethyl group in methanol-d$_4$ solutions were different than those obtained in chloroform-d solutions, indicating the presence of hemiacetalic structures at C-3. However, it is important to note that these hemiacetalic structures are not the direct product of the oleuropein and ligstroside transformations. They are probably formed when the phenolic fraction of olive oil is dissolved in methanol just before the HPLC analysis. The structure elucidation of new epimeric metabolites of oleuropein glucoside isolated from methanol/acetone extracts of green olive fruits was carried out by Bianco and co-workers (Bianco et al., 1999a). The identification of the two isomers of oleuropeindials (**4a** and **4b** of Figure 5.1) at C-4, postulated but not identified in a previous study, was achieved by two-dimensional NMR spectroscopy. These compounds were isolated by flash chromatography on a silica gel column with chloroform/methanol as eluent.

In order to understand the oleuropein glucoside (and ligstroside) biotransformation pathway, several groups have investigated its enzymatic degradation *in vitro* using β-glucosidases or yeasts. The enzymatic degradation of oleuropein glucoside under biomimetic conditions was monitored *in situ* by NMR spectroscopy (Limiroli et al., 1995; Bianco et al., 1999b). An important observation was that the hydrolysis products of **1** and their lifetimes depend on the medium in which hydrolysis occurs. The first product of the hydrolytic conversion of **1** in D$_2$O with β-glucosidase was the oleuropein hemiacetal or oleuropein aglycon (**2** in Figure 5.1) resulting from the removal of the attached glucose moiety. This compound undergoes a fast chemical conversion in water solution leading to a mixture of two isomers of the aldehyde **5** or oleuropeindial gem diols. The two isomers **5a** and **5b** (Figure 5.1) differ in their relative stereochemistry at C-4. An analogous enzymatic hydrolysis performed in a D$_2$O/chloroform-d mixture showed the presence of oleuropeinenol **3** (Figure 5.1) in equilibrium with the diastereomeric aldehydes **4a** and **4b** (Figure 5.1). Aldehydes **4** were also obtained as an equilibrium mixture from acetal **2** by straightforward acid-catalyzed hydrolysis. Finally, aldehydes **3** or **5** were transformed, at room temperature and 60°C, respectively, into the ultimate hydrolysis product, the aldehydic form of oleuropein **6**. Metabolites such as elenolic acid and its methyl ester as well as the various decarboxylated compounds reported in previous studies (see above) were not detected in the biomimetic investigations.

One- and two-dimensional ^{1}H NMR spectroscopy was also used to investigate the *in situ* hydrolytic conversion of oleuropein glucoside during the industrial debittering process of table olives (Capozzi et al., 2000). The reactivity of **1** was investigated by performing alkaline hydrolysis with NaOD/D$_2$O in the NMR tube at different times, pH values, and molar ratios of the reactants following technological procedures applied for table olive processing. In the aqueous medium with pH

12.7 and 5 min after the addition of NaOD, the ^{1}H NMR signals of compound **1** started diminishing, whereas new signals appeared. After 40 min the hydrolysis of **1** was nearly complete as indicated by the absence of the original signals in the ^{1}H NMR spectrum, while the spectrum revealed signals from free hydroxytyrosol and the sodium salt of 11-methyl oleoside (**10**), which was confirmed by two-dimensional NMR spectroscopy and also by reference to the previously reported spectrum of this compound (Gariboldi et al., 1986). Further addition of NaOD induced a fast hydrolysis of the less reactive estereal group of **10** at C-7 leading to the loss of a methyl group and the formation of the sodium salt of the oleoside (**11**).

   ^{1}H and ^{13}C NMR spectroscopy were very useful to identify new phenolic components isolated from olive fruits and oils. A series of compounds depicted in Scheme 5.2 were obtained from cornoside (**12**), which was transformed by enzymatic hydrolysis with β-glucosidase into the less polar cornoside aglycon (**13**), which is partially converted to another less polar compound, the halleridone (**14**) (Bianco et al., 1993). The molecular structures of three new monoglucosides of hydroxytyrosol in olive leaves, fruits, and oils from two Italian cultivars were fully determined by ^{1}H and ^{13}C NMR spectroscopy (Bianco et al., 1998) and the use of semi-preparative HPLC for their purification. The relative position of the glucose unit in each of these three phenolic molecules was confirmed by one-dimensional NOE experiments. Irradiation of the well-separated anomeric proton of the glucose moiety resulted in a significant positive NOE effect of the respective neighboring aromatic or aliphatic protons. The full characterization of a new compound and its distribution in different parts of olive fruit (peel, pulp, and seed) were carried out by employing one- and two-dimensional NMR spectroscopy (Servili et al., 1999b). The new compound, known by the empirical name nüzhenide (**15** in Scheme 5.3), was isolated from three Italian cultivars. Contrary to oleuropein, demethyloleuropein, and verbascoside, which are present in all of the constitutive parts of the olive fruit, nüzhenide was detected exclusively in the seed of the fruit. New tyrosol derivatives were isolated and identified from two fractions with different polarities obtained from olive leaves and fruits from several cultivars of Calabria (Bianco et al., 2004). In the more polar fraction the tyrosol glucoside (**16** in Scheme 5.4) (salidroside) was found together with cornoside and its cyclic aglycon halleridone (see above). The main component present in the less polar fraction was the ester of tyrosol with

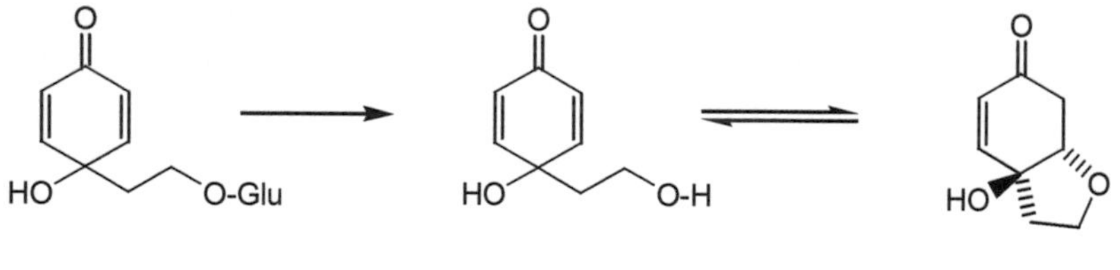

| 12 | 13 | 14 |

SCHEME 5.2

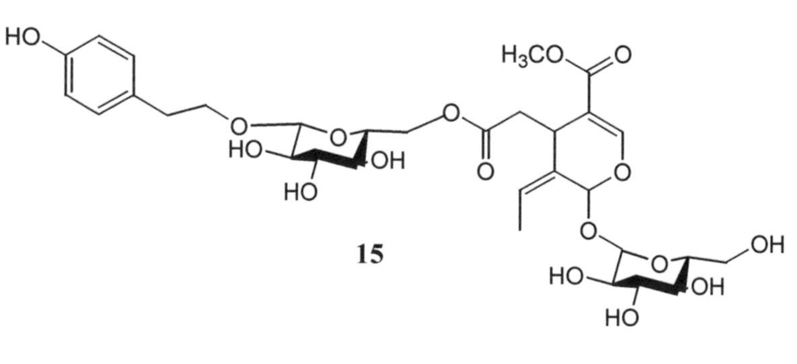

15

SCHEME 5.3

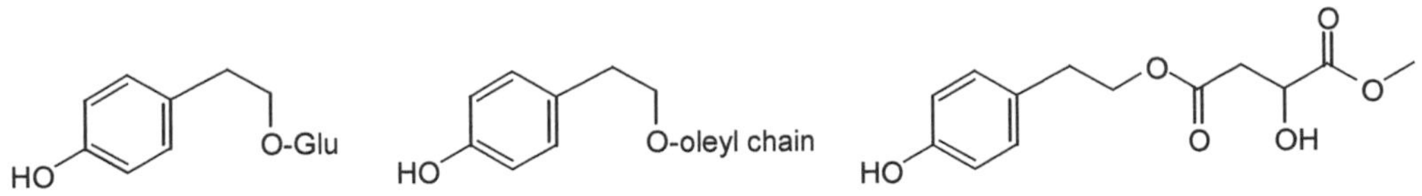

SCHEME 5.4

cis-oleic acid (1-oleyltyrosol) (**17**). The chemical structure of the first compound was determined by ^1H and ^{13}C NMR spectroscopy, whereas the structure of the second compound was determined by chemical (alkaline hydrolysis) and spectroscopic methods.

Recently, two new hydroxytyrosol and tyrosol derivatives were isolated from green olive fruits belonging to the Hojiblanca cultivar (Bianco et al., 2006). The first compound was the methyl acetal of the ligstroside aglycon, probably formed from ligstroside during the extraction process by exchange with methanol. The second derivative was the β-hydroxytyrosyl ester of methyl maleate (**18**), which may be related to the occurrence of malic acid and Krebs cycle acids in olive pulp. Full characterization of these compounds was obtained by one-dimensional ^1H and ^{13}C NMR and two-dimensional NMR experiments. Their presence in table olives may be correlated with the texture and organoleptic properties of the food product.

The occurrence of polyphenols in fresh and processed olive fruits was examined by Bianco and co-workers as a function of olive fruit variety, olive ripeness, and pedoclimatic conditions (Bianco and Uccella, 2000; Bastoni et al., 2001) in an attempt to predict olive oil quality from olives. Four different protocols were employed to estimate the concentration of the various classes of polyphenols in olive fruits from Italy, Spain, Greece, and Portugal. The first protocol allowed for the estimation of the total concentration of simple phenolic compounds, the second for soluble polyphenols and soluble esterified derivatives, the third for the quantitative determination of cytoplasmatic soluble phenolic content, and the fourth for the determination of soluble glucosidic, esterified, and cell-wall–bound polyphenols. These experimental procedures produced four different fractions of the phenolic components that were checked by column chromatography and HPLC, and structurally identified by NMR spectroscopy. The comparison of each of these fractions gave very useful information about the phenolic composition in olive samples harvested from several environments and cultivars at different ripening stages. It is worth mentioning that very good agreement was observed among data obtained from ^1H NMR with those measured by HPLC for each fraction (Bastoni et al., 2001), suggesting that ^1H NMR spectroscopy may be an alternative methodology for the rapid determination of phenolic content in olives.

5.3.3 IDENTIFICATION OF POLYPHENOLS BY ^{31}P NMR SPECTROSCOPY

To avoid the shortcomings of the ^1H and ^{13}C NMR spectroscopy mentioned previously for the determination of polyphenols in olive fruits and oil, an alternative methodology was proposed recently (Spyros and Dais, 2000). This method is based on the derivatization of the labile hydrogens of the hydroxyl and carboxyl groups of polyphenols by the phosphorous reagent 2-chloro-4,4,5,5-tetramethyldioxaphospholane (**I**) according to the reaction scheme shown in Scheme 5.5, and the use of ^{31}P NMR spectroscopy to identify the labile centers (compound **II**). Compound **I** reacts rapidly (~15 min) and quantitatively under mild conditions (within the NMR tube) with the hydroxyl and carboxyl groups. The wide range of ^{31}P chemical shifts (~1000 ppm), and the single resonances for each phosphitylated hydroxyl and/or carboxyl group under proton decoupling simplify the analysis of the ^{31}P NMR spectra. Moreover, the 100% natural abundance of the ^{31}P nucleus and its high sensitivity, which is only ~15 times less than that of the proton nucleus, make

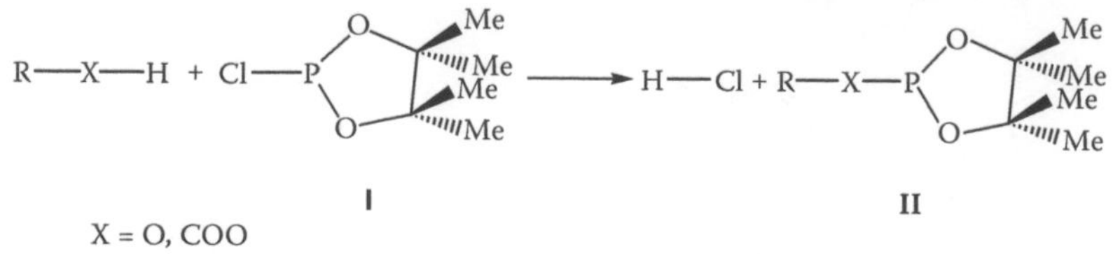

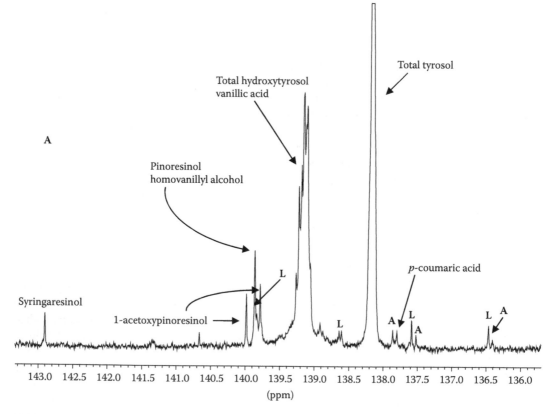

SCHEME 5.5

the ^{31}P NMR experiments a reliable analytical tool to determine amounts of the order of μmol, or lower, depending on the available instrumentation. Another advantage of the ^{31}P NMR method is the introduction of an internal standard of known amount (usually cyclohexanol) in the reaction mixture, which allows the determination of the absolute concentration of the phosphitylated product **II**, thus avoiding normalization conditions.

Figure 5.3A and Figure 5.3B show the ^{31}P NMR spectrum of the polar part of an extra virgin olive oil sample in the regions where the aromatic and aliphatic phosphitylated hydroxyl groups of phenolic compounds are resolved, respectively (Christophoridou and Dais, 2006). The assignment of the ^{31}P chemical shifts reported in Figures 5.3A and 5.3B was based on the chemical shifts of the appropriate model compounds determined by employing one- and two-dimensional NMR techniques and by spiking the sample with pure compounds when necessary (Christophoridou et al., 2001; Christophoridou and Dais, 2006). Polyphenol-containing olive oil model compounds were purchased, synthesized, or extracted from olive oil. In the spectrum of Figure 5.3A, the

FIGURE 5.3 202.2 MHz ^{31}P NMR spectrum of the phosphitylated polar fraction of a virgin olive oil sample from Messinia in chloroform/pyridine solution. (A) Aromatic region. A = apigenin, L = luteolin.

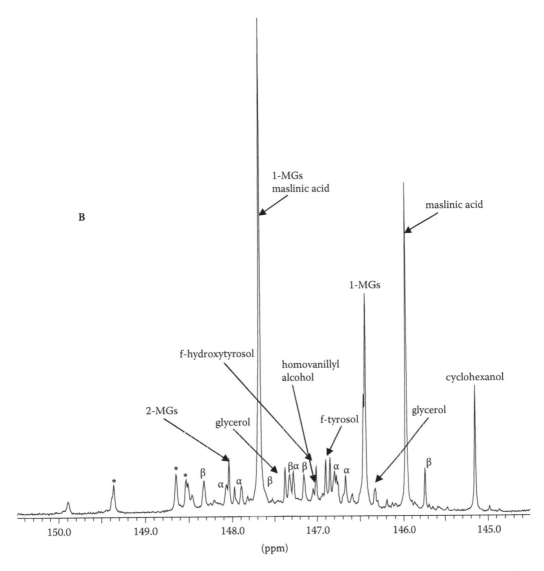

B

FIGURE 5.3 (continued) 202.2 MHz ^{31}P NMR spectrum of the phosphitylated polar fraction of a virgin olive oil sample from Messinia in chloroform/pyridine solution. (B) Aliphatic region. 1-MGs = 1-monoacyl-glycerols, 2-MGs = 2-monoacylglycerols, f-hydroxytyrosol = free hydroxytyrosol, f-tyrosol = free tyrosol, α = α-D-glucopyranose, β = β-D-glucopyranose. Unidentified signals of hydrolysis products of oleuropein glucoside (and ligstroside) are denoted by asterisks.

strong signals at δ 138.19 and δ 139.20 reflect the total amount of tyrosol and hydroxytyrosol contained in olive oil, respectively, since the phosphitylated aromatic hydroxyl groups of these compounds in their free and esterified forms are expected to show about the same chemical shifts. The esterified hydroxytyrosol and tyrosol involve their acetate derivatives and the hydrolysis products of oleuropein and ligstroside that were mentioned previously. Free and esterified hydroxytyrosol constitute an important class of phenolic compounds that contributes to the stability of extra virgin olive oil against oxidation and benefits human health. The signal at δ 142.89 was attributed to the lignan syringaresinol (**19**) depicted in Scheme 5.6, which was detected for the first time in Greek olive oils (see below). Another polyphenol, which was detected for the first time in Greek olive oils, was homovanillyl alcohol (**20**). The signals of the aromatic phosphitylated hydroxyl groups of homovanillyl alcohol and those of the lignan (+) pinoresinol overlap at δ 139.84 in the ^{31}P NMR spectrum (Figure 5.3A). Fortunately, both compounds can be quantified, since the concentration of homovanillyl alcohol can be calculated from the signal of its phosphitylated aliphatic hydroxyl group that resonates at δ 142.89 (Figure 5.3B). Other simple polyphenols, e.g., *o*-coumaric acid, vanillin, gallic acid, *p*-hydroxybenzoic acid, caffeic acid, ferulic acid, etc., were not detected in the spectrum presumably because of their absence and/or their low concentration. Spiking of olive oil with these pure substances resulted in new peaks in the spectrum.

On the basis of the known ^{31}P chemical shifts of model compounds (Christophoridou and Dais, 2006), the strong signals at δ 146.47 and 147.66 are attributed to 1-monoacylglycerol and at δ 148.05 to 2-monoacylglycerol. Maslinic acid (**21** in Scheme 5.6) is detected from signals at δ 145.95 and 147.66, the latter being overlapped by the strong signal of 1-monoacylglycerols. The presence of these signals in the polar part of olive oil indicates that monoacylglycerols and maslinic acid were co-extracted with polyphenols by the liquid-liquid extraction procedures used in this study. A number of signals denoted by α and β (Figure 5.3B) were attributed to the two tautomers α-D- and β-D-glucopyranose, respectively, produced by hydrolysis of the various polyphenol glucosides. The complete assignment of phenolic compounds, as well as for those compounds contained in the polar fraction of olive oil, has been described in detail in Christophoridou and Dais (2006).

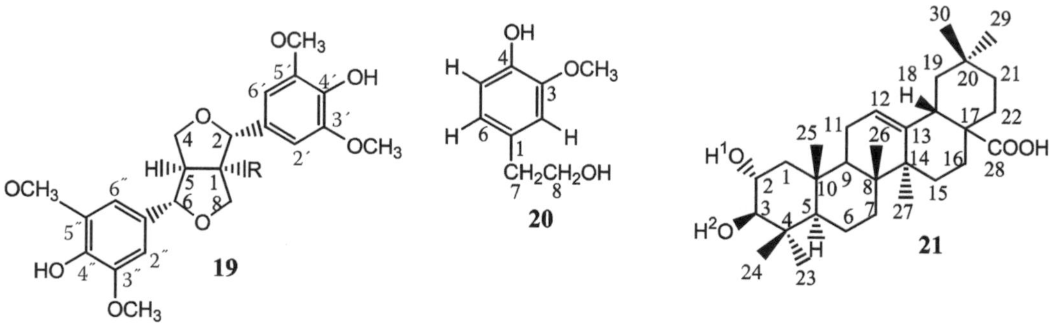

SCHEME 5.6

5.3.4 IDENTIFICATION OF POLYPHENOLS BY LC-NMR

We have seen in the previous paragraph that the traditional and time-consuming ways of studying polyphenols in the polar fraction of olive fruit and oil by using one-dimensional ^{1}H and ^{13}C NMR spectroscopy include fractionation of the crude extract, and separation and isolation of the individual components using liquid chromatography. It would be advantageous to be able to speed up this part of the work by performing the separation and structure elucidation online. Such an approach requires the combination of the most powerful separation technique of liquid chromatography (LC) with the most information-rich spectroscopic technique (NMR) for structure elucidation.

Some practical and theoretical aspects of this coupling technique, including the development of special flow through probes, and other technical details concerning the physical connection of LC and NMR (e.g., control and transport of the analyte from LC detector to NMR probe) are given elsewhere (Albert, 2002). Currently, several LC-NMR systems and modes of operation exist, and their use depends on the nature of the sample being studied. It is worth mentioning that significant improvement to LC-NMR sensitivity has been obtained by adding a post-column solid-phase extraction (SPE) system to replace loop collection. S/N improvements up to a factor of 4 could be demonstrated with this new technology (Corcoran et al., 2002; Exarchou et al., 2005). The use of individual SPE cartridges after chromatographic separation and prior to NMR analysis allows significant enrichment of the analyte concentration and the performance of one- and two-dimensional

NMR experiments of less sensitive nuclei, such as carbon-13. In addition, deuterated solvents are required only for the transport of the analyte from the SPE unit to the NMR probe. Therefore, chromatographic separation can use the less expensive protonated solvents, thereby decreasing considerably the cost of the analysis.

LC-NMR has been used in recent years for the analysis of natural products and plant metabolites (Cavin et al., 1998; Exarchou et al., 2003, 2005), including lignans, flavonoids, and tocopherol derivatives. Separation and identification of phenols in olive oil by employing the LC-SPE-NMR technique has been reported recently (Christophoridou et al., 2005). Separation was achieved by HPLC using as a mobile phase a mixture of water and acetonitrile; both solvents were acidified with 0.1% trifluoroacetic acid. One- and two-dimensional NMR spectra were recorded on a 600-MHz spectrometer equipped with a ^1H-^{13}C inverse detection flow probe. Figure 5.4 shows selections of 600-MHz LC-SPE-^1H NMR spectra indicating the presence of different oleuropein metabolites in olive oil. These spectra were recorded for HPLC fractions transferred to a peak-trapping unit equipped with solid-phase cartridges after UV detection and water addition for temporary storage, dried with nitrogen gas, and transferred to the NMR probe with deuterated acetonitrile. The first ^1H NMR spectrum (Figure 5.4A) is consistent with the dialdehydic form of oleuropein lacking a carboxymethyl group, whereas the spectrum in Figure 5.4B is more interesting because it reveals the existence of two coeluted isomers of the aldehydic form of oleuropein (**4a** and **4b** in Figure 5.1), namely, 5S, 8R, 9S and 5S, 8S, 9S, the latter isomer being detected for the first time in olive oil. The presence of the second isomer was confirmed by performing a TOCSY experiment (Christophoridou et al., 2005). Figure 5.4C illustrates the spectrum of the hemiacetal at C-3 of the dialdehydic form of oleuropein lacking a carboxymethyl group, formerly detected by Montedoro and co-workers (Montedoro et al., 1993). Another example indicating the potential of this technique is shown

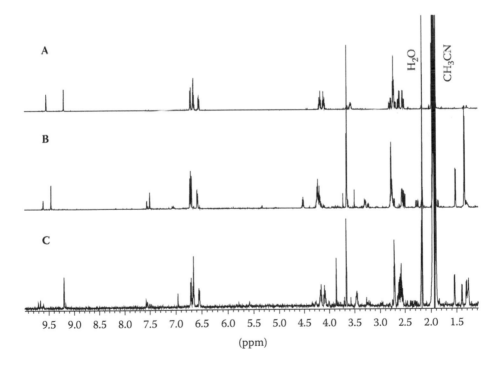

FIGURE 5.4 600 MHz LC-SPE-1H-NMR spectra of oleuropein derivatives; (A) dialdehydic form of oleuropein lacking a carboxymethyl group; (B) the coeluted two isomers of the aldehydic form of oleuropein; (C) hemiacetal of the dialdehydic form of oleuropein. The suppressed signals of H_2O and CH_3CN solvents give spikes at ~ δ 1.95 and δ 2.18.

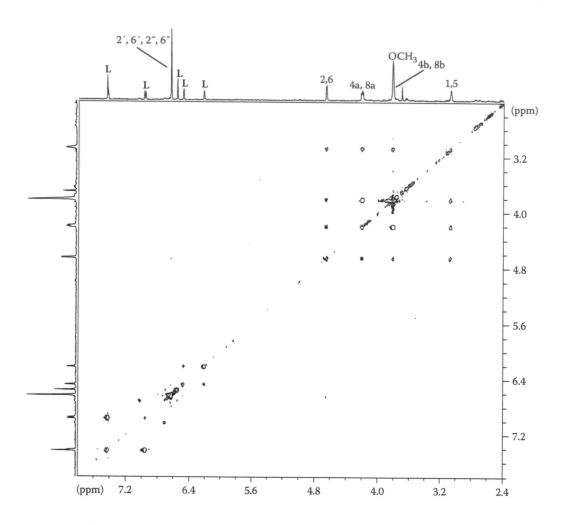

FIGURE 5.5 600 MHz TOCSY spectrum indicating the presence of the lignan syringaresinol. The signals denoted by L belong to luteolin. Protons were numbered as in compound 19 in Scheme 5.6.

in Figure 5.5, which depicts the 600-MHz TOCSY spectrum of a peak in the chromatogram corresponding to the flavanol luteolin. Apart from the signals of luteolin (indicated by L), several additional signals were discovered, reflecting the presence of an unknown phenolic compound coeluted with luteolin. The chemical shifts and coupling constant pattern of the signals at high magnetic field strength were similar to those observed for the bicyclic skeleton of the lignans (+)-pinoresinol and (+)-1-acetoxypinoresinol bearing two aryl groups, whereas the signal intensity of the singlet at δ 3.81 corresponded to 12 protons, and it was assigned to four equivalent methoxy groups. These data along with the singlet in the aromatic region (δ 6.61) corresponding to four equivalent aromatic protons supported the structure of a new compound, namely, the lignan syringaresinol (**19**) detected for the first time in olive oil.

The presence of homovanillyl alcohol (**20** in Scheme 6) in olive oil has been confirmed by the LC-SPE-^{1}H NMR spectrum displayed in Figure 5.6, which is similar to that of hydroxytyrosol with an additional singlet at δ 3.82 owing to the OCH_3 group. While examining the LC-SPE-^{1}H NMR spectra at long retention times of the HPLC chromatogram at 280 nm, a peak eluting at 37.1 min gave a complex ^{1}H NMR spectrum with the characteristics of maslinic acid (**21** in Scheme 5.6)

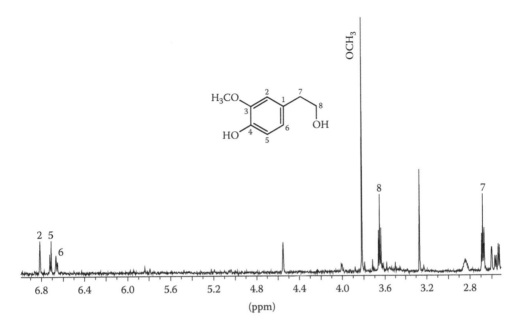

FIGURE 5.6 600 MHz LC-SPE-^{1}H-NMR spectrum indicating the presence of homovanillyl alcohol.

(Figure 5.7). Complete assignment of the spectrum was not possible due to severely overlapped signals even at 600 MHz. However, the TOCSY experiment assisted with the assignment of a few signals of the triterpenic skeleton in addition to those reported in earlier experiments at weaker magnetic field strengths. In summary, the use of LC-SPE-NMR methodology made possible the detection and structure elucidation of 27 constituents in the phenolic fraction of olive oil. Five phenolic compounds out of 27 had not been reported previously, namely, syringaresinol, homovanillyl alcohol, the 5S, 8S, 9S isomer of the aldehydic form of oleuropein, and the dialdehydic form of free elenolic acid lacking a carboxymethyl group. The presence of ligstroside aglycon and the two isomers of the aldehydic form of ligstroside were also confirmed by the technique (Christophoridou et al., 2005).

5.3.5 CONCLUSIONS

Multinuclear and multidimensional NMR spectroscopy offers new opportunities for determining a large number of phenolic compounds contained in olive fruit and oil. The advantages of using high-resolution ^{1}H NMR spectroscopy for the analysis of the polar fraction of olive fruit and oil have been demonstrated by concrete examples from the literature. The structure-specific analysis of different components in a single experiment provides a rapid and reliable analytical tool to be used in conjunction with other recognized analytical methods (GC, HPLC) for the detection and quantification of polyphenols. The coupling of HPLC with ^{1}H NMR (and ^{13}C NMR) spectroscopy provided new capabilities in polyphenols analysis. This technique avoided the time-consuming off-line identification of polyphenols, and assisted the search for new phenolic compounds and for a rapid identification of known compounds.

Other nuclei can also be used for polyphenol analysis. In particular, ^{31}P NMR spectroscopy in combination with the phosphitylation reaction provides complementary information, and it is very useful in cases where ^{1}H and ^{13}C NMR spectroscopy are unable to offer a straightforward analysis.

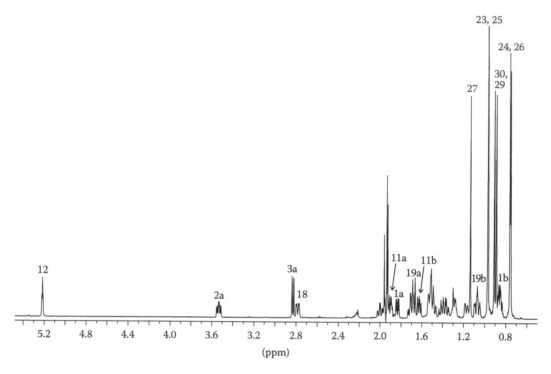

FIGURE 5.7 600 MHz LC-SPE-¹H-NMR spectrum indicating the presence of maslinic acid. Protons were numbered as in compound 21 in Scheme 5.6.

5.4 MASS SPECTROMETRY

5.4.1 INTRODUCTION

MS is a powerful analytical technique that is used to identify unknown compounds, to quantify known compounds, and to elucidate the structure and chemical properties of molecules. It had its beginnings in the pioneer work of J.J. Thomson (1906 Nobel Laureate in physics), who studied the effects of electric and magnetic fields on ions generated in a cathode ray tube, and observed that ions move through parabolic trajectories proportional to their mass-to-charge ratio (m/z). Since then several important advances in this technique were attained, having a significant impact on its capabilities for routine and especially for sophisticated applications. One of the main advantages of MS is the use of different physical principles for sample ionization and separation of the generated ions. For this reason, MS is different from other spectroscopic methods, and it provides considerable flexibility in the detection, quantification, and structural determination of compounds.

The mass spectrometer can be divided into three fundamental parts. The first part is the ionization chamber, where sample ions are formed by an ionization source; the second part is the mass analyzer, where the ions are sorted according to their m/z ratios; and the third part is a detector. The output of the detector is an electronic signal, the magnitude of which is proportional to the ion flux that hits the detector. The magnitude of these signals as a function of m/z is the mass spectrum. The three parts of the mass spectrometer are maintained under high vacuum to decrease collisions of the ions with air molecules, and thereby increasing their lifetime. The entire operation of the mass spectrometer is under computer control.

The ionization method to be used depends on the type of sample under investigation and the mass spectrometer used. There are several ionization methods, ranging from the classical electron impact and chemical ionization methods, which are suitable for producing ions in the gas phase upon ionization of small nonpolar and nonvolatile molecules, to the more sophisticated matrix-assisted laser desorption ionization method, which is applicable to biochemical analyses involving large molecules. Other ionization techniques, such as thermospray ionization, electrospray ionization, and atmospheric pressure ionization, are well suited for liquid chromatography coupled with MS. With most ionization procedures ions with positive charge, H $[M+1]^+$, and/or negative charge, H $[M-1]^-$, are created depending on the proton affinity of the neutral sample molecule M, and/or salt cationization, e.g., Na $[M+23]^+$, K $[M+39]^+$, NH_4 $[M+18]^+$. Therefore, the user of the mass spectrometer has the possibility to detect ions in the positive and/or negative mode.

There are a number of mass analyzers currently available. The simplest type of mass analyzer is the time of flight (TOF), which is very fast and has very high sensitivity at a virtually unlimited mass range. Although the time of flight mass spectrometry (TOF-MS) was developed about 50 years ago, only recently was it implemented in high resolution MS instruments. Other mass analyzers include quadrupoles, quadrupole ion traps, and the more sophisticated Fourier transform ion cyclotron resonance (FT-ICR). There are excellent references in the literature and Websites, where the interested reader can find useful information about theory, instrumentation, and applications of MS.

The application of MS to the analysis of phenolic compounds in olive fruit and olive oil has grown along with the new developments in MS, the so-called soft ionization techniques that favor the detection of these polar, nonvolatile, and thermally labile compounds. The structural information obtained by MS could be enhanced by using the so-called tandem MS with different experimental approaches classified according the ionization setup used. Moreover, the high sensitivity and possibilities of use with gas and liquid chromatographic techniques have made MS one of the most appropriate physicochemical methods for the study of natural products from biological materials at very low concentrations (10 pg for a compound of mass equal to 1 kDa). It should be noted that the fragmentation pathways in mass spectrometric measurements and the relative abundance of the various fragment ions are largely dependent on the ionization mode and the type of the mass analyzer used. Applications of MS to identification and structural determination of plant phenolic compounds have been reviewed recently (Ryan et al., 1999a). Also, excellent reviews (Stobiecki, 2000; Frański et al., 2005; de Rijke at al., 2006; Willfor et al., 2006) describe mass spectrometric techniques used for the characterization of lignans and flavonoids in plants, food, drinks, and biological fluids. Careri, Bianchi, and Corradini presented a review on applications of MS-based techniques for the analysis of organic compounds occurring in foods, including antioxidant phenols in olive oil (Careri et al., 2002). Finally, various analytical methods, including MS, used for the detection of phenolic compounds in olives have been discussed critically (Ryan and Robards, 1998).

5.4.2 Ionization Methods for Simple Mass Spectra of Phenolic Compounds

The traditional mode of MS involves electron impact ionization (EI) with electron energies ranging from 10–100 eV, and chemical ionization (CI) with ionized reagent gases (usually methane, ammonia, and noble gases) for the production of charged sample ions via charge transfer and proton transfer reactions (Mark and Dunn, 1985; Harrison, 1999). These hard ionization methods were not suitable for MS analysis of underivatized phenolic compounds, since both methods require the analyte to be in the gas phase for ionization, and thus derivatization of the hydroxyl groups (methylation, trimethysilylation, or acetylation) especially for the phenolic glucosides was mandatory (Willfor et al., 2006). Chemical derivatization appears to overcome the limitation of restricted volatility and thermal stability. The procedure may increase the molecular mass of the analyte beyond the capability of the mass analyzer; as a result poor resolution and limited structural information are obtained (Ryan et al., 1999a; Harrison, 1999).

The advent of desorption ionization techniques, in which ionization of thermolabile and low volatility molecules occurs directly from the condense phase, made the analysis of phenolic compounds feasible without derivatization. The most successful desorption techniques were the fast atom bombardment (FAB) (Barber et al., 1982) and the liquid secondary ion mass spectrometry

(LSIMS) (Aberth and Burlingame, 1984). These techniques involve the bombardment of the analyte solubilized in a solid or liquid nonvolatile matrix (e.g., glycerol, thioglycerol, 3-nitrobenzyl alcohol), with a particle beam thereby inducing desorption and ionization. In FAB, the particle beam consisted of neutral inert gas, typically xenon or argon, at bombardment energies of 4–10 keV, whereas the particle beam in LSIMS comprises an ion, typically Cs^+, at bombardment energies of 2–30 keV. The particle beam hits the mixture (analyte + matrix) surface and transfers much of its energy to the surroundings, inducing instant collisions and eventually molecular fragmentation. Both FAB and LSIMS methods produce strong peaks in the mass spectrum for the pseudo-molecular species $[M+H]^+$ (positive ion mode) and $[M-H]^-$ (negative ion mode), along with structurally important fragment ions. Matrix-assisted laser desorption ionization (MALDI) (Karas and Hillenkamp, 1988) is another desorption ionization method employing laser light (usually a pulsed nitrogen laser of wavelength 337 nm) to bring about sample ionization. Again the sample is pre-mixed with a viscous matrix, which transforms the laser energy into excitation energy for the sample, thus sputtering the analyte and matrix ions from the surface of the mixture in the form of positive and negative ions. This technique finds application mainly in biochemical areas for the analysis of large molecules, such as polysaccharides, proteins, peptides, and oligonucleotides. Drawbacks of the desorption ionization methods could be the dependence of MS data on the choice of matrix, and the appearance in the mass spectra signals owing to matrix ionization, thus complicating their interpretation.

Apart from the aforementioned developments, additional ionization techniques were invented and applied especially to combined systems of MS and HPLC. These techniques were applied in cases where FAB and LSIMS methods were not so effective because of the low sample concentration and the relatively high flow rates in the liquid chromatograph. Soft ionization techniques, such as thermospray ionization (TSI), electrospray ionization (ESI), nanospray ionization, atmospheric pressure ionization (API), and atmospheric pressure chemical ionization (APCI) allowed the exploitation of the tremendous potential inherent in the combination of MS with GC and LC. These ionization techniques will be presented briefly in Section 5.4.4.

5.4.3 MULTIDIMENSIONAL MASS SPECTROMETRY

To improve the effectiveness of MS in full structural analysis of unknown substances, coupling two or more stages of mass analysis $(MS)^n$ has been introduced (McLafferty, 1980; Niessen, 1998). The exponent n represents the number of generations of fragment ions being analyzed. The so-called tandem (in space) mass spectrometer has two or more mass analyzers, in practice usually two, abbreviated as $(MS)^2$ or (MS/MS). The two analyzers are separated by a collision cell, in which an inert gas (e.g., xenon, argon) is admitted to collide with the sample ions (usually molecular ions in the positive or negative mode) that are user-specified and selected in the first mass analyzer. The secondary fragment ions, resulting upon bombardment of the precursor ions, are separated according to their m/z ratios by the second analyzer, which has been set to monitor specific fragment ions. In most studies, the multidimensional MS is used to confirm unambiguously the presence of a compound in a matrix, e.g., substances in biological fluids. The tandem $(MS)^n$ method is superior to the single-stage MS detection because of the much better selectivity, the higher sensitivity, and the wide range of structural information that can be obtained. Figure 5.8 shows the principle underlying the operation of tandem mass spectrometry. In several instances, tandem mass spectrometry has been combined with liquid chromatography to facilitate the structural determination of phenolic compounds.

5.4.4 MASS SPECTROMETRY COUPLED TO SEPARATION TECHNIQUES

Mass spectrometry coupled to gas chromatography (GC-MS) and especially with liquid chromatography (LC-MS) is of enormous potential in instrumental analysis; it combines the advantages of the most effective separation techniques with the ability of MS for identification and structural characterization of unknown compounds. For GC-MS or LC-MS combinations, the results are shown as

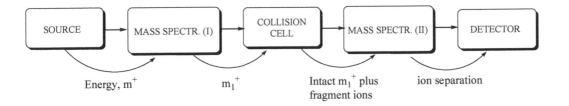

FIGURE 5.8 Schematic representation of the tandem mass spectrometry setup.

a series of mass spectra that are acquired sequentially in time. To obtain this information, the mass spectrometer scans the appropriate mass range repetitively during the chromatographic run. This information may be displayed in several ways, as shown in Figure 5.9. One way is to sum up the intensities of all the ions in each spectrum, and this sum is plotted as a function of chromatographic retention time to give a total ion chromatogram or current (TIC) (Figure 5.9A). The resulting plot is similar to the output of a conventional chromatographic UV detector. Each peak in the TIC represents an eluting compound that can be identified by interpretation of the mass spectra recorded for the peak. Finding the compound of interest by the TIC method can be difficult, inasmuch as many compounds may have the same mass. Another way is the diagonal display shown in the lower part of Figure 5.9A. According to this presentation, the intensity at a single m/z over the course of a chromatographic run can be displayed to yield a selected ion current profile or mass chromatogram. Another mode of obtaining LC-MS data is the selected ion monitoring (SIM), in which the mass analyzer scans selectively a small mass range, typically one mass unit (Figure 5.9B). Therefore, only compounds with selected mass are detected and plotted. Selected reaction monitoring (SRM) or multiple reaction monitoring (MRM) is the method used preferably by the majority of scientists conducting mass spectrometric quantitation. SRM is sensitive and allows specific quantitation, since it delivers a unique fragment ion from a complex matrix that can be monitored and quantified (Figure 5.9C). In summary, the combination techniques are valuable whenever identification of unknown compounds in a complex mixture is sought without having to examine each individual mass spectrum.

The subtle point of interfacing a mass spectrometer to a separation system like a gas or liquid chromatograph is to maintain the required vacuum in the mass spectrometer while introducing flow from the chromatograph. Interfaces developed commercially over the last decade have solved the problem of eliminating the gas load from the separation system by using combinations of heating and pumping, sometimes with the assistance of a drying gas stream. The inlets for higher flow rates (as in analytical HPLC) employed in LC-MS systems in routine use today belong to the API technology (Niessen, 1998). The latter comprises two different interfaces based mainly on ESI and APCI, although TSI has been used in a few cases (Wolfender et al., 1995). The ESI technique and its version at low flow rate, the nanospray ionization, produce gaseous ionized molecular ions directly from a liquid solution. It operates by creating a fine spray of highly charged droplets in the presence of an electric field (1–4 kV). Evaporation of the solvent from each droplet of the spray at atmospheric pressure is achieved by dry gas, heat, or both. The ionized sample molecules that are free from solvent are then swept into the mass analyzer of the mass spectrometer. When APCI interface is used in a coupled mode, the eluant from HPLC is evaporated completely and the mixture of solvent and sample vapor is then ionized by chemical ionization. This involves proton transfer, cationization, and charge exchange reactions in positive ion mode or proton abstraction, anion attachement, and electron capture reactions in the negative mode. The APCI procedure is compatible with 100% aqueous or 100% organic mobile phases at flow rates up to 2 ml/min, and therefore ideal for normal or reverse-phase operation with a conventional HPLC column. The API interphases may be coupled to different mass spectrometric analyzers and, thus, different designs

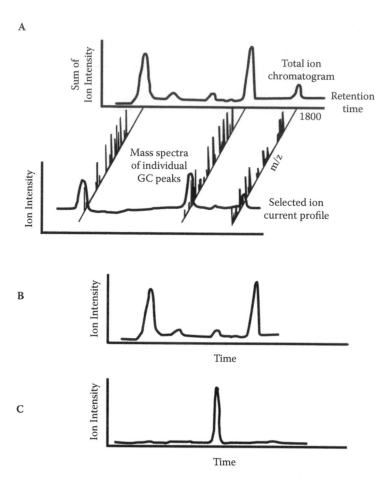

FIGURE 5.9 Modes of LC-MS monitoring. (A) Total ion chromatogram (TIC) and mass spectra of individual HPLC peaks; (B) Selected ion monitoring (SIM); (C) Selected reaction monitoring (SRM) or multiple reaction monitoring (MRM).

of API for all kinds of instruments are available (Niessen, 1998, 1999). Both GC-MS and LC-MS are now well-established techniques, and the choice between the two depends on the system under study. However, because of limited volatility, phenolic compounds and in particular their glucosides cannot be easily analyzed by GC-MS, unless hydrolysis of their glucosides to their corresponding aglycons and/or derivatization is performed prior to analysis.

5.4.5 Applications

On rare occasions, normal MS provides sufficient data leading to complete structural analysis of phenolic compounds. It is rather used to determine molecular mass and to establish the substitution pattern of the phenolic rings (Stobiecki, 2000). Analysis by employing single-stage MS requires isolation of phenolic compounds from olives and/or olive oil either by liquid-liquid or solid-phase extraction. ESI-MS in the positive and negative mode has been used for fast fingerprint characterization of the methanol/water (60:40 v/v) extracts of the edible oils of soybean, corn, canola, sunflower, cottonseed, and olive oil to detect aging and possible adulteration of olive oil (Catharino et al., 2005). The sample preparation with the methanol/water mixture permitted the simultaneous detection of the fatty acids and the polar polyphenols. Application of the principal component analysis (PCA) to ESI-MS data obtained in the positive and negative modes allowed the differentiation among the six edible oils. Also, olive oil adulteration with soybean was estimated semiquantitatively by comparing the relative intensities of the ions observed in the ESI(-)-MS spectra of admixtures with those of pure olive oil. Structural information can be improved considerably by using tandem mass spectrometry (MS/MS). Ionspray ionization with the MS/MS methodology was applied to detect and quantify oleuropein in virgin olive oil (Perri et al., 1999). An acetonitrile solution of standard oleuropein containing ammonium acetate was ionized, mainly producing the species [M + NH$_4$]$^+$ at m/z 558. The latter was transmitted by the first mass filter into the second quadrupole of a triple quadrupole instrument and there was allowed to react with an inert gas, producing the MS/MS spectrum shown in Figure 5.10 through the scanning of the last mass analyzer. The inset of Figure 5.10 depicts the structure of the daughter ions resulting from a series of consecutive and competitive unimolecular fragmentations of the initially formed ammoniated species. Although identification of all ions in the spectrum was not reported (e.g., at m/z 329 and 225), the most intense fragments at m/z 137 and 361 attributed to hydroxytyrosol and oleuropein aglycon, respectively, were used as reference peaks for a quantitative determination of oleuropein in olive oil.

GC coupled to MS was applied for the first time to the analysis of phenolic compounds in olive oil by Angerosa and co-workers (Angerosa et al., 1995, 1996). They found that tyrosol and hydroxytyrosol were the main simple phenols present in olive oil. Furthermore, it was observed (Angerosa et al., 1995) that fragmentation of aglycons produced by EI brought about a main peak at m/z 280 (hydroxytyrosol trimethysilyl derivative) or m/z 192 (tyrosol trimethysilyl derivative). By using a soft ionization with NH$_3$ as the reactant gas, they were able (Angerosa et al., 1996) to detect the parent ions of these peaks, which were the aglycons from oleuropein and ligstroside occurring in olive oil. Also, the authors pointed out the problem associated with derivatization leading to the formation of several derivatives from a single analyte. Phenolic compounds in Spanish virgin olive

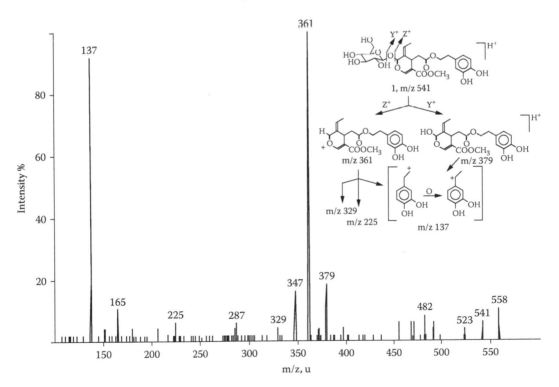

FIGURE 5.10 ISI-MS/MS spectrum of oleuropein glucoside (1 in Figure 5.1) and the structure of the main fragment.

oil were analyzed by GC-MS after solid-phase extraction and clean-up procedure and posterior derivatization to trimethylsilyl ethers (Rios et al., 2005). By using reference commercial products and fractions collected from phenolic extracts by semipreparative HPLC, several phenolic compounds were detected and 21 of them were identified. In addition, GC-MS was employed for the first time to gain insight into the structures of the oxidation products of elenolic acid, oleuropein, and ligstroside aglycons, thus making this technique a useful tool to monitor oxidation in olive oil (Rios et al., 2005). Single-stage MS and GC-MS and HPLC were used for the quantitative determination of the phenolic constituents in extra virgin olive oil (EVOO), refined olive oil (ROO), and refined hask oil (RHO) in order to study the interrelation between reactive oxygen species generated by the fecal matrix and dietary antioxidants (Owen et al., 2000a). EVOO contained significantly higher quantities of phenolic compounds, including secoiridoids, lignans, and flavonoids, than either ROO or RHO, which was reflected in its overall higher antioxidant activity; this proves that the refining process caused partial loss of the preservative action of the natural antioxidants.

Technical developments in coupling liquid chromatography with mass spectrometry during the last decades, and in particular introduction of the ESI and API techniques, facilitated the separation, identification, and structural determination of phenolic compounds in olive fruits and oils. Table 5.1 summarizes applications of HPLC coupled to mass spectrometry in the analysis of olive fruits and oils for the detection and quantification of phenolic compounds. Also, Table 5.1 lists the ionization methodologies used, the extraction method employed to obtain the phenolic fraction, and the mobile phase utilized in HPLC chromatography. LC-ESI-MS in the positive and negative ion modes was used to characterize phenolic compounds in Italian cultivars (Ryan et al., 1999b,c,d). This methodology confirmed the presence of oleuropein as the major phenolic in olive fruits. Other compounds detected by LC-MS were tyrosol, syringic, ferulic and homovanilic acids, quercetin-3-rhamnoside, elenolic acid, elenolic acid glucoside, ligstroside, and two isomers of verbascoside. The structures of the later isomers were determined by employing LS-MS/MS (Ryan et al., 1999d). Ryan and co-workers studied (Ryan et al., 1999b) the concentration changes of phenolic compounds during olive maturation. They observed that oleuropein was the principal phenolic compound that underwent significant changes in its concentration during fruit development. Robards and co-workers (McDonald et al., 2001) assessed the antioxidant activity of the phenolic content in olive extracts by employing LC-MS with ESI and APCI ionization systems. The kinetics of the oxidation process studied in olive extract was found to be complex, suggesting that no simple relationship exists between antioxidant activity and chemical structure. A great number of simple biophenols were detected and quantified in olive fruits collected in Spain (hojiblanca cultivar) at two different ripening stages (green and black) and brine samples by using LC-API-MS/MS in the negative ion mode (Bianco et al., 2001a). Figure 5.11 shows the LC-MS/MS chromatogram of a sample of green olives for the analysis of phenolic compounds, derivatives of benzoic and cinnamic acids. The analysis of the spectra was facilitated upon obtaining LC-MS/MS chromatograms of a standard mixture of benzoic and cinnamic acids and vanillin (1 ng/l). The results of the analyses showed that brine olive samples had a higher level of phenolic compounds than olive fruits, and black brine olives and olive fruits higher than the respective green olives. LC-MS with electrospray ionization in the negative ion mode was employed along with a specific extraction procedure for the identification of a new phenolic compound, namely, hydroxytyrosol-4-β-D-glucoside, in olive fruit (Romero et al., 2002c). The mass spectrum of this compound displayed major signals at m/z 153 and 315, corresponding to hydroxytyrosol and hydroxytyrosol glucoside molecular ions, respectively. LC-MS and LC-MS/MS systems have been applied for screening of phenolic compounds in olive oils extracted from various types of olive varieties. Simple phenols, such as the derivatives of cinamic acid, derivatives of p-hydrobenzoic acid, derivatives of p-hydrophenylacetic acid, phenylalcohols, etc., have been detected and quantified in several instances by employing ESI and/or API technologies in both positive and negative ionization (Bianco et al., 2001a, 2003; Murkovic et al., 2004; de la Torre-Carbot et al., 2005). Qualitative and quantitative determination of polyphenols in virgin olive oil was carried out by optimizing the extraction and purification procedure (Bianco et al., 2003). Depending on

TABLE 5.1
Applications of LC-MS and LC-MS/MS for the Determination of Phenolic Compounds in Olives and Olive Oil

Cultivars	Phenolic Compounds Detected	Ionization Mode	Extraction Method	LC Eluents	Comments	Ref.
Olive fruits						
Manzanillo, Cusso	Homovanillic acid, ferulic acid, syringic acid, elenolic acid, quercetin-3-rhamnoside, tyrosol, ligstroside, oleuropein, verbascoside	ESI(+), ESI(−)	SPE	H_2O-CH_3OH		Ryan et al., 1999b
Unknown	Oleuropein, isomers of verbascoside	ESI(+), ESI(−)	Semipreparative HPLC	CH_3OH-CH_3CN	Determination of oleuropein fragmentation; structural assignment of verbascoside	Ryan et al., 1999c
Manzanillo, Cusso	Homovanillic acid, ferulic acid, syringic acid, elenolic acid, quercetin-3-rhamnoside, ligstroside, oleuropein, isomers of verbascoside, tyrosol, elenolic acid, elenolic acid glucoside	ESI(+), ESI(−)	SPE	H_2O-CH_3OH	Changes in polyphenol content during olive maturation	Ryan et al., 1999d
Manzanillo	Tyrosol, oleuropein, verbascoside, dialdehyde form of oleuropein	ESI(+), ESI(−), APCI(+), APCI(−)	H_2O-CH_3OH	H_2O-CH_3OH	Studies on the antioxidant activity of phenolic fractions	McDonald et al., 2001
Manzannillo, Picual	Hydroxytyrosol-4-glucoside	ESI(−)	H_2O-CH_3OH	H_2O-CH_3OH	Determination of hydroxytyrosol-4-glucoside in olive pulp, vegetation water, and pomace olive oil; this compound was not found in olive oil	Romero C. et al., 2002
Hojiblanca at two different ripening stages (green and black olives)	14 polyphenols were detected and quantified (see Table 3 of this reference)	API(−)	H_2O-CH_3OH	H_2O-CH_3OH	Phenolic content of black and green olive fruits and brines	Bianco et al., 2001a
Olive oil						
Home-made and commercial oils	Tyrosol, hydroxytyrosol, elenolic acid, deacetoxyligstroside aglycon, diacetoxyoleuropein aglycon, ligstroside aglycon, oleuropein aglycon	APCI(−)	H_2O-CH_3OH	H_2O-CH_3OH	Single MS, LC-MS, and LC-MS/MS were used; quantitative determination of oleuropein aglycon	Caruso et al., 2000

(continued)

TABLE 5.1 (continued)
Applications of LC-MS and LC-MS/MS for the Determination of Phenolic Compounds in Olives and Olive Oil

Cultivars	Phenolic Compounds Detected	Ionization Mode	Extraction Method	LC Eluents	Comments	Ref.
Commercial EVOO (Hojiblanca)	18 polyphenols were detected in extra virgin olive oil (see Table 4 of this reference)	API(−)	H_2O-CH_3OH	H_2O-CH_3OH	Not all polyphenols were quantified	Bianco et al., 2001a
Farchioni, frantoio, della Rocca	Hydroxyl-isochromans	API(−)	H_2O-CH_3OH	H_2O-CH_3OH	New class of phenolic compounds of unknown origin	Bianco et al., 2001b
20 EVOO samples from Picual, Hojiblanca, and Cornicabra	Structural confirmation of dialdehydic forms of oleuropein and ligstroside, and the aldehydic forms of oleuropein and ligstroside	ESI(+)-CID	SPE	H_2O-CH_3OH-CH_3CN	Sensory analysis for olive oil bitterness	Gutierrez-Rosales et al., 2003
Italian cultivars and soybean oil	Large number of phenolic compounds (see Tables 5 and 6 of this reference)	API-CID(−)	H_2O-CH_3OH, SPE		The phenolic content of soybean oil was also determined	Bianco et al., 2003
EVOO from Greek cultivars	Tyrosol, vanillic acid, luteolin, apigenin	Not mentioned	CH_3OH	H_2O-CH_3OH		Murkovic et al., 2004
LOO, OPO, SCOO	4-Ethylphenol and other phenolic acids	ESI(−)	DMF	H_2O-CH_3OH	Detection of 4-ethylphenol, high concentrations of polyphenols after olive paste storage for 8 months	Brenes et al., 2004
Picual and arbequina	20 out of 23 phenolic compounds detected were characterized	ESI(−), CID	SPE	H_2O-CH_3CN	Structural characterization of secoiridoids	De la Torre-Carbot et al., 2005
Picual	21 polyphenols and oxidation products were detected and quantified (see Table 1 of this reference)	EI(+) for GC-MSAPCI(+) for LC-MS	SPE	H_2O-CH_3OH-CH_3C	Polyphenols and oxidation products were detected by GC-MS; the identity of oxidation products was confirmed by LC-MS	Rios et al., 2005
Picual, hojiblanca, lechin de Sevilla	Phenolic alcohols, secoiridoids and the lignans pinoresinol and 1-acetoxypinoresinol	ESI(+), APCI (+)	SPE	H_2O-CH_3CN	Capillary electrophoresis–MS (CE-MS) was used; a biochemical mechanism for the formation of secoiridoids was proposed	Carrasco-Pancorvo et al., 2006

Note: EVOO = extra virgin olive oil, LOO = lampante olive oil, COPO = crude olive pomace oil, SCOO = second centrifugation olive oil.

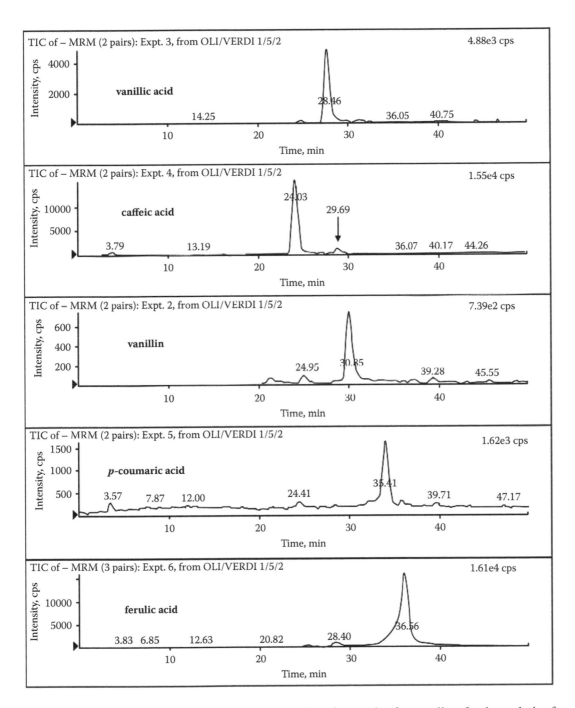

FIGURE 5.11 MRM chromatogram in negative ionization of a sample of green olives for the analysis of derivatives of hydroxybenzoic and sinapic acids.

the liquid-liquid extraction method the phenolic content was divided into two groups: A (extraction with a mixture of methanol/water, 80:20 v/v) and B (extraction with a phosphate buffer at pH = 8). Figure 5.12 shows the TICs in the negative ionization mode of virgin olive oil extract for group B, whereas Figure 5.13 illustrates a series of TIC mass spectra of selected ions of hydroxytyrosol, tyrosol, and oleoside methyl ester acquired during the first 35 min of the chromatogram of Figure 5.12 in a successive LC-MS/MS experiment (Bianco et al., 2003). Additional phenolic compounds were detected but not quantified in this extract, such as oleuropein glucoside and elenolic acid.

Apart from simple phenolic acids and phenyl alcohols, olive oil contains secoiridoids, mostly the hydrolysis products of oleuropein glucoside and ligstroside; the lignans, (+)pinoresinol, (+)1-acetoxypinoresinol, and syringaresinol; the flavanols, apigenin, luteolin, quercetin, and traces of

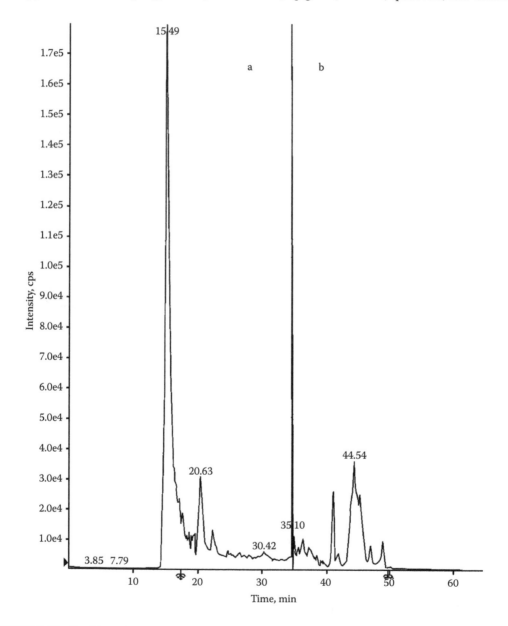

FIGURE 5.12   Total ion chromatogram (TIC) in MRM in negative ionization of a virgin olive oil extract of group B. Acquisition period indicated respectively as a (0–35 min) and b (35–65 min).

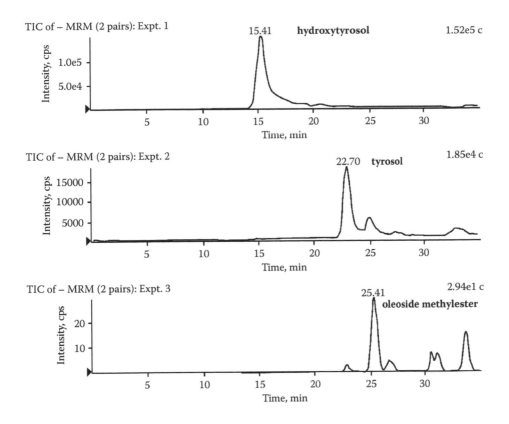

FIGURE 5.13 TIC of the compounds of group B acquired in the fast acquisition period a of Figure 5.12.

their glucosidic derivatives. Structural information for the oleuropein and ligstroside metabolites was provided by several authors using LC-MS and LC-MS/MS with ESI, API, and APCI ionization methodologies (Brenes et al., 2000; Caruso et al., 2000; Bianco et al., 2003; Gutierrez-Rosales et al., 2003; de la Torre-Carbot et al., 2005). Caruso and co-workers (Caruso et al., 2000) demonstrated that LC-APCI-MS and single-stage APCI-MS and APCI-MS/MS were very useful techniques to obtain the profile of phenolic components of oil from methanolic extracts of crude olive oil; tyrosol, hydroxytyrosol, elenolic acid, oleuropein and ligstroside aglycons, deacetoxyligstroside and deacetoxyoleuropein aglycons, and 10-hydroxy-oleuropein were clearly identified in the MS spectra shown in Figure 5.14.

In a thorough study (de la Torre-Carbot et al., 2005), application of LC-MS in the full scan mode to the phenolic fraction of olive oil resulted in several compounds with the same m/z, namely, 553, 335, 377, 319, 361, 365, and 393, which were attributed to oleuropein and ligstroside derivatives. Because no standards were available for comparison, identification of these compounds was attempted by employing LC-MS/MS experiments. The fragmented ions produced by collision-activated dissociation of selected precursors and detected in the second mass analyzer of the instrument were evaluated on the basis of secoiridoids found in the literature. Table 2 of de la Torre-Carbot et al. (2005) summarizes possible models and corresponding structures of derivatives of aglycons of oleuropein, ligstroside, and elenolic acid detected in olive oil. Recently, capillary electrophoresis (CE) in combination with MS has been employed as an alternative or complementary to the LC-MS separation technique to identify and characterize phenolic compounds in the polar fraction of olive oil (Carrasco-Pancorbo et al., 2006a).

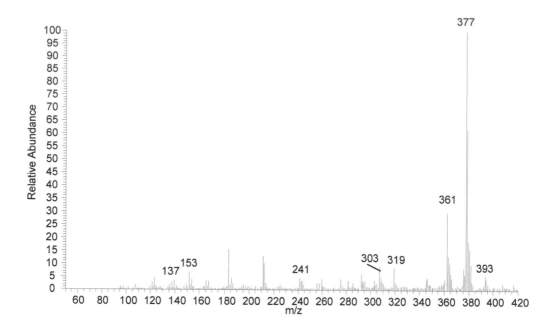

FIGURE 5.14 LC-APCI-MS of a virgin olive oil extract: ion at m/z 137 = tyrosol; m/z 153 = hydroxytyrosol; m/z 241 = elenolic acid; m/z 303 = deacetoxyligstroside aglycon; m/z 319 = deacetoxyoleuropein aglycon; m/z 361 = ligstroside aglycon; m/z 377 = oleuropein aglycon; m/z 393 = 10-hydroxy-oleuropein.

A new phenolic compound, namely, 4-ethylphenol, was detected, while the phenolic composition of lampante olive oils (LOO), crude olive pomace oils (COPO), and second centrifugation olive oils (SCOO) was examined by LC-ESI-MS (Brenes et al., 2004). 4-Ethylphenol was found at relatively high concentrations in LOO, COPO, and SCOO, the latter oil being the richest source of this compound. It appears that 4-ethylphenol was formed during olive paste storage and reached the highest concentration after 8 months of paste storage. Another important finding of this study is that these low quality olive oils intended for refining contain a significant concentration of phenolic compounds, which is high enough to make their recovery attractive.

5.4.6 CONCLUSION

Single-stage and/or tandem mass spectrometry with various ionization methods have rapidly evolved as a very useful instrumental method for the study of the various polyphenols in olive fruits and oils. After the development of the combined setups of GC-MS and in particular HPLC-MS or HPLC-MS/MS techniques, the potential for identification and structural characterization of polyphenols in the crude extracts at nanogram levels increased considerably, although for a complete structure elucidation of conjugates, the complementary information from LC-NMR is indispensable. Finally, it has to be added that quantification of analytes still requires calibration with standards that are not always available.

5.5 ELECTRON SPIN RESONANCE

5.5.1 INTRODUCTION

The technique of electron spin resonance (ESR) may be regarded as an extension of the Stern-Gerlach experiment, which is considered as one of the most fundamental experiments on the structure of matter. Their discovery, that the electron magnetic moment can take only discrete orientations within a magnetic field, and the radical idea (proposed by Uhlenbeck and Goudsmit) that the electron magnetic moment is due to electron spin, were the basis of ESR spectroscopy. ESR spectroscopy is applicable only to systems with net electron spin angular momentum, such as radicals, biradicals, systems with two unpaired electrons (triplet state), or systems with three or more unpaired electrons. The magnitude and the orientation of the electron magnetic moment of a single electron within a magnetic field are quantized quantities. The magnitude is governed by the spin quantum number, s, whereas the orientations along the direction (z-axis) of the magnetic field strength, B_0, are restricted by the magnetic spin quantum number m_s, according to the following simple equations:

$$\mu_e = g\hbar\sqrt{s(s+1)} \tag{5.1}$$

$$\mu_z = gm_s\hbar \tag{5.2}$$

s takes a single value of ½, whereas m_s 2s+1 values, +½ and −½, when the magnetic moment orients assume antiparallel and parallel to magnetic field strength, respectively. These two orientations specify two energy levels. The higher energy level is that with m_s = +½, whereas that with m_s = −½ is characterized by lower energy. g is the so-called g-factor (for the free electron g_e = 2.00232) and β is the Bohr magneton (β = 9.2741 × 10^{-21} erg gauss^{-1}).

Molecules containing unpaired electrons interact with a beam of electromagnetic radiation, and the ESR spectrometer measures its attenuation as the electrons at the lower energy level absorb energy and are excited to the level of higher energy. The electromagnetic radiation energy or frequency depends on the energy gap ΔE between the two energy levels,

$$\Delta E - h\nu = g\beta B_0 \tag{5.3}$$

The frequency required for ESR transitions between the two energy levels is in the microwave region and it is expressed in GHz.

Apart from the interaction of electrons with an external magnetic field, what is more important to chemists is the further interaction between the electron spin and internal local magnetic fields induced by the chemical environment of the electron. In particular, the magnetic interaction between the electron spins and nuclear spins results in the ESR spectrum that consists of a number of lines rather than a single line. The splitting of the electron single line and the arrangement of the resulting group of lines in the ESR spectrum is called the hyperfine structure of the spectrum. The number of lines (multiplicity) and their relative intensities depend on the magnetic spin quantum number (I) of the nearby nonequivalent nuclei (the multiplicity is equal to $2I + 1$) and the selection rules for the allowed transitions. The magnetic moments of the nuclei concerned and the strength of interactions between the electron and nuclear spins determine the separation between the lines (hyperfine splitting constant [denoted by α]), which is measured in gauss. The position of the lines in the spectrum is stated in terms of the g-factor. Finally, the appearance of the lines in the ESR spectrum is that shown in Figure 5.15. Contrary to NMR spectroscopy, ESR spectrometers almost always provide the derivative of the absorption signal.

Figure 5.16 shows the typical ESR spectrum of the methyl radical $\overset{\bullet}{C}H_3$ at 25°C in aqueous solution. The signal is split into a quartet with relative intensities 1:3:3:1 and hyperfine splitting constant of 23.0 Gauss. The splitting is due to the interaction between the unpaired electrons with the magnetic moments of the three equivalent hydrogen nuclei with I = ½. ESR spectroscopy has been used

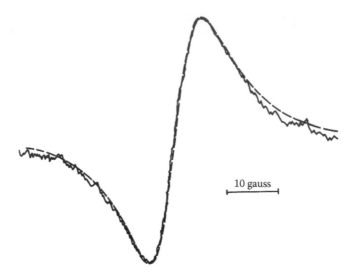

FIGURE 5.15   Derivative of a typical ESR absorption signal.

with great success to evaluate the oxidative stability of extra virgin olive oil and other edible oils, and the radical scavenging capability of their natural antioxidants.

5.5.2   ANALYSIS OF LIPID OXIDATION IN OLIVE OIL BY ESR SPECTROSCOPY

Oxidative stability is of paramount importance in assessing the quality of EVOO. This quality parameter reflects the susceptibility of EVOO to oxidative degeneration, which is the major cause for the rancidity development, resulting from the autoxidation of unsaturated fatty acids (Velasco and Dobarganes, 2002; Boskou, 2006). This process takes place in the presence of atmospheric oxygen generating unstable free radicals, which are very reactive and are able to modify the sensory and nutritional characteristics of EVOO, thus leading to product spoilage. Nevertheless, EVOO has constituents that delay the oxidation process by preventing the propagation of lipid peroxidation or removing free radicals, and thereby increasing its stability. In EVOO, different classes of compounds characterized by antioxidant activity are present, namely, tocopherols, carotenoids, chlorophylls, and in particular phenolic compounds (Boskou, 2006). These natural antioxidants exert their antioxidant activity through various mechanisms preventing free radical initiation by scavenging initially formed radicals, decreasing the localized oxygen concentration, and decomposing peroxides.

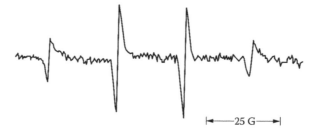

FIGURE 5.16   ESR spectrum of the methyl radical $\overset{\bullet}{C}H_3$ at 25°C in aqueous solution.

Oxidative stability is known as the resistance to oxidation under well-defined conditions and is expressed as the period of time required to reach an end point, which can be selected following different criteria, but usually corresponds to an abrupt increase of the oxidation rate, the so-called induction period (IP). Numerous chemical and physical methods, under accelerated oxidation conditions, have been suggested for the evaluation of oxidative stability. Among these are those widely used in the oil industry: the Rancimat method introducing the oil stability index (OSI), differential scanning calorimetry (DSC), the active oxygen method, the analytical indices such as the peroxide value (PV), the thiobarbituric acid index (TBA), the anisidine value, and others. The Rancimat and DSC methods are indicative of the onset of advanced oxidation, whereas the analytical indices account for relatively stable compounds formed in the propagation and termination steps of the chain reaction producing the free radicals.

None of these methods, however, is sensitive enough to detect directly free radicals produced during the oxidation process, since the free radical concentration is kept at very low levels. This is achieved by using ESR spectroscopy and the spin-trapping technique. The ESR spin-trapping technique is very useful as a method employing milder conditions, thus avoiding the loss of volatile components and shorter times, and it can be applied for the evaluation of oxidative stability of turbid oils. It is based on the reaction of radicals with diamagnetic compounds (spin traps) added to the system to form more stable radicals (spin adducts), which accumulate at detectable concentrations ($>10^{-7}$–10^{-6} M). Detection of these new radical species allows the indirect detection and quantification of radicals involved in lipid oxidation. Since this method is sensitive to low radical concentration and detects free radicals formed at the early stages of oxidation, the corresponding induction period, defined as the resistance to the formation of radicals, is very short compared to the induction periods shown by other methods. The Rancimat and DSC methods are based on generation of volatiles and thermal release, respectively, which are indicative of the onset of advanced oxidation. The ESR induction period is expressed as the period of time during which radicals are formed very slowly before a sharp linear increase is observed. As an example, the IPs provided by the Rancimat method, DSC, and ESR spectroscopy, while monitoring the oxidative stability of sunflower oil, were 12.90 h, 7.36 h, and 122.78 min, respectively (Valavanidis et al., 2004). Despite these differences, results obtained by the ESR spin-trapping technique correlated nicely with those measured by Rancimat and DSC (Velasco et al., 2004; Papadimitriou et al., 2006).

Several spin traps have been used in combination with ESR spectroscopy to assess the oxidative stability of olive oils, the most popular of them being α-phenyl-N-tert-butyl nitrone (PBN), which forms adduct according to the reaction in Scheme 5.7. This spin trap was preferred due to its lipophilic character and the stability of the spin adducts it forms with transient radicals. The ESR spectrum of PBN spin adducts in EVOO is illustrated in Figure 5.17 after 6 and 24 h of incubation in 70oC (Papadimitriou et al., 2006). The ESR peak appears as a triplet due to coupling (α_N = 14.73 G) of the unpaired electron with the nitrogen nucleus (14N, I = 1), although computer simulation of the ESR spectra is commensurate with a triplet of doublet due to coupling (α_H = 2.50 G) with the hydrogen nucleus (1H, I = ½). Broadening effects due to restricted tumbling of the radicals in the

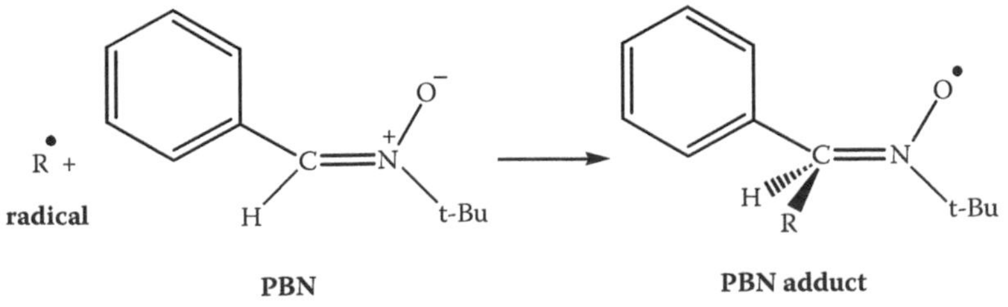

PBN   PBN adduct

SCHEME 5.7

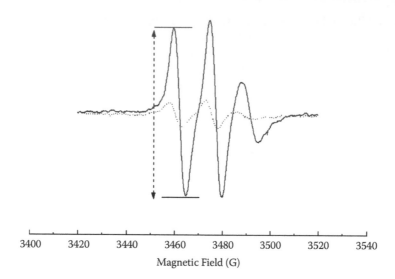

FIGURE 5.17 ESR spectra of PBN spin-adduct in EVOO samples after 6 h (dotted line) and 24 h (solid line) of incubation at 70°C.

lipid matrix are likely to hide the smaller splitting with hydrogen (Velasco et al., 2005; Papadimitriou et al., 2006).

Quantification of radical concentrations was achieved by comparing the intensities of the ESR spectra from oil solutions with external standard solutions of stable radicals, such as 2,2,6,6-tetra-methylpiperidine-1-oxyl (TEMPO) (Ottaviani et al., 2001; Velasco et al., 2005), or 5,5-dimethyl-1-pyroline-*N*-oxide (DMPO) (Valavanidis et al., 2004).

The ESR spin-trapping technique has been used in several investigations for determining the antioxidant capacity of edible oils, including olive oil, under different conditions that influence the type and the amount of radicals formed. From the data analysis in various studies (Ottaviani et al., 2001; Quiles et al., 2002; Valavanidis et al., 2004; Velasco et al., 2005), several useful conclusions were drawn:

1. The extraction system may play a role in radical concentrations. Olive oils produced by continuous centrifugation and aged for 1 year showed an increase by 25–30% in radical concentration compared to fresh olive oil obtained by the same extraction system. On the contrary, 1-year olive oil produced by pressure showed no difference in radical concentration with the non-aged olive oil.
2. The heating of olive oils at high temperatures favored radical formation, owing to oxidation and disruption of the unsaturated fatty acids. Among edible oils, EVOO and, second, soybean and sunflower oil, showed the highest antioxidant capacity. This was explained on the basis of the highest content of phenolic compounds in EVOO.
3. N_2 bubbling led to a decrease in radical concentration. It appears that nitrogen bubbling expels oxygen responsible for the radical formation in olive oil, and simultaneously speeds up the molecular motion favoring collisions among radicals or between radicals and the natural antioxidants of the olive oil.
4. UV irradiation of olive oil resulted in an increase of radical concentration up to a maximum, and then decreased to a constant value. This behavior may be related to the olive oil age, and the concentration and type of natural antioxidants.
5. Air bubbling increased the radical concentration, since oxygen promotes oxidation. However, bubbling may cause the opposite effect favoring collisions among radicals and antioxidants.

5.5.3 Radical Scavenging Activity

As mentioned above, the antioxidant potential of olive oil and other vegetable oils is the result of a direct scavenging effect of their natural antioxidants, dominated by polar phenolic compounds and tocopherols. The scavenging activity of these compounds toward radicals has been assessed spectrophotometrically using various solutions of stable free radicals (Perez-Bonilla et al., 2006). The most used stable radicals were the galvinoxyl radical (2,6-di-*tert*-butyl-α-(3,5-di-*tert*-butyl-4-oxo-2,5-cyclohexadiene-1-ylidene)-*p*-tolyoxy) (Papadimitriou et al., 2006), DPPH$^\bullet$ (2,2-diphenyl-1-picrylhydrazyl), and the radical cation ABTS$^{\bullet+}$ (2,2'-azino-*bis*(3-ethylbenzothiazoline-6-sulfonate) (Perez-Bonilla et al., 2006). The concentration of these radicals is expected to decrease upon addition of EVOO in their solution due to the scavenging effect induced by the EVOO antioxidant compounds. The scavenging activity of EVOO polyphenol or tocopherol indicated as A-OH against the stable radicals, e.g., galvinoxyl radical, can be described by the following simplified reaction (Papadimitriou et al., 2006):

$$Galv - O^\bullet + A - OH \rightarrow Galv - OH + A - O^\bullet \qquad (5.4)$$

Galv $- O^\bullet$ is the galvinoxyl free radical, a sterically protected, resonance-stabilized, synthetic radical, and A $- O^\bullet$ is the resulting unstable radical. Usually the oil is diluted in ethanol, and the ethanolic solution is assessed for its ability to reduce an equivalent amount of galvinoxyl radical. In this study (Papadimitriou et al., 2006), 20–80 mg of EVOO was added to a 0.12-mM solution of Galv $- O^\bullet$ in isooctane and the mixture was transferred into an ESR sample tube for analysis. The depletion of galvinoxyl radicals was monitored by a Bruker ER 200D spectrometer operating at the X-band at 25°C. Figure 5.18 shows the rapid decrease of the ESR signal intensity of the Galv $- O^\bullet$ radical upon addition of 2% EVOO at different incubation times. After 30 min of incubation, about 60% of the galvinoxyl radicals were quenched by the EVOO samples with the highest amount of polyphenols and tocopherols. In the same study, both oxidative stability and radical scavenging activity of EVOO samples were correlated to their content in polyphenols and tocopherols. Valavanidis et al. (2004) studied the radical scavenging activity of the phenolic fraction of EVOO, corn, sunflower, and soybean oils, as well as that of pure hydroxytyrosol, tyrosol, and oleuropein,

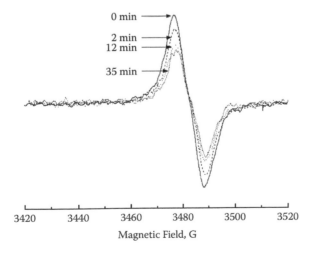

FIGURE 5.18 ESR spectra of galvinoxyl radicals in the presence of 2% (v/v) EVOO at different incubation times: (solid line) 0 min, (dashed line) 2 min, (dotted line) 12 min, (short dashed line) 35 min.

toward the most important oxygen-free radicals, superoxide anion ($O_2^{\bullet-}$) and hydroxyl ($OH^\bullet$) radicals, by employing ESR spectroscopy. They found that the antioxidant activity of the various oils toward the $O_2^{\bullet-}$ and $OH^\bullet$ radicals was proportional to phenolic content. The EVOO with more than 200 mg/kg of polyphenols showed the highest antiradical activity among the edible oils studied. Also, hydroxytyrosol was found to be the most active scavenger *in vitro* toward the $O_2^{\bullet-}$ and $OH^\bullet$ radicals, second was oleuropein but equally active, whereas tyrosol had a much lower antiradical activity.

It is worthwhile to mention the use of ESR spectroscopy and galvinoxyl radicals to evaluate the antioxidant capacity of a number of flavonoids present in a wide range of vegetables, nuts, beverages, and fruits, including olive fruit (McPhail et al., 2003). The kinetic treatment and determination of the stoichiometry of the reaction between each flavonoid and the galvinoxyl radical according to Equation 5.4 disclosed the influence of the flavonoids' molecular structures on their antioxidant activity, although no simple correlation between kinetic rates and stoichiometries was found.

5.5.4 CONCLUSIONS

The ESR spin-trapping technique is very useful as a method to assess the oxidative stability of olive oil and to estimate the scavenging activity of its natural antioxidants polyphenols and tocopherols. Although ESR spin-trapping, Rancimat, and DSC techniques do not differ significantly in their prediction of olive oil oxidative stability, the ESR method appears to be more sensitive, simpler, and directly detects free radicals produced during the oxidation process. An important finding of ESR applications is that the oxidative stability of olive oil correlates with its content in polyphenols and tocopherols.

5.6 ANALYSIS OF BIOLOGICAL FLUIDS

To understand the impact of olive oil polyphenols on human health, it is essential to give definite answers to several questions: To what extent are olive oil polyphenols absorbed by the human body? What is the bioavailability of the ingested polyphenols and how can it be measured? What factors influence their bioavailability (e.g., chemical structure, dietary origin)? What are the metabolic pathways followed by polyphenols ingested in the various human organs (e.g., small intestine, liver, and colon)? What are the conversion rates of the various polyphenols, and what are the structures of the resulting metabolites? What enzymes are involved in polyphenol metabolism? What are the mechanisms of interactions with cell receptors? What are the effects of their metabolites on the antioxidant capacity of plasma? Some answers to these questions have been given in other chapters of this book, and especially in Chapter 6.

Intensive research has been carried out in the past decade on these subjects, especially on ingestion and bioavailability. Direct evidence on bioavailability of olive oil phenolic compounds has been obtained by measuring the concentration of a few phenols and their metabolites in body fluids after ingestion. These measurements require careful study designs (e.g., preparation of subjects, duration and settings of studies, daily dosing of olive oil with known content of polyphenols or polyphenol supplements), and sensitive and rapid analytical techniques for screening a large number of samples. A variety of analytical techniques, which are presented briefly in the following paragraphs, have been used to measure the concentration of polyphenols in biological fluids. Emphasis will be given to studies dealing with the metabolism and bioavailability of olive oil polyphenols.

5.6.1 ANALYSIS OF POLYPHENOLS IN HUMANS AND LABORATORY ANIMALS BY HIGH-PERFORMANCE LIQUID CHROMATOGRAPHY

HPLC with different detection systems has been applied to the analysis of olive oil polyphenols in urine and blood. Determination of hydroxytyrosol in rat plasma was carried out by HPLC with a mobile phase consisting of 3% acetic acid in deionized water and a mixture of acetonitrile/methanol (50:50 v/v), and UV detection at 280 nm (Ruiz-Gutierrez et al., 2000). Pure hydroxytyrosol was orally administered to rats at a dose of 20 mg/kg, whereas hydroxytyrosol from plasma was purified initially by solid-phase extraction. HPLC methodology was modified for the simultaneous quantification of both hydroxytyrosol and oleuropein glucoside in rat plasma (Tan et al., 2003). The chromatographic analysis was performed using an isocratic elution of acidified water and acetonitrile with fluorescence detection at 281 and 316 nm for excitation and emission, respectively. HPLC equipped with a spectrofluorometer was employed to study the bioavailability of oleuropein glucoside in plasma after absorption on an isolated perfused rat intestine (Edgecombe et al., 2000). The conclusion derived from this study was that oleuropein was poorly absorbed from an aqueous solution. Simultaneous determination of oleuropein and its metabolites hydroxytyrosol and tyrosol in human plasma was achieved by using an HPLC method with a diode array detection system (Tsarbopoulos et al., 2003). This method includes a clean-up solid-phase extraction procedure. HPLC with radiometric detection was used to examine the bioavailability of radiolabeled (with tritium) hydroxytyrosol and tyrosol administered to rats intravenously (in saline) and orally (in oil and water-based solutions) (Tuck et al., 2001). Oral and intravenous bioavailability of both phenolic compounds in rats' urine was found to be higher when administered in an olive oil solution than dosed as an aqueous solution. Moreover, the amounts of both hydroxytyrosol and tyrosol determined in rats' urine after 24 h were similar, indicating that the intravenous and oral oil-based methods were equally effective; oral bioavailability estimates of hydroxytyrosol were 99 and 75% when it was administered in an olive oil solution and when dosed as an aqueous solution, respectively. These estimates for tyrosol were 98 and 71%, respectively. HPLC methodology has also been used in the analysis of human plasma and urine, while assessing the bioavailability of phenolic compounds in foodstuffs other than olive oil, e.g., tea, onions, etc. (Lee et al., 1995; Hollman et al., 1996). Finally, a method for HPLC equipped with a coulometric electrode array detection system was developed to measure plant and mammalian lignans in human urine (Nurmi et al., 2003).

The toxicity and more interestingly the metabolism of hydroxytyrosol in rats were studied by using HPLC and radioactivity measurements (D'Angelo et al., 2001). When orally administered to rats, hydroxytyrosol does not show appreciable toxicity up to 2 g/kg body wt. The preparation of the labeled [^{14}C] hydroxytyrosol allowed the monitoring of the rate of absorption and the metabolic pathways of this molecule in rats. The measured radioactivity in blood showed that less than 8% of the administered radioactive hydroxytyrosol is still present in the animal blood after 5 min, its amount being decreased gradually; only 0.1% of the administered dose (1 mg/kg body wt) was detectable 5 h after the treatment. The highest ^{14}C radioactivity associated with liver, kidney, and lung was measured 5 min after injection followed by a rapid decrease. A similar behavior of the exogenously administered hydroxytyrosol was observable for other investigated tissues. Characterization of the various hydroxytyrosol metabolites extracted from rat plasma and urine and the various organs was made by HPLC. In all investigated tissues, hydroxytyrosol was enzymatically converted into four oxidized and/or methylated derivatives, namely, 3,4-hydroxyphenylacetaldehyde, 3,4-hydroxy-phenylacetic acid (homoprotocatechuic acid), 4-hydroxy-3-methoxy-phenylethanol (homovanillyl alcohol, HValc), and 4-hydroxy-3-methoxy-phenylacetic acid (homovanillic acid, HVA), whereas a significant amount of sulfo-conjugated derivatives of hydroxytyrosol and its derivatives was identified. On the basis of the reported results an intracellular metabolic pathway was proposed. Recently, a reversed-phase HPLC method with UV detection for the simultaneous determination of oleuropein and tyrosol in plasma has been proposed (Grizis et al., 2003). Isolation of plasma was carried out by liquid extraction with ethyl acetate after addition of Na_2SO_4. Chromatographic analysis was performed using a C8 column with CH_3OH/CH_3COOH 2% in water as the mobile phase. Although this methodology appears to be simple, rapid, sensitive, accurate, and shows good linearity, it has not been tested yet in bioavailability studies.

5.6.2 Analysis of Polyphenols in Humans and Laboratory Animals by Mass Spectrometry

Although certain detection systems of HPLC methodologies appear to be more sensitive than others, and despite the advantages of the low cost of the analysis and ease of operation, these techniques suffer from low sensitivity and poor selectivity. In this respect, the development of more effective analytical techniques was sought in recent years. The analytical potential of tandem mass spectrometry (MS/MS) in identifying olive oil polyphenols in biological fluids has been evaluated recently (Tuck et al., 2002). The authors of this study were able to identify conclusively three out of five hydroxytyrosol metabolites excreted in rat urine. These metabolites were reported in an older study by using the HPLC analytical technique (Tuck et al., 2001), but their identification was not attempted in that study. These metabolites, the structure of which was confirmed by ^{1}H NMR spectroscopy, were hydroxytyrosol monosulfate (at m/z 233 and its fragment after the loss of a sulfate group at m/z 153), 3-O-glucuronide conjugate (at m/z 329 and its fragment at m/z 153 after the loss of a glucuronide group), and homovanillic acid. A fourth metabolite, although not confirmed, has been attributed to the glucuronide conjugate of homovanillic acid. MS/MS has also been applied to the determination of the citrus flavanones naringenin and hesperitin in human urine after oral ingestion of these flavones (Weintraub et al., 1995). Among the three ionization modes of operation (EI, positive and negative chemical ionization), positive chemical ionization was superior to EI for identification of these citrus flavonoids scanning in the selective reaction monitoring. The m/z 153 daughter ion, resulting from the pyrone ring fragmentation of the aglycon flavanone via a retro-Diels-Alder reaction, was the basic diagnostic ion in searching for naringenin and hesperitin.

A wide variety of epidemiological and biological studies associated with olive oil polyphenols have utilized exclusively combined GC and HPLC techniques with mass spectrometry for the analysis of urine and blood from both humans and laboratory animals. These methodologies, which have been optimized for the examination of polyphenols in biological fluids, are characterized by superior sensitivity, and ability to analyze rapidly and precisely multiple analytes in one run. LC-MS or LC-MS/MS is considered to be more advantageous than GC-MS or GC-MS/MS, since the latter requires large volumes of sample and complex sample preparation, which involves multistage purification procedures and derivatization of the analytes prior to analysis. An assay has been developed recently using low volumes of urine (200 µl) and a simple sample preparation procedure (one solid-phase extraction stage) that found application to the analysis of phytoestrogens (isoflavones and lignans) with GC-MS (Grace et al., 2003).

Table 5.2 summarizes bioavailability studies by employing combined GC and HPLC with mass spectrometry for the analysis of biological fluids. Also, Table 5.2 lists sources and quantities of the ingested olive oil polyphenols, the polyphenols detected in plasma and/or urine, and their maximum concentration measured. It should be noted that the total amount of phenolic compounds mentioned in Table 5.2 includes their conjugated forms, which were determined by subjecting the biological samples to acidic (HCl) or enzymatic (β-glucuronidase) hydrolysis.

One of the first bioavailability studies of olive oil polyphenols in humans was performed by Visioli and co-workers (Visioli et al., 2000) using GC-MS analysis. They reported that absorption of olive oil phenolic compounds, namely, hydroxytyroso and tyrosol by humans after ingestion, depends on the doses delivered to the human subjects. Moreover, they found that these polyphenols are excreted in urine as glucuronide conjugates, and that the proportion of conjugation increases with increasing dose of phenolics. In a subsequent publication, the same authors succeeded in elucidating the metabolic fate of hydroxytyrosol after ingestion of virgin olive oil enriched in hydroxytyrosol (Caruso et al., 2001). By employing GC-MS analysis, they identified in human urines the

TABLE 5.2

Bioavailability in Humans and Laboratory Animals of Polyphenols Consumed in Olive Oil or Alone

Method of Analysis	Source of Polyphenols	Biological Fluid	Quantity of Polyphenols Injested	Maximum Concentration in Plasma	Excretion in Urine (% of Administered Amount)	Reference
MS/MS	Aqueous and oil solutions of tritiated Htyr[a]	Rat urine	(a) 25 mg/1300 mg water (b) 23.5 mg/1300 mg EVOO[a]		Htyr[a] sulphate: 48.42% (oral), 24.24% (iva) Htyr glucuronide: 9.53% (oral), 3.58% (ivb) Free Htyr: 4.60 (oral), 2.35 (iv) HVA:[a] 10.26% (oral), 18.26% (iv) Other metabolites: 20.27% (oral), 30.87% (iv) (after 24 h)	Tuck et al., 2002
GC-MS	Synthetic Htyr	Rat plasma	10 mg/ml	0.89–3.26 µg/L (after 10 min)		Bai et al., 1998
GC-MS	Olive oil enriched with phenolic extracts	Human urine	Total pherols: 487.5–1950 mg/L Htyr: 20–84 mg/L Tyr: 36–140 mg/L		Htyr glucuronide: 21–24% Tyra glucuronide: 29–40%	Visioli et al., 2000
GC-MS	Olive oil enriched with phenolic extracts	Human urine	Total Htyr: 7–23.2 mg/50 mL		Htyr: 16.8–23.7 µg/L HVA: 53.9–61.8 µg/L HVAlc:[a] 22.0–22.4 µg/L (after 24 h)	Caruso et al., 2001
GC-MS	Olive oil		50 mL (1650 µg of Tyr)		Tyr conjugates : 17–43%	Miró-Casas et al., 2001a
GC-MS	Olive oil	Human urine	50 mL (Htyr: 1055 µg, Tyr: 655 µg)		Total Htyr: 32–98.8% Total Tyr: 12.1–52%; total free Htyr and Tyr: ~15%	Miró-Casas et al., 2001b
GC-MS	Polyphenol supplements from olive oil		Nonpolar phenols:[c] 371 and 382 µmol polar phenols:[c] 498 and 526 µmol oleuropein:[c] 190 and 0 µmol		Nonpolar phenols:[c] 12% and 6% µmol polar phenols:[c] 6% and 5% µmol oleuropein:[c] 16% and 0%	Vissers et al., 2002
GC-MS	Virgin olive oil	Human urine and plasma	Total Htyr: 7–23.2 mg/50 mL virgin olive oil	Htyr conjugate: 25.83 µg/L HVAlc: 3.94 µg/L	Htyr glucuronide: 65% HVAlc: 69% other conjugated forms: 35%	Miró-Casas et al., 2003a

(continued)

TABLE 5.2 (continued)

Bioavailability in Humans and Laboratory Animals of Polyphenols Consumed in Olive Oil or Alone

Method of Analysis	Source of Polyphenols	Biological Fluid	Quantity of Polyphenols Injested	Maximum Concentration in Plasma	Excretion in Urine (% of Administered Amount)	Reference
GC-MS	EVOO		Rats:Total Htyr: 201 µg/kg Humans: Total Htyr 45.7 µg/kg		Rats: Htyr + HValc: 7.6% Humans: Htyr + HValc: 44.2%	Visioli et al., 2003
GC-MS/MS	EVOO Oleuropein	Rat urine	EVOO 50 g/kg; oleuropein 0.15 g/kg		See Table 4 of this reference	Bazoti et al., 2005
LC-MS/MS	Oleuropein	Rat plasma and urine	Oleuropein 100 mg/kg	Oleuropein: 200 ng/ml (after 2 h)	Oleuropein glucuronide::91% Htyr glucuronide:: 97%	Del Boccio et al., 2003
LC-MS/MS	Polyphenol-rich diet (fruits, vegetables, and coffee)	Human urine			See Table 4 of this reference	Gonthier et al., 2003
LC-MS/MS	EVOO	Human blood[d]	50 mL EVOO			de la Tore-Carbot et al., 2006, 2007
LC/MS/MS	Olive oil, ROO,[a] BOO[a]	Human urine and plasma[e]				Hillestrom et al., 2006

[a] Htyr = hydroxytyrosol, Tyr = tyrosol, HVAlc = homovanillyl alcohol, HVA = homovanillic acid, EVOO = extra virgin olive oil, ROO = refined olive oil, BOO = blended olive oil.

[b] Intravenous administration.

[c] First and second percentage correspond to ileostomy subjects and subjects with a colon, respectively.

[d] Detection of olive oil metabolites in LDL.

[e] Detection of etheno-DNA adducts.

hydroxytyrosol metabolites homovanillic acid (HVA) and homovanillyl alcohol (HValc) resulting from hydroxytyrosol oxidation by catechol-O-methyl transferase enzymes. A major limitation of these studies is that they employed olive oil samples artificially enriched with phenolic extracts, and therefore extrapolation of these results to typical olive oil consumption may not be realistic. It should be noted that the hydroxytyrosol metabolite HValc was reported by Manna and co-workers (Manna et al., 2000) in human Caco-2 cells incubated with hydroxytyrosol (see below).

The bioavailability of tyrosol in humans after administration of virgin olive oil was studied by using GC-MS operating in the single-ion monitoring mode (Miró-Casas et al., 2001a). This technique allowed the detection of the derivatized tyrosol (bis-trimethylsilyl-tyrosol) recovered in urine during 24 h after ingestion of 50 ml of virgin olive oil by eight volunteers. Tyrosol was excreted mainly in its conjugated form, and only 6–11% of the total tyrosol (obtained after chemical hydrolysis) was in its free form. The fate of both hydroxytyrosol and tyrosol in humans after ingestion of virgin olive oil was monitored quantitatively in urine of human subjects by employing capillary GC-MS (Miró-Casas et al., 2001b). All reference materials in this study were prepared in synthetic urine in order to avoid the basal levels of hydroxytyrosol and tyrosol derived from other dietary sources and the production of hydroxytyrosol through dopamine metabolism. To obtain information about the rates of hydrolysis of the conjugated forms of these phenolic compounds in the gastrointestinal tract, olive oil extracts were submitted to different experimental conditions (treatment with concentrated hydrochloric acid), similar to those occurring as a response to food intake in the gastrointestinal tract. This bioavailability study showed that hydroxytyrosol and tyrosol were mainly excreted in conjugated form, and only a small fraction of the total amount of these polyphenols excreted in urine was found in free form. Further investigation using GC-MS revealed the presence of an additional metabolite in human plasma, 3-O-methyl hydroxytyrosol, after consumption of a single dose of raw virgin olive oil (Miró-Casas et al., 2003a).

The absorption of tyrosol and hydroxytyrosol by humans was studied after moderate and sustained doses of virgin olive oil consumption (Miró-Casas et al., 2003b). This study aimed to assess the bioavailability of these important olive oil polyphenols following a single dose (50 ml) and sustained doses (25 ml/day) of virgin olive oil, the latter being equal to the average dose consumed daily according to the Mediterranean diet. Urinary recoveries for tyrosol were similar after a single dose and after sustained doses of virgin olive oil, whereas the mean recovery values for hydroxytyrosol after sustained doses were 1.5 times higher than those measured after a single dose.

An advanced GC method coupled with tandem mass spectrometry has been proposed recently for the simultaneous determination of hydroxytyrosol, tyrosol, and elenolic acid in rat urine after administration of sustained oral intakes of extra virgin olive oil and/or pure oleuropein (Bazoti et al., 2005). An SPE extraction system with 80% analytical recovery for all compounds was performed followed by derivatization reaction prior to GC-MS/MS analysis. The employment of MS/MS analysis allowed a better selectivity than the single GC-MS methods. Selection of a specific precursor ion for each compound at its characteristic chromatographic retention time, and the selection of specific product ions generated by the fragmentation of each precursor ion introduced a three-level specificity. This methodology applied to the analysis of rat urine was able to detect and quantify free and conjugated hydroxytyrosol and tyrosol in the picogram range. It is worth mentioning that no elenolic acid was detected in samples of rat urine following sustained dose protocol.

APCI and ESI techniques have been used to introduce the sample into the mass spectrometer while measuring the bioavailability of polyphenols in humans and in laboratory animals by using HPLC coupled to mass spectrometry. Both SIM and SRM modes were utilized, although no general consensus exists in the literature as to whether positive or negative ion analysis yields higher sensitivity. Few studies using LC-MS or LC-tandem mass spectrometry for the detection and quantification of olive oil phenolic compounds in biological fluids are reported in the literature. Most applications are referred to bioavailability and biotransformation studies in urine and plasma for ingested polyphenols originating from different sources other than olive oil, such as dietary flavonoids (Nielsen et al., 2000; Barnes et al., 2006), tea catechins (Li et al., 2001), dietary polyphenols

(Gonthier et al., 2003; Ito et al., 2004), and plant and mammalian lignans (Smeds and Hakala, 2003; Smeds et al., 2004, 2005; Knust et al., 2006). Finally, main dietary sources of polyphenols, their daily intake, distribution, metabolism, pharmacokinetics, and excretion in human biofluids were reviewed in recent references (Scalbert and Williamson, 2000; Manach et al., 2004).

LC-tandem mass spectrometry analysis of rat plasma and urine was carried out after administration of pure oleuropein (Del Boccio et al., 2003). This methodology was found very useful for the simultaneous measurement of oleuropein and hydroxytyrosol in plasma and urine by monitoring the ion transitions m/z 539 $\rightarrow$ 275 for oleuropein, and m/z 153 $\rightarrow$ 123 for hydroxytyrosol in the negative ion mode. Only oleuropein was detected in plasma in the form of glucoside, whereas hydroxytyrosol was found in traces. Contrary to plasma results, oleuropein and hydroxytyrosol were both recovered in urine mainly as glucuronides and in very low concentrations as free forms.

A recent study (de la Tore-Carbot et al., 2006) presented a novel analytical method for the detection and quantification of metabolites of olive oil polyphenols (glucuronide and sulfate metabolites of hydroxytyrosol, tyrosol, and homovanillic acid) in low-density lipoprotein (LDL), based on a cleanup with solid-phase extraction and the use of LC-ESI-MS/MS. In a subsequent publication (de la Tore-Carbot et al., 2007) the LDL isolation method was improved by using a short second-step ultracentrifugation, thus leading to a better recovery for antioxidant compounds in LDL.

Vissers and co-workers, in an attempt to gain more insight into the metabolism of olive oil polyphenols in humans, measured their absorption and urinary excretion in healthy ileostomy subjects and subjects with a colon (Vissers et al., 2002). By using LC-MS/MS as the analytical technique for the detection and quantification of tyrosol and hydroxytyrosol in urine, they concluded that only a fraction of ingested olive oil phenols was recovered in human urine. They found that 55–56 mol/100 mol of ingested olive phenols was absorbed and that 5–16 mol/100 mol was excreted as tyrosol and hydroxytyrosol. This finding supports the conclusion that humans absorb a major fraction of the polyphenols of olive oil that they consume. Moreover, an important conclusion was drawn about the metabolism of olive oil polyphenols in the human body by measuring urinary excretion in ileostomy subjects. More than 55 mol/100 mol of olive oil polyphenols was absorbed in ileostomy subjects, whereas smaller amounts of tyrosol and hydroxytyrosol were detected in urine of the subjects with a colon; this implies that olive oil polyphenols are absorbed mainly by the small intestine. A further step in the elucidation of the metabolism of olive oil polyphenols in the human body was the possibility that both oleuropein glucoside and oleuropein aglycon were biotransformed into hydroxytyrosol, whereas ligstroside and ligstroside aglycon were metabolized into tyrosol. Metabolism was considered to occur either in the gastrointestinal tract before they were absorbed or in the intestinal cells, blood, or liver after they were absorbed. In accord with other studies, the authors confirmed the presence of hydroxytyrosol and tyrosol conjugates with glucuronic acid in urine, although the O-methylated hydroxytyrosol mentioned in other studies was not detected.

The metabolism of olive oil polyphenols in humans was studied by using Caco-2 cell monolayers as a model system of the human intestinal epithelium (Manna et al., 2000). The only metabolite identified was homovanillic acid, which accounted for only 10% of the total radioactivity of the administered radioactive [^{14}C]-hydroxytyrosol. This finding indicated the limited metabolism of hydroxytyrosol by Caco-2 cells in contrast with the extensive conjugation of olive oil phenols observed *in vivo*. From these results, it was concluded that biotransformation of absorbed hydroxytyrosol may occur in the liver.

The metabolism of hydroxytyrosol, tyrosol, and hydroxytyrosyl acetate in the liver was modeled by using human hepatoma cells (HepG2) (Mateos et al., 2005). Hepatic metabolism of these three polyphenols was monitored at short (2-h) and long (18-h) incubation times. At short incubation time, hydroxytyrosol and tyrosol were found almost intact, whereas hydroxytyrosyl acetate lost its acetyl group forming the deacetylated hydroxytyrosol with small amounts of four more metabolites. At long incubation time (18 h), five metabolites were observed when cells were incubated with hydroxytyrosol. The same five metabolites together with a sixth one, and minor amounts of free hydroxytyrosyl acetate were detected when cells were treated with this acetylated phenol. Conversely, tyrosol appeared to be poorly metabolized and only one metabolite was formed after 18 h of incubation with HepG2 cells. Identification of the various metabolites was achieved by *in vitro* conjugation of pure standards, i.e., methylation, glucuronidation, and sulfation and hydrolysis with β-glucuronidase and sulfatase of metabolites formed by HepG2 cells, and confirmation by LC-ESI-MS. Quantification of metabolites showed that after 18 h of incubation 75% of hydroxytyrosol was metabolized, with 25% of free nonmetabolized phenol. The extent of glucuronidation (32%) was comparable to that of methylation (26%), with up to 18% of methylglucuronides. On the other hand, hydroxytyrosyl acetate was metabolized more effectively and rapidly by HepG2 cells. Only 57 and 9% of nonmetabolized hydroxytyrosyl acetate were detected in the culture medium after 2 and 18 h, respectively. Contrary to previous polyphenols, tyrosol was poorly metabolized. Less than 10% of this olive oil phenol was found as glucuronidated metabolite after 18 h in culture with HepG2 cells.

LC-MS/MS used to detect etheno-DNA adducts in human urine formed as a result of the reaction between DNA bases and intermediates (mainly *trans*-4-hydroxy-2-nonenal) resulted from lipid peroxidation of PUFAs (Hillestrom et al., 2006). Etheno-DNA modifications have miscoding base-repairing properties upon replication or transmission; they can accumulate in DNA after chronic carcinogen exposure and are considered as highly mutagenic lesions. The urinary excretion of the DNA adducts before and after consumption of virgin olive oil did not differ significantly, indicating that consumption of olive oil polyphenols did not modify to a significant degree the urinary excretion of etheno-DNA biomarkers, and therefore did not protect the cells from oxidation. On the other hand, significant association between ethane-DNA adduct excretion rate and the dietary intake of linoleic acid was observed in healthy men (Hillestrom et al., 2006). In this respect, it appears that olive oil, which contains the highest amount of monounsaturated oleic acid among edible oils, does not favor harmful lipid oxidation.

5.6.3 ANALYSIS OF POLYPHENOLS IN HUMANS AND LABORATORY ANIMALS BY OTHER ANALYTICAL TECHNIQUES

Recently, a novel analytical technique — time-resolved fluoroimmunoassay (TR-FIA) — has been developed for the determination of isoflavones and lignans in human plasma and sera using an europium chelate as a label (Adlercreuth et al., 1998; Stumpf et al., 2000; Wang et al., 2000; L'Homme et al., 2002). This technique is highly sensitive and rapid in analysis time, but it is less specific than other techniques (e.g., mass spectrometry) leading to substantial errors. Recent measurements (Kilkkinen et al., 2001) have shown that TR-FIA overestimated the serum concentration of certain lignans. The TR-FIA method has not been applied to the detection of olive oil polyphenols in biological fluids.

NMR spectroscopy has not been used so far in the exploration of human and animal biofluid composition after olive oil ingestion despite the fact that this spectroscopic technique is very powerful in elucidating the structure of small molecules in a multicomponent mixture. This is probably due to the presence of intense broad signals from lipoproteins in plasma and lipids in tissues, which eventually severely overlap the signals from the small metabolites. It appears that these problems have been overcome lately by using one- and two-dimensional editing techniques exploiting differences in spin relaxation times. Spin relaxation–edited NMR spectra can be obtained by inserting a "relaxation filter" prior to detection to eliminate the lipoprotein and lipid signals having relatively short relaxation times, thus leaving the signals from the small metabolite molecules characterized by longer relaxation times (Tang et al., 2004). Also, the study of biochemical profiles in biofluids and tissues may be more effective by using the rapidly expanding method of metabonomics based primarily on NMR spectroscopy (Nicholson et al., 2002).

5.6.4 Conclusions

A variety of analytical techniques have been used to quantify the low levels of polyphenols and their metabolites in biological fluids of humans and laboratory animals. Due to inherent sensitivity and selectivity, direct spectrometric detection (single MS or tandem MS) or preferably indirect detection by coupling mass spectrometry with separation techniques has been used extensively. A drawback of this methodology may be the lack of proper standards for quantification of certain analytes. Instead, standards exhibiting the greatest possible similarity to the analytes have been utilized. The use of NMR spectroscopy alone or in LC-NMR will certainly expand the range of analytical techniques and yield a unique metabolic fingerprint of complex biological fluids.

REFERENCES

Aberth, W. and Burlingame, A.L., 1984, Comparison of three geometries for a cesium primary beam liquid secondary ion mass spectrometry source, *Anal. Chem.*, 56, 2915–2918.

Adlercreuth, H., Wang, G.J.J., Lapcik, O., Hampl, R., Wähälä, K., Mäkelä, T., et al., 1998, Time-resolved fluoroimmunoassay for plasma enterolactone, *Anal. Biochem.*, 265, 208–215.

Albert, K., Ed., 2002, *On-Line LC-NMR and Related Techniques*, John Wiley & Sons, Chichester.

Andary, C., Wylde, R., Laffite, C., Privat, G., and Winternitz, F., 1982, Structures of verbascoside and oroban-choside, caffeic acid sugar esters from Orobanche rapum-genistae, *Phytochemistry*, 21, 1123–1127.

Angerosa, F., d'Alessandro, N., Konstantinou, P., and Di Giancinto, L., 1995, GC-MS evaluation of phenolic compounds in virgin olive oil, *J. Agric. Food Chem.*, 43, 1802–1807.

Angerosa, F., d'Alessandro, N., Corana, F., and Mellerio, G., 1996, Characterization of phenolic and secoiri-doid aglycons present in virgin olive oil by gas chromatography–chemical ionization mass spectrometry, *J. Chromatogr. A*, 736, 195–203.

Angerosa, F., 2006, Analysis and authentication, in *Olive Oil, Chemistry and Technology*, Boskou, D., Ed., AOCS Press, Champaign, IL, 113–172.

Armaforte, E., Mancebo-Campos, V., Bendini, A., Desaparados Salvador, M., Fregapane, G., and Cerretani, L., 2007, Retention effects of oxidized polyphenols during analytical extraction of phenolic compounds of virgin olive oil, *J. Sep. Sci.*, 30, 2401–2406.

Artajo, L.S., Romero, M.P., and Moltiva, M.J., 2006, Enrichment of olive oil: antioxidant capacity functional-ized with phenolic compounds, *4th EuroFed Lipid Congress, Madrid*, Book of Abstracts, p. 471.

Bai, C., Yan, X., Takenaka, M., Sekiya, K., and Nagata, T., 1998, Determination of synthetic hydroxytyrosol in rat plasma by GC-MS, *J. Agric. Food Chem.*, 46, 3998–4001.

Barber, M., Bordoli, R.S., Elliot, J., Sedwick, R.D., and Tyler, A., 1982, Fast atom bombardment mass spectrometry, *Anal. Chem.*, 54, 645A–657A.

Barnes, S., Prasain, J.K., Wang, C.-C., and Moore, D.R. II, 2006, Applications of LC-MS in the study of the uptake, distribution, metabolism and excretion of bioactive polyphenols from dietary supplements, *Life Sci.*, 78, 2054–2059.

Bastoni, L., Bianco, A., Piccioni, F., and Uccella, N., 2001, Biophenolic profile in olives by nuclear magnetic resonance, *Food Chem.*, 73, 145–151.

Bazoti, F.N., Gikas, E., Puel, C., Coxam, V., and Tsarbopoulos, A., 2005, Development of a sensitive and specific solid phase extraction–gas chromatography–tandem mass spectrometry method for the determination of elenolic acid, hydroxytyrosol, and tyrosol in rat urine, *J. Agric. Food Chem.*, 53, 6213–6221.

Bendini, A., Bonoli, M., Cerretani, L., Biguzzi, B., Lercker, G., and Gallina Toschi, T., 2003, Liquid-liquid and solid-phase extractions of phenols from virgin olive oil and their separation by chromatographic and electrophoretic methods, *J. Chromatogr.*, 985, 425–433.

Bendini, A., Cerretani, L., Carrasco-Pancorbo, A., Gomez-Caravaca, A.M., Segura-Carretero, A., Fernandez-Gutierrez, A., and Lerker, G., 2007, Phenolic molecules in virgin olive oils: a survey of their sensory properties, health effects, antioxidant activity and analytical methods. An overview of the last decade, *Molecules*, 12, 1679–1719.

Bianco, A. and Uccella, N., 2000, Biophenolic components of olives, *Food Res. Int.*, 33, 475–485.

Bianco, A., Lo Scalzo, R., and Scarpati, M.L., 1993, Isolation of cornoside from *Olea europaea* and its trans-formation into halleridone, *Phytochemistry*, 32, 455–457.

Bianco, A., Mazzei, R.A., Melchioni, C., Romeo, G., Scarpati, M.L., Soriero, A., and Uccella, N., 1998, Micro-components of olive oil. III. Glucosides of 2(3,4-dihydroxy-phenyl)ethanol, *Food Chem.*, 63, 461–464.

Bianco, A.D., Muzzalupo, I., Piperno, A., Romeo, G., and Uccella, N., 1999a, Bioactive derivatives of oleuropein from olive fruits, *J. Agric. Food Chem.*, 47, 3531–3534.

Bianco, A.D., Piperno, A., Romeo, G., and Uccella, N., 1999b, NMR experiments of oleuropein biomimetic hydrolysis, *J. Agric. Food Chem.*, 47, 3665–3668.

Bianco, A., Buiarelli, F., Cartoni, G., Coccioli, F., Muzzalupo, I., Polidori, A., and Uccella, N., 2001a, Analysis by HPLC-MS/MS of biophenolic components in olives and oils, *Anal. Lett.*, 34, 1033–1051.

Bianco, A., Coccioli, F., Guiso, M., and Marra, C., 2001b. The occurrence in olive oil of a new class of phenolic compounds: hydroxy-isochromans, *Food Chem.*, 77, 405–411.

Bianco, A., Buiarelli, F., Cartoni, G., Coccioli, F., Jasionowska, R., and Margherita, P., 2003, Analysis by liquid chromatography–tandem mass spectrometry of biophenolic compounds in virgin olive oil. II, *J. Sep. Sci.*, 26, 417–424.

Bianco, A., Melchioni, C., Ramunno, A., Romeo, G., and Uccella, N., 2004, Phenolic components of *Olea europaea* — isolation of tyrosol derivatives, *Nat. Prod. Res.*, 18, 29–32.

Bianco, A., Chiaccho, M.A., Grassi, G., Iannazzo, D., Piperno, A., and Romeo, R., 2006, Phenolic components of *Olea europaea*: isolation of new tyrosol and hydroxytyrosol derivatives, *Food Chem.*, 95, 562–565.

Blekas, G., Psomiadou, E., Tsimidou, M., and Boskou, D., 2002, On the importance of total polar phenols to monitor the stability of Greek virgin olive oil, *Eur. J. Lipid Sci. Technol.*, 104, 340–346.

Bonoli, M., Montanucci, M., Toschi, T.G., and Lercker, G., 2003, Fast separation and determination of tyrosol, hydroxytyrosol and other phenolic compounds in extra virgin olive oil by capillary zone electrophoresis with ultraviolet diode array detection, *J. Chromatogr. A*, 1011, 163–172.

Boskou, D., 2006, *Olive Oil: Chemistry and Technology*, AOCS Press, Champaign, IL.

Brenes, M., Garcia, A., Garcia, P., Rios, J.J., and Garrido, A., 1999, Phenolic compounds in Spanish olive oils, *J. Agric. Food Chem.*, 47, 3535–3540.

Brenes, M., Hidalgo, F.J., Garcia, A., Rios, J.J., Garcia, P., Zamora, R., et al., 2000, Pinoresinol and 1-acetoxypinoresinol, two new phenolic compounds identified in olive oil, *J. Amer. Oil Chem. Soc.*, 77, 715–719.

Brenes, M., Garcia, A., and Dobarganes, M.C., 2002, Influence of thermal treatments simulating cooking processes on the polyphenol content in virgin olive oil, *J. Agric. Food Chem.*, 50, 5962–5967.

Brenes, M., Romero, C., Garcia, A., Hidalgo, F.J., and Ruiz-Méndez, M.V., 2004, Phenolic compounds in olive oils intended for refining: formation of 4-ethylphenol during olive paste storage, *J. Agric. Food Chem.*, 52, 8177–8181.

Busch, J., Hrncirik, E., Bulukin, E., Hermanns, G.G.H., Boucon, C., and Mascini, M., 2006, Biosensor measurements of polyphenols for the assessment of bitterness and pungency of virgin olive oil, *J. Agric. Food Chem.*, 54, 4371–4376.

Capozzi, F., Piperno, A., and Uccella, N., 2000, Oleuropein site selective hydrolysis by technomimetic nuclear magnetic resonance experiments, *J. Agric. Food Chem.*, 48, 1623–1629.

Careri, M., Bianchi, F., and Corradini, C., 2002, Recent developments in application of mass spectrometry in food-related analysis, *J. Chromatogr. A*, 970, 3–64.

Carrasco-Pancorbo, A., Cruces-Blanco, C., Carretero, A.S., and Gutierrez, F., 2004, Sensitive determination of phenolic acids in extra virgin olive oil by capillary zone electrophoresis, *J. Agric. Food Chem.*, 52, 6687–6693.

Carrasco-Pancorbo, A., Arraez-Roman, D., Segura-Carretero, A., and Fernandez-Gutierrez, A., 2006a, Capillary electrophoresis–electrospray ionization–mass spectrometry method to determine the phenolic fraction of extravirgin olive oil, *Electrophoresis*, 27, 2182–2196.

Carrasco-Pancorbo, A., Cerretani, L., Segura-Carretero, A., Gallina-Toschi, T., Lercker, G., and Fernandez-Gutierrez, A., 2006b, Evaluation of individul antioxidant activity of single phenolic compounds on virgin olive oil, *Prog. Nutr.*, 8, 28–39.

Caruso, D., Colombo, R., Patelli, R., Giavarini, F., and Galli, G., 2000, Rapid evaluation of phenolic component profile and analysis of oleuropein aglycon in olive oil by atmospheric pressure chemical ionization–mass spectrometry (APCI-MS), *J. Agric. Food Chem.*, 48, 1182–1185.

Caruso, D., Visioli, F., Patelli, R., Galli, C., and Galli, G., 2001, Urinary excretion of olive oil phenols and their metabolites in humans, *Metabolism*, 50, 1426–1428.

Catharino, R.R., Haddad, R., Giroto-Cabrini, L., Cunha, I.B.S., Sawaya, A.C.H.F., and Eberlin, M.N., 2005, Characterization of vegetable oils by electrospray ionization mass spectrometry fingerprinting: classification, quality, adulteration, and aging, *Anal. Chem.*, 77, 7429–7433.

Cavin, A., Potterat, O., Wolfender, J.-L., Hostettman, K., and Dyatmyko, W., 1998, Use of on-flow LC/^{1}H NMR for the study of an antioxidant fraction from *Orophea enneandra* and isolation of a polyacetylene, lignans, and a tocopherol derivative, *J. Nat. Prod.*, 61, 1497–1501.

Cert, A., Moreda, W., and Perez-Camino, M.V., 2000, Chromatographic analysis of minor constituents in vegetable oils, *J. Chromatogr. A*, 881, 131–148.

Christophoridou, S., Dais, P., Tseng, L.-H., and Spraul, M., 2005, Separation and identification of phenolic compounds in olive oil by coupling high-performance liquid chromatography with post column solid-phase extraction to nuclear magnetic resonance spectroscopy (LC-SPE-NMR), *J. Agric. Food Chem.*, 53, 4667–4679.

Christophoridou, S. and Dais, P., 2006, Novel approach for detection and quantification of phenolic compounds in olive oil based on ^{31}P NMR spectroscopy, *J. Agric. Food Chem.*, 54, 656–664.

Christophoridou, S., Spyros, A., and Dais, P., 2001, ^{31}P nuclear magnetic resonance spectroscopy of polyphenol-containing olive oil model compounds, *Phosphorus Sulfur Silicon Related Elements*, 170, 139–157.

Corcoran, O., Wilkinson, P.S., Godejohann, M., Brauman, U., Hoffman, M., and Spraul, M., 2002, Advanced sensitivity for flow NMR spectroscopy: LC-SPE-NMR and capillary scale LC-NMR, *Amer. Lab. Chromatogr. Perspect.*, 5, 18–21.

Cortesi, N., Azzolini, M., and Rovellini, P., 1995, Determination of minor polar components in virgin olive oil, *Riv. Ital. Sostanze Grasse*, 74, 411–414.

D'Angelo, S., Manna, C., Migliardi, V., Mazzoni, O., Morrica, P., Capasso, G., et al., 2001, Pharmacokinetics and metabolism of hydroxytyrosol, a natural antioxidant from olive oil, *Drug Metab. Disp.*, 29, 1492–1498.

De la Torre-Carbot, K., Jauregui, O., Gimeno, E., Castellote, A.I., Lamuela-Raventos, R.M., and Lopez-Sabater, M.C., 2005, Characterization and quantification of phenolic compounds in olive oil by solid-phase extraction, HPLC-DAD, and HPLC-MS/MS, *J. Agric. Food Chem.*, 53, 4331–4340.

De la Torre-Carbot, K., Jauregui, O., Castellote, A.I., Lamuela-Raventos, R.M., Covas, M.-I., Casals, I., and Lopez-Sabater, M.C., 2006, Rapid high–performance liquid chromatography–electrospray ionization mass spectrometry method for qualitative and quantitative analysis of virgin olive oil phenolic metabolites in human low-density lipoproteins, *J. Chromatogr. A*, 1116, 69–75.

De la Torre-Carbot, K., Chavez-Servin, J.L., Jáuregui, O., Castellote, A.I., Lamuela-Raventos, R.M., Fito, M., et al., 2007, Presence of virgin olive oil phenolic metabolites in human low density lipoprotein fraction: determination by high–performance liquid chromatography–electrospray ionization tandem mass spectrometry, *Anal. Chim. Acta*, 583, 402–410.

Del Boccio, P., Di Deo, A., De Curtis, A., Celli, N., Iacoviello, L., and Rotilio, D., 2003, Liquid chromatography–tandem mass spectrometry analysis of oleuropein and its metabolite hydroxytyrosol in rat plasma and urine after oral administration, *J. Chromatogr. B*, 785, 47–56.

Del Carlo, M., Ritelli, R., Diocida, G., Murmura, F., and Cichelli, A., 2006, Characterization of extra virgin olive oils obtained from different cultivars, *Pomologia Croatica*, 12, 29–41.

De Rijke, E., Out, P., Niessen, W.M., Ariese, F., Gooijer, C., and Brinkman, U.A.Th., 2006, Analytical separation and detection methods for flavonoids, *J. Chromatogr. A*, 1112, 31–63.

Edgecombe, S.C., Stretch, G.L., and Hayball, P.J., 2000, Oleuropein, an antioxidant polyphenol from olive oil, is poorly absorbed from isolated perfused rat intestine, *J. Nutr.*, 130, 2996–3002.

Exarchou, V., Godejohann, M., van Beek, T.A., Gerothanassis, I.P., and Vervoot, J., 2003, LC-UV-solid-phase extraction-NMR-MS combined with a cryogenic flow probe and its application to the identification of compounds present in Greek oregano, *Anal. Chem.*, 75, 6288–6294.

Exarchou, V., Krucker, M., van Beek, T.A., Vervoort, J., Gerothanassis, I.P., and Albert, K., 2005, LC-NMR coupling technology: recent advancements and applications in natural products analysis, *Magn. Reson. Chem.*, 43, 681–687.

Fogliano, V., Ritieni, S., Monti, S., Gallo, M., Madaglia, D.D., Ambrosino, M.L., and Sacchi, R., 1999, Antioxidant activity of virgin olive oil phenolic compounds in a micellar system, *J. Sci. Food Agric.*, 79, 1803–1808.

Frański, R., Bednarek, P., Wojtaszek, P., and Stobiecki, M., 2005, Identification of flavonoid diglycosides in yellow lupin (*Lupinus luteus* L.) with mass spectrometric techniques, *J. Mass Spectrom.*, 34, 486–495.

Garcia-Mesa, J.A. and Mateos, R., 2007, Direct automatic determination of bitterness and total phenolic compounds in virgin olive oil using a pH-based flow injection analysis system, *J. Agric. Food Chem.*, 55, 3863–3868.

Gariboldi, P., Jommi, G., and Verrota, L., 1986, Secoiridoids from *olea europaea*, *Phytochemistry*, 25, 865–869.

Georgiou, C.A., Komaitis, E.M., Vasiliou, E.G., Kremmydas, G., and Georgakopoulos, G., 2007, Response of *Vibrio fischeri* whole cell biosensors to olive oil phenolics, *5th EuroFed Lipid Congress, Oils Fat and Lipids: From Science to Applications, Gothenburg,* Book of Abstracts, p. 43.

Gikas, E., Papadopoulos, N., and Tsarbopoulos, A., 2006, Kinetic study of the acidic hydrolysis of oleuropein, the major bioactive metabolite of olive oil, *J. Liquid Chromatogr. Related Technol.*, 29, 497–508.

Gomez-Alonso, S., Fregapane, G., Salvador, M.D., and Gordon, M.H., 2003, Changes in phenolic composition and antioxidant activity of virgin olive oil during frying, *J. Agric. Food Chem.*, 51, 667–672.

Gonthier, M.-P., Rios, L.Y., Verny, M.-A., Remesy, C., and Scalbert, A., 2003, Novel liquid chromatography-electrospray ionization mass spectrometry method for the quantification in human urine of microbial aromatic acid metabolites derived from dietary polyphenols, *J. Chromatogr. B*, 789, 247–255.

Grace, P.B., Taylor, J.I., Botting, N.P., Fryatt, T., Oldfield, M.F., and Bingham, S.A., 2003, Quantification of isoflavones and lignans in urine using gas chromatography/mass spectrometry, *Anal. Biochem.*, 315, 114–121.

Grigoriadou, D., Androulaki, A., Psomiadou, E., and Tsimidou, M.Z., 2007, Solid phase extraction in the analysis of squalene and tocopherols in olive oil, *Food Chem.*, 105, 675–680.

Grizis, C., Atta-Politou, J., and Koupparis, M.A., 2003, Simultaneous determination of oleuropein and tyrosol in plasma using high performance liquid chromatography with UV detection, *J. Liquid Chromatogr. Related Technol.*, 26, 599–616.

Gutierrez-Rosales, F., Rios, J.J., and Gomez-Rey, M.L., 2003, Main polyphenols in the bitter taste of virgin olive oil. Structural confirmation by on-line high-performance liquid chromatography electrospray ionization mass spectrometry, *J. Agric. Food Chem.*, 51, 6021–6025.

Harrison, A.G., 1999, *Chemical Ionization Mass Spectrometry*, Franklin Book Company, Elkins Park, PA.

Hillestrom, P.R., Covas, M.-I., and Poulsen, H.E., 2006, Effect of dietary virgin oil on urinary excretion of etheno-DNA adducts, *Free Radiat. Biol. Med.*, 41, 1133–1138; and references therein.

Hollman, P.C.H., Gaag, M.V.D., Mengelers, M.J.B., van Trijp, J.M.P., de Vries, J.H.M., and Katan, M.B., 1996, Absorption and disposition kinetics of the dietary antioxidant quercetin in man, *Free Radiat. Biol. Med.*, 21, 703–707.

Hrncirik, K. and Fritsche, S., 2004, Comparability and reliability of different techniques for the determination of phenolic compounds in virgin olive oil, *Eur. J. Lipid Sci. Technol.*, 106, 540–549.

Ito, H., Gonthier, M.-P., Manach, C., Morand, C., Menneti, L., Remesy, C., and Scalbert, A., 2004, High throughput profiling of dietary polyphenols and their metabolites by HPLC-ESI-MS-MS in human urine, *Biofactors*, 22, 241–243.

Karas, M. and Hillenkamp, F., 1988, Laser desorption ionization of proteins with molecular masses exceeding 10,000 Daltons, *Anal. Chem.*, 60, 2299–2301.

Kilkkinen, A., Stumpf, K., Pietinen, P., Valsta, L.M., Tapanainen, H., and Adlercreutz, H., 2001, Determinants of serum enterolactone concentration, *Am. J. Clin. Nutr.*, 73, 1094–1100.

Knust, U., Hull, W.E., Spiegelhalder, B., Bartsch, H., Strowitzki, T., and Owen, R.W., 2006, Analysis of entero-lignan glucuronides in serum and urine by HPLC-ESI-MS, *Food Chem. Toxicol.*, 44, 1038–1049.

Lee, M.-J., Wang, Z.-Y., Li, H., Chen, L., Sun, Y., Gobbo, S., Balentine, D., and Yang, C.S., 1995, Analysis of plasma and urinary tea polyphenols in human subjects, *Cancer Epidemiol. Biomarkers Prevention,* 4, 393–399.

L'Homme, R., Brouwers, E., Al-Maharik, N., Lapcik, O., Hampl, R., Mikola, H., et al., 2002, Time-resolved fluoroimmunoassay of plasma and urine O-desmethylangolensin, *J. Steroid Biochem. Mol. Biol.*, 81, 353–361.

Li, C., Meng, X., Winnik, B., Lee, M.-J., Lu, H., Sheng, S., Buckley, B., and Yang, C.S., 2001, Analysis of urinary metabolites of tea catechins by liquid chromatography/electrospray ionization mass spectrometry, *Chem. Res. Toxicol.*, 14, 702–707.

Liberatore, L., Procida, G., d'Alesandro, N., and Cichelli, A., 2001, Solid-phase extraction and gas chromatographic analysis of phenolic compounds in virgin olive oil, *Food Chem.*, 73, 119–124.

Limiroli, R., Consonni, R., Ottolina, G., Marsilio, V., Bianchi, G., and Zetta, L., 1995, ^1H and ^{13}C NMR characterization of new oleuropein aglycones, *J. Chem. Soc. Perkin Trans.*, 1, 1519–1523.

Manach, C., Scalbert, A., Morand, C., Remesy, C., and Jimenez, L., 2004, Polyphenols: food sources and bioavailability, *Am. J. Clin. Nutr.*, 79, 727–747.

Manna, C., Galletti, C., Maisto, G., Cucciola, V., D'Angelo, S., and Zappa, V., 2000, Transport mechanism and metabolism of olive oil 3,4-dihydroxyphenylethanol in Caco-2 cells, *FEBS Lett.*, 470, 341–344.

Mark, T.D. and Dunn, G.H., 1985, *Electron Impact Ionization*, Springer Verlag, Vienna.

Mateos, R., Espartero, J.L., Trujillo, M., Rios, J.J., Leon-Camacho, M., Alcudia, F., et al., 2001, Determination of phenols, flavones and lignans in virgin olive oils by solid-phase extraction and high performance liquid chromatography with diode array ultraviolet detection, *J. Agric. Food Chem.*, 49, 2185–2192.

Mateos, R., Goya, L., and Bravo, L., 2005, Metabolism of the olive oil phenols hydroxytyrosol, tyrosol, and hydroxytyrosol acetate by human hepatoma HepG2 cells, *J. Agric. Food Chem.*, 53, 9897–9905.

McDonald, S., Prenzler, P.D., Antonovich, M., and Robards, K., 2001, Phenolic content and antioxidant activity of olive extracts, *Food Chem.*, 73, 73–84.

McLafferty, F.W., 1980, Tandem mass spectrometry (MS/MS): a promising new analytical technique for specific component determination in complex mixture, *Acc. Chem. Res.*, 13, 33–39.

McPhail, D.B., Hartley, R.C., Gardner, P.T., and Duthie, G.G., 2003, Kinetic and stoichiometric assessment of the antioxidant activity of flavonoids by electron spin resonance spectroscopy, *J. Agric. Food Chem.*, 51, 1684–1690.

Miró-Casas, E., Farre-Albaladejo, M., Covas-Planells, M.I., Fito-Colomer, M., Lamuela-Raventos, R.M., and de la Torre-Fornell, R., 2001a, Tyrosol bioavailability in humans after ingestion of virgin olive oil, *Clin. Chem.*, 47, 341–343.

Miró-Casas, E., Farre-Albaladejo, M., Covas, M.-I., Ortuno-Rodriguez, J.O., Colomer, E., Lamuela-Raventos, R.M., and de la Torre, R., 2001b, Capillary gas chromatography–mass spectrometry quantitative determination of hydroxytyrosol and tyrosol in human urine after olive oil intake, *Anal. Biochem.*, 294, 63–72.

Miró-Casas, E., Covas, M.-I., Farre, M., Fito, M., Ortuno, J., Weinbrenner, T., Roset, P., and de la Torre-Fornell, R., 2003a, Hydroxytyrosol disposition in humans, *Clin. Chem.*, 49, 945–952.

Miró-Casas, E., Covas, M.-I., Fito, M., Farre-Albaladejo, M., Marrugat, J., and de la Torre, R., 2003b, Tyrosol and hydroxytyrosol are absorbed from moderate and sustained doses of virgin olive oil in humans, *Eur. J. Clin. Nutr.,* 57, 186–190.

Montedoro, G., Servili, M., Baldioli, M., and Miniati, E., 1992, Simple and hydrolysable phenolic compounds in virgin olive oil. I. Their extraction, separation and quantitative and semiquantitative evaluation by HPLC, *J. Agric. Food Chem.*, 40, 1571–1576.

Montedoro, G., Servili, M., Baldioli, M., Selvaggini, R., Miniati, E., and Macchioni, A., 1993, Simple and hydrolysable compounds in virgin olive oil. III. Spectroscopic characterizations of secoiridoids derivatives, *J. Agric. Food Chem.*, 41, 2228–2234.

Monti, S.M., Ritieni, A., Sacchi, R., Skog, K., Borgen, E., and Fogliano, V., 2001, Characterization of phenolic compounds in virgin olive oil and their effect on the formation of carcinogenic/mutagenic heterocyclic amines in a model system, *J. Agric. Food. Chem.*, 49, 3969–3975.

Mosca, L., DeMarco, C., Visioli, F., and Canella, C., 2000, Enzymatic assay for the determination of olive oil polyphenol content: assay conditions and validation of the method, *J. Agric. Food Chem.,* 48, 297–301.

Murkovic, M., Lechner, S., Pietzka, A., Bratacos, M., and Katzogiannos, E., 2004, Analysis of minor components in olive oil, *J. Biochem. Biophys. Methods,* 61, 155–160.

Nicholson, J.K., Connelly, J., Lindon, J.C., and Holmes, E., 2002, Metabonomics: a platform for studying drag toxicity and gene function, *Nat. Rev. Drug Discov.*, 1, 153–161.

Nielsen, S.E., Freese, R., Cornett, C., and Dragsted, L.O., 2000, Identification and quantification of flavonoids in human urine samples by column-switching liquid chromatography coupled to atmospheric pressure chemical ionization mass spectrometry, *Anal. Chem.*, 72, 1503–1509.

Niessen, W.M.A., 1998, Advances in instrumentation in liquid chromatography–mass spectrometry and related liquid-introduction techniques, *J. Chromatogr. A,* 794, 407–435.

Niessen, W.M.A., 1999, *Liquid Chromatography–Mass Spectrometry,* 2nd ed., Marcel Dekker, New York.

Nurmi, T., Voutilainen, S., Nyyssonen, K., Adlercreutz, H., and Salonen, J.T., 2003, Liquid chromatography method for plant and mammalian lignans in human urine, *J. Chromatogr. B,* 798, 101–110.

Ottaviani, M.F., Spallaci, M., Cangiotti, M., Bacchiocca, M., and Ninfali, P., 2001, Electron paramagnetic resonance investigations of free radicals in extra virgin olive oils, *J. Agric. Food Chem.*, 49, 3691–3696.

Owen, R.W., Mier, W., Giacosa, A., Hull, W.E., Spiegelhalder, B., and Bartsch, H., 2000a, Identification of lignans as major components in the phenolic fraction of olive oil, *Clin. Chem.*, 46, 976–988.

Owen, R.W., Giacosa, A., Hull, W.E., Haubner, R., Mier, W., Spiegelhalder, B., and Bartsch, H., 2000b, The antioxidant/anticancer potential of phenolic compounds isolated from olive oil, *Eur. J. Cancer*, 36, 1235–1247.

Owen, R.W., Haubner, R., Mier, W., Giacosa, A., Hull, W.E., Spiegelhalder, B., and Bartsch, H., 2003, Isolation, structure elucidation and antioxidant potential of the major phenolic and flavonoid compounds in brined olive drupes, *Food Chem. Toxicol.*, 41, 703–717.

Papadimitriou, V., Sotiroudis, T.G., Xenakis, A., Sofikiti, N., Stavyiannoudaki, V., and Chaniotakis, N.A., 2006, Oxidative stability and radical scavenging activity of extra virgin olive oils: an electron paramagnetic resonance spectroscopy study, *Anal. Chim. Acta*, 573, 453–458.

Pellegrini, N., Visioli, F., Buratti, S., and Brighenti, F., 2001, Direct analysis of total antioxidant activity of olive oil and studies on the influence of heating, *J. Agric. Food Chem.*, 49, 2532–2538.

Pereira, J.A., Pereira, A.P., Ferreira, I.F.R., Valentino, P., Andrade, P.B., Seabra, R., et al., 2006, Table olives from Portugal: phenolic compounds, antioxidant potential, and antiradical activity, *J. Agric. Food Chem.*, 54, 8425–8431.

Perez-Bonilla, M., Salido, S., van Beek, T.A., Linares-Palomino, P.J., Altrarejos, J., Nogueras, M., and Sanchez, A., 2006, Isolation and identification of radical scavengers in olive tree (*Olea europaea*) wood, *J. Chromatogr.*, 1112, 311–318.

Perez-Camino, M.C. and Cert, A., 1999, Quantitative determination of hydroxyl pentacyclic triterpene acids in vegetable oils, *J. Agric. Food Chem.*, 47, 1558–1562.

Perri, E., Raffaelli, A., and Sindona, G., 1999, Quantitation of oleuropein in virgin olive oil by ionspray mass spectrometry–selected reaction monitoring, *J. Agric. Food Chem.*, 47, 4156–4160.

Pirisi, F.M., Cabras, P., Falqui, C.C., Migliorini, M., and Mugelli, M., 2000, Phenolic compounds in virgin olive oil. Reappraisal of the extraction, HPLC separation and quantification procedures, *J. Agric. Food Chem.*, 48, 1191–1196.

Quiles, J.L., Ramirez-Tortosa, M.C., Gomez, J.A., Huertas, J.R., and Mataix, J., 2002, Role of vitamin E and phenolic compounds in the antioxidant capacity, measured by ESR, of virgin olive, olive and sunflower oils after frying, *Food Chem.*, 76, 461–468.

Rios, J.J., Gil, M.J., and Gutierez-Rosales, F., 2005, Solid-phase extraction gas chromatography–ion mass spectrometry qualitative method for evaluation of phenolic compounds in virgin olive oil and structural confirmation of oleuropein and ligstroside aglycons and their oxidation products, *J. Chromatogr. A*, 1093, 167–176.

Romani, A., Mulinacci, N., Pinelli, P., Vincieri, F.F., and Cimato, A., 1999, Polyphenolic content in five Tuscany cultivars of *Olea europaea* L., *J. Agric. Food Chem.*, 47, 964–967.

Romero, C., Brenes, M., Garcia, P., and Garrido, A., 2002, Hydroxytyrosol 4-β-D-glucoside, an important phenolic compound in olive fruits and derived products, *J. Agric. Food Chem.*, 50, 3835–3839.

Romero, M.P., Tovar, M.J., Girona, J., and Motilva, M.J., 2002, Changes in the HPLC phenolic profile of virgin olive oil from young trees (*Olea europaea* L. cv. *Arbequina*) grown under different deficit irrigation strategies, *J Agric. Food Chem.*, 50, 5349–5354.

Rotondi, A., Bendini, A., Cerretani, L., Mari, M., Lercker, G., and Toschi, T.G., 2004, Effect of olive ripening degree on the oxidative stability and organoleptic properties of CV Nostrana di Brisighela extra virgin olive oil, *J. Agric. Food Chem.*, 52, 3649–3654.

Ruiz-Gutierrez, V., Juan, M.E., Cert, A., and Planas, J.M., 2000, Determination of hydroxytyrosol in plasma by HPLC, *Anal. Chem.*, 72, 4458–4461.

Ruiz-Mendez, M.V. and Dobarganes, C., 2005, Triterpenic acids from olive pomace, *26th World Congress, Int. Soc. Fat Research, Modern Aspects of Fats and Oils, Prague*, Book of Abstracts, p. 92.

Ryan, D. and Robards, K., 1998, Phenolic compounds in olives, *Analyst*, 123, 31R–44R.

Ryan, D., Robards, K., Prenzler, P., and Antolovich, M., 1999a, Applications of mass spectrometry to plant phenols, *Trends Anal. Chem.*, 18, 362–372.

Ryan, D., Robards, K., and Lavee, S., 1999b, Determination of phenolic compounds in olives by reversed-phase chromatography and mass spectrometry, *J. Chromatogr. A*, 832, 87–96.

Ryan, D., Robards, K., Prenzler, P., Jardine, D., Herlt, T., and Antolovich, M., 1999c, Liquid chromatography with electrospray ionization mass spectrometric detection of phenolic compounds from *Olea europaea*, *J. Chromatogr. A*, 855, 529–537.

Ryan, D., Robards, K., and Lavee, S., 1999d, Changes in phenolic content of olive during maturation, *Int. J. Food Sci. Technol.*, 34, 265–274.

Scalbert, A. and Williamson, G., 2000, Dietary intake and bioavailability of polyphenols, *J. Nutr.*, 130, 2073S–2085S.

Selvaggini, R., Servili, M., Urbani, S., Esposto, S., Taticchi, A., and Montedoro, G., 2006, Evaluation of phenolic compounds in virgin olive oil by direct injection in high-performance liquid chromatography with fluorescent detection, *J. Agric. Food Chem.*, 54, 2832–2838.

Servili, M., Baldioli, M., Savaggini, R., Miniati, E., Macchioni, A., and Montedoro, G., 1999a, High-performance liquid chromatography evaluation of phenols in olive fruit, virgin olive oil, vegetation waters and pomace and 1D- and 2D-nuclear magnetic resonance characterization, *J. Amer. Oil Chem. Soc.*, 76, 873–882.

Servili, M., Baldioli, M., Selvaggini, R., Macchioni, A., and Montedoro, G., 1999b, Phenolic compounds of olive fruit: one- and two-dimensional nuclear magnetic resonance characterization of nüzhenide and its distribution in the constitutive parts of fruit, *J. Agric. Food Chem.*, 47, 12–18.

Silva, S., Gomez, L., Leitao, F., Coelho, A.V., and Vilas Boas, L., 2006, Phenolic compounds and antioxidant activity of *Olea europea* L. fruits and leaves, *Food Sci. Technol. Int.*, 12, 385–395.

Smeds, A. and Hakala, K., 2003, Liquid chromatography–tandem mass spectrometric method for the plant lignan 7-hydroxymatairesinol and its potential metabolites in human plasma, *J. Chromatogr. B*, 793, 297–308.

Smeds, A.I., Saarinen, N.M., Hurmerinta, T.T., Penttinen, P.E., Sjöholm, R.E., and Mäkelä, S.I., 2004, Urinary excretion of lignans after administration of isolated plant lignans to rats: the effect of single dose and ten-day exposures, *J. Chromatogr. B*, 813, 303–312.

Smeds, A.I., Saarinen, N.M., Eklund, P.C., Sjöholm, R.E., and Mäkelä, S.I., 2005, New lignan metabolites in urine, *J. Chromatogr. B*, 816, 87–97.

Spyros, A. and Dais, P., 2000, Application of ^{31}P NMR spectroscopy in food analysis. Quantitative determination of the mono- and diglyceride composition of olive oils, *J. Agric. Food Chem.*, 48, 802–805.

Stobiecki, M., 2000, Application of mass spectrometry for identification and structural studies of flavonoid glucosides, *Phytochemistry*, 54, 237–256.

Stumpf, K., Uehara, M., Nurmi, T., and Adlercreuth, H., 2000, Changes in the time-resolved fluoroimmunoassay of plasma enterolactone, *Anal. Biochem.*, 284, 153–157.

Tan, H.-W., Tuck, K.L., Stupans, I., and Hayball, P.J., 2003, Simultaneous determination of oleuropein and hydroxytyrosol in rat plasma using liquid chromatography with fluorescence detection, *J. Chromatogr. B*, 785, 187–191.

Tang, H., Wang, Y., Nicholson, K., and Lindon, C., 2004, Use of relaxation-edited one-dimensional and two-dimensional nuclear magnetic resonance spectroscopy to improve detection of small metabolites in blood plasma, *Anal. Biochem.*, 325, 260–272.

Torrecilla, J.S., Mena, M.L., Yanez-Sedeno, P., and Gacia, J., 2007, Quantification of phenolic compounds in olive oil mill wastewater by artificial neural network/laccase biosensor, *J. Agric. Food Chem.*, 55, 7418–7426.

Tsarbopoulos, A., Gikas, E., Papadopoulos, N., Aligiannis, N., and Kafatos, A., 2003, Simultaneous determination of oleuropein and its metabolites in plasma by high performance liquid chromatography, *J. Chromatogr. B*, 785, 157–164.

Tsimidou, M., 1999, Analysis of virgin olive oil polyphenols, *Semin. Food Anal.*, 4, 13–29.

Tuck, K.L., Freeman, M.P., Hayball, P.J., Stretch, G.L., and Stupans, I., 2001, The *in vivo* fate of hydroxytyrosol and tyrosol, antioxidant phenolic constituents of olive oil, after intravenous and oral dosing of labeled compounds to rats, *J. Nutr.*, 131, 1993–1996.

Tuck, K.L., Hayball, P.J., and Stupans, I., 2002, Structural characterization of the metabolites of hydroxytyrosol, the principal phenolic component in olive oil, in rats, *J. Agric. Food Chem.*, 50, 2404–2409.

Valavanidis, A., Nisiotou, C., Papageorgiou, Y., Kremli, I., Satravelas, N., Zinieris, N., and Zygalaki, H., 2004, Comparison of the radical scavenging potential of polar and lipidic fractions of olive oil and other vegetable oils under normal conditions and under thermal treatment, *J. Agric. Food Chem.*, 52, 2358–2365.

Velasco, J. and Dobarganes, C., 2002, Oxidative stability of virgin olive oil, *Eur. J. Lipid Sci. Technol.*, 104, 661–676.

Velasco, J., Andersen, M.L., and Skibsted, L.H., 2004, Evaluation of oxidative stability of vegetable oils by monitoring the tendency to radical formation. A comparison of electron spin resonance spectroscopy with the Rancimat method and differential scanning calorimetry, *Food Chem.*, 85, 623–632.

Velasco, J., Andersen, M.L., and Skibsted, L.H., 2005, Electron spin resonance spin trapping for analysis of lipid oxidation in oils: inhibiting effect of the spin trap α-phenyl-*N-tert*-butylnitrone on lipid oxidation, *J. Agric. Food Chem.*, 53, 1328–1336.

Vinha, A.F., Silva, B.M., Andrade, P.B., Seabra, R.M., Pereira, J.A., and Oliveira, M.B., 2002, Development and evaluation of an HPLC/DAD method for the analysis of phenolic compounds from olive fruits, *J. Liquid Chromatogr. Related Technol.*, 25, 151–160.

Vinha, A.F., Ferreres, F., Silva, B.M., Valentao, P., Goncalves, A., Pereira, J.A., et al., 2005, Phenolic profiles of portugese olive fruits (*Olea europaea* L.): influences of cultivar and geographical origin, *Food Chem.*, 89, 561–568.

Visioli, F., Galli, C., Bornet, F., Mattei, A., Patelli, R., Galli, G., and Caruso, D., 2000, Olive oil phenolics are dose-dependently absorbed in humans, *FEBS Lett.*, 468, 159–160.

Visioli, F., Gali, C., Galli, G., and Varuso, D., 2002, Biological activities and metabolic fate of olive oil phenols, *Eur. J. Lipid Sci. Technol.*, 104, 677–684.

Visioli, F., Galli, C., Grande, S., Colonnelli, K., Patelli, C., Galli, G., and Caruso, D., 2003, Hydroxytyrosol excretion differs between rats and humans and depends on the vehicle of administration, *J. Nutr.*, 133, 2612–2615.

Vissers, M.N., Zock, P.L., Roodenburg, A.J.C., Leenen, R., and Katan, M.B., 2002, Olive oil phenols are absorbed in humans? *J. Nutr.*, 132, 409–417.

Wang, G.J., Lapcik, O., Hampl, R., Uehara, M., Al-Maharik, N., Stumpf, K., et al., 2000, Time-resolved fluoroimmunoassay of plasma daidzein and genistein, *Steroids,* 65, 339–348.

Weintraub, R.A., Ameer, B., Johnson, J.V., and Yost, R.A., 1995, Trace determination of naringerin and hesperitin by tandem mass spectrometry, *J. Agric. Food Chem.*, 43, 1966–1968.

Willfor, S.M., Smeds, A.I., and Holmbon, B.R., 2006, Chromatographic analysis of lignans, *J. Chromatogr. A,* 1112, 64–77.

Wolfender, J.-L., Hostettmann, K., Abe, F., Nagao, T., Pkabe, H., and Yamauchi, T., 1995, Liquid chromatography combined with thermospray and continuous flow atom bombardment mass spectrometry of glucosides in crude plant extracts, *J. Chromatogr. A,* 712, 155–168.

Zabaras, Z. and Gordon, M.H., 2004, Detection of pressed hazelnut oil in virgin olive oil by analysis of polar components: improvement and validation of the method, *Food Chem.*, 84, 475–483.

6 Bioavailability and Antioxidant Effect of Olive Oil Phenolic Compounds in Humans

María-Isabel Covas, Olha Khymenets,
Montserrat Fitó, and Rafael de la Torre

CONTENTS

6.1 BIOAVAILABILITY OF OLIVE OIL PHENOLIC COMPOUNDS IN HUMANS

6.1.1 BACKGROUND

Epidemiological studies have shown that the incidence of coronary heart disease and certain cancers is lower in the European Mediterranean regions than in the Northern or other Western countries (Trichopoulou et al., 2003). This has been attributed to the high consumption of olive oil in the Mediterranean diet, which contains phenolic compounds with antioxidant activity. The most abundant of these are hydroxytyrosol (HT) and tyrosol (T) derivatives, present mainly in the form of secoiridoid aglycons (Tsimidou, 1998; Mateos et al., 2001; Servili et al., 2004; Carrasco-Pancorbo et al., 2006; see also Chapter 3). HT is the most potent phenolic antioxidant of olive oil and olive mill waste water (Owen et al., 2000).

The biological activities of olive oil phenols have stimulated research on their potential role in cardiovascular protection. Although many *in vitro* studies have been performed to elucidate the mechanisms by which these compounds may act, there are few reports related to their fate after ingestion.

Dietary intake of olive oil polyphenols has been estimated to be around 9 mg, based on a consumption of 25–50 ml of olive oil per day; at least 1 mg of them is derived from free HT and T, and 8 mg is related to their elenolic acid (EA) esters and also to the oleuropein- and ligstroside-aglycons (Vissers et al., 2004). The ingestion of HT as oleuropein is probably the highest, given that oleuropein is broken down in the gastrointestinal tract (GI) into HT and EA, as will be discussed later in the chapter. Several clinical and animal studies have provided evidence that phenolic compounds are absorbed and exert their biological effects in a dose-dependent manner (Visioli et al., 2001; Weinbrenner et al., 2004a, b). However, some authors caution that the attained concentrations after their ingestion are too low to explain the observed biological activities in *in vitro* and *in vivo* models at higher doses/concentrations (Vissers et al., 2004).

6.1.2 Bioavailability Studies in Experimental Models

6.1.2.1 Absorption in the Gastrointestinal Tract

Once olive oil has been ingested, HT and T as well as their glucosides and aglycons, such as oleuropein, undergo rapid hydrolysis under gastric conditions, resulting in a significant increase in the levels of free HT and T entering the small intestine (Corona et al., 2006).

Several authors have performed experiments with polyphenols that were administered in oil-based or aqueous dosing. The purpose of these studies was to have a better understanding of the role of the biological matrix surrounding the phenol compounds in relation to their absorption. If these compounds are ever used in nutraceutical preparations this is an issue to be taken into consideration.

In *in vitro* models, both HT and T are able to cross human Caco-2 cell monolayers and rat segments of jejunum and ileum (Manna et al., 2000; Corona et al., 2006). In an experiment performed in Caco-2 cell monolayers using [^{14}C]HT, kinetic data showed that transport occurs via a bidirectional passive diffusion mechanism; the calculated apparent permeability coefficient indicates that the molecule is quantitatively absorbed at the intestinal level.

In a study performed in rats where HT and T were administered intravenously (in saline) and orally (in oil- and water-based solutions), the intravenously and orally administered oil-based dosing promoted a greater recovery of the phenolics in 24-h urine in comparison to that obtained with the oral aqueous dosing method. There was no significant difference in the amount of phenolic compounds eliminated in urine between the intravenous and the oral oil-based dosing methods for either T or HT. Oral bioavailability estimates of HT and T were 25% higher when administered in an olive oil solution compared to an aqueous solution (Tuck et al., 2001). These results were further confirmed in humans where HT bioavailability was compared by administering this compound in different matrices (olive oil, spiked refined oil, and yogurt). It was found that HT recovery (measured as urinary HT) was much higher after HT administration as a natural component of olive oil (44.2% of HT administered) than after HT addition to refined olive oil (23% of HT administered), or to a yogurt (5.8% of dose or approximately 13% of that recorded after virgin olive oil intake) (Visioli et al., 2003).

The absorption of oleuropein, one of the major bioactive phenols present in olive oil, has always been elusive. By applying an *in situ* intestinal perfusion technique, the absorption of oleuropein was studied under both iso-osmotic and hypotonic luminal conditions. Under iso-osmotic conditions oleuropein was absorbed, but the mechanism of absorption is still unclear; it may involve transcellular transport (SGLT1) or paracellular movement. The permeability of oleuropein was significantly greater under hypotonic conditions. This fact may be due to an increase in the paracellular movement facilitated by the opening of paracellular junctions in response to hypotonicity. Overall, oleuropein can be absorbed, albeit poorly, from isolated perfused rat intestine. It is therefore possible that oleuropein exerts its biological activities through its conversion to HT due to a poor absorption in the GI tract (Edgecombe et al., 2000). This idea is supported by the results of bioavailability studies in rats, in which peak plasma concentrations, reached after high doses of oleuropein (100 mg/kg), were in the nanogram range, suggesting an oleuropein conversion to HT in the GI tract and a poor absorption of oleuropein itself (Del Boccio et al., 2003; Bazoti et al., 2005). These observations made in rat models have been further confirmed in humans (Vissers et al., 2002; Visioli et al., 2003).

6.1.2.2 First Pass Metabolism

In the process of crossing epithelial cells of the GI tract, phenolic compounds from olive oil are subject to a classic phase I/II biotransformation and, therefore, subjected to an important first pass metabolism. From data of *in vitro* studies, about 10% of HT is converted into homovanillyl alcohol (HVAL) by the catechol-*O*-methyltransferase (Manna et al., 2000). Other authors (Corona et al., 2006), in addition to the *O*-methylated derivative of HT, found glucuronides of HT and T and a novel glutathionylated conjugate of HT. In contrast, there was no absorption of oleuropein as it was rapidly degraded by the colonic microflora to HT (Corona et al., 2006).

6.1.2.3 Hepatic Metabolism

The hepatic metabolism of the olive oil phenols (HT, HT acetate, and T) has been studied in human hepatoma HepG2 cells. After incubation, culture media and cell lysates were hydrolyzed with β-glucuronidase and sulfatase. Methylated and glucuronidated forms of HT were detected after 18 h of incubation, together with methyl-glucuronidated metabolites. Hydroxytyrosyl acetate was largely converted into free HT and subsequently metabolized, although small amounts of glucuronidated hydroxytyrosyl acetate were detected. T was poorly metabolized, with <10% of the phenol glucuronidated after 18 h. Minor amounts of free or conjugated phenols were detected in cell lysates. No sulfated metabolites were found (Mateos et al., 2005). In experiments made with human liver microsomes, HT, T, and HVAL are preferentially glucuronidated in the position 4′ of the benzene ring, although in the case of HT conjugation at the 3′ position is possible but at a lower rate (Khymenets et al., 2006).

The pharmacokinetics of HT intravenously administered to rats (D'Angelo et al., 2001) indicates a fast and extensive uptake of the molecule by the organs and tissues, with a preferential renal uptake. In urine collected up to 5 h after injection of the phenolics, 90% of the administered dose was recovered, and about 5% was detectable in feces and gastrointestinal content. HT was metabolized to four oxidized and/or methylated derivatives. The HT recovered was sulfo-conjugated forms representing major urinary excretion products. The recovery of HT in urine was about 6% of the dose administered: 0.3% recovered as HVAL (3-methoxy-4-hydroxy-phenylethanol, MOPET), 12.3% as DOPAC (3,4-dihydroxy-phenylacetic acid), 23.6% as homovanillic acid (3-methoxy-4-hydroxy-phenylacetic acid, HVA), and 26% as DOPAL (3,4-dihydroxy-phenylacetaldehyde) (D'Angelo et al., 2001). It is noteworthy that some of the reported metabolites of HT are common to dopamine (DOPAC, HVA, DOPAL, MOPET); this is not surprising as HT itself can be renamed DOPET, a well-known dopamine metabolite (de la Torre et al., 2006). Although there is no disagreement in findings between studies, some authors question the rat model as being adequate for this type of study, given that rats display an extremely high HT basal metabolism (30-fold greater than humans) (Visioli et al., 2003). Additionally, some metabolic studies on the disposition of HT may be cross-contaminated with or through the catecholamine disposition pathways (Visioli et al., 2003). Absence of the 3-*O*-glucuronide of HT reported in some studies is probably due to the administration route used. As stated earlier, HT administered by the oral route is subject to an extensive first-pass metabolism, where the contribution of intestinal metabolism is quite relevant. When HT is administered intravenously only hepatic contribution to its disposition is seen (Tuck et al., 2002).

6.1.2.4 Are Metabolites Biologically Active?

Studies *in vivo* performed on rats on the metabolic disposition of phenolic compounds from olive oil suggest that they are well absorbed but extensively metabolized. Most biological activities attributed to HT are associated with preservation of the catechol group and its antioxidant activity. Those metabolic processes leading to conjugates (glucuronides, sulfates, methyl) with phenol groups of catechol may give rise to a loss of HT biological activity. It has been reported that the radical scavenging potency of 3-*O*-glucuronide conjugate is higher than that of HT itself, whereas the monosulfate conjugate is almost devoid of radical scavenging activity (Tuck et al., 2002). Thus, glucuronides of HT appeared to be more active than HT. Under this hypothesis, dietary HT is bioactivated in the body. This makes *in vitro* and *in vivo* findings more compatible in terms of doses/concentrations. In addition, poor bioavailability of HT appears to be biologically less relevant when taking into account its bioactivation. However, these results have not been reproduced in other studies and chemical mechanisms behind scavenging activities of metabolites remain an enigma.

Alternatively, it may be considered that some conjugates of phenolic compounds may behave as carriers of free forms of phenolic compounds to target tissues — the "depot hypothesis." Within this hypothesis, determination of bioavailability of phenol metabolites in tissues may be more relevant than that in plasma. Data are still very scarce, even in animals, and perhaps the nature of tissue metabolites may be different from that of blood metabolites. The proportion of free aglycons in some tissues can differ from that observed in blood (D'Angelo et al., 2001); this may be explained by a specific uptake of aglycon or intracellular deconjugation. This last hypothesis implies that anionic conjugates could be transported across plasma membranes via carrier systems, as has been shown for acyl-glucuronides (Sallustio et al., 2000). Furthermore, β-glucuronidase is located in the lumen of the endoplasmic reticulum in various organs, which could be reached by phenol glucuronides. β-Glucuronidase is also present in lysosomes of several cells, from which the enzyme can be released under some particular conditions such as an oxidative stress situation. Situations that decrease pH promote hydrolysis of phenol glucuronides because the activity of β-glucuronidase is optimal at pH 4–5 and it is reduced ninefold at neutral pH (Sperker et al., 1997). β-Glucuronidase activity can increase in some physiopathologic states, such as inflammation or cancer, with a concomitant *in situ* deconjugation of phenol metabolites.

6.1.3 Metabolic Disposition in Humans

In a pioneering experiment on the bioavailability and disposition of olive oil phenolic compounds in humans (Visioli et al., 2000b), HT and T were spiked to a poor-phenolic content olive oil and administered to healthy volunteers. Preliminary conclusions, later confirmed, were that phenolic compounds are dose-dependently absorbed in humans after olive oil ingestion and that their bioavailability is extremely poor, most phenolic compounds being recovered in biological fluids as conjugates. In Visioli's study, an increase in the dose of administered phenolics increased the proportion of their conjugation with glucuronic acid. Phenolic compounds, particularly those bearing a catechol group, are typically biotransformed by three enzymatic systems: catechol-*O*-methyltransferase (COMT), sulfatases (SULT), and glucuronosyltransferases (UDGPT). Depending on the dose and the availability of co-factors the proportion of methyl, sulfate, and glucuronide conjugates varies among subjects.

Preliminary studies were performed, as stated earlier, with olive oils spiked with free phenols; further studies on the olive oil phenolic compound bioavailability (Miró-Casas et al., 2001, 2003a, b) were performed with extra virgin olive oil. After administering 25 ml of extra virgin oil (with an estimated content of HT of 49.3 mg/l or 1.2 mg administered), HT plasma concentrations peaked at 30 min and those of HVAL at 50 min. Plasma peak concentrations were about 25 ng/ml for HT and 4 ng/ml for HVAL. The estimated half-life for HT was 3 h after fitting plasma concentrations with a mono-compartimental model. Plasma concentrations declined, most probably following a bi-compartimental model (some missing data points prevented the application of this model), and at 8 h HT concentrations could not be distinguished from background. It cannot be discarded that there is a partial enterohepatic recirculation of HT conjugates. HT and HVAL were analyzed in their free and conjugated forms (both in plasma and urine), and it was estimated that more than 98% of these compounds were in their conjugated forms, mainly glucuronides, confirming previous findings. In urine, HT and HVAL concentrations peaked in the collection period 0–2 h (Miró-Casas et al., 2003a). Figure 6.1 displays results obtained after ingestion of a single dose of high-phenolic-content olive oil.

In a second experiment, extra virgin olive oil (25 ml) with three increasing concentrations of polyphenols — high (486 mg/kg of olive oil), moderate (133 mg/kg), and low (10 mg/kg) — were administered on 4 consecutive days. Plasma and urinary levels of phenolic compounds (HT, T, and HVAL) increased significantly in a dose-dependent manner. An increase in plasma concentrations of T and HT was observed from day 1 and 4, mainly at postprandial state, which could reflect an increased "pool" of phenolic compounds (Weinbrenner et al., 2004b). This observation was reproduced in a clinical trial where healthy volunteers were administered with a single dose of 50 ml extra virgin olive oil, and later with repeated doses of 25 ml of the same oil during a 1-week period. The mean recovery values for HT after sustained doses were 1.5-fold higher than those obtained after a single 50-ml dose (Miró-Casas et al., 2003b).

Most bioavailability studies on olive oil phenols have measured total HT and T concentrations in blood or urine after acidic or enzymatic treatment of the samples. There is a lack of studies in which glucuronide and sulfate conjugates of HT and T in biological samples were measured. Recently, our group has succeeded in the synthesis of the main HT, T, and HVAL glucuronide conjugates using porcine liver microsomes, and quantitative analytical methods are under development for their detection in biological fluids (Khymenets et al., 2006).

6.1.4   OLIVE OIL PHENOLIC COMPOUNDS AS BIOMARKERS OF OLIVE OIL INGESTION

The potential of using urinary concentrations of phenolic compounds as biomarkers of olive ingestion, and more interestingly as biomarkers of treatment compliance in nutritional intervention

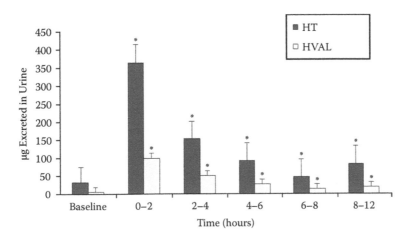

FIGURE 6.1   Hydroxytyrosol and homovanillyl alcohol in urine after the ingestion of 40 ml of an olive oil with high phenolic content (366 mg/kg). * = P < 0.05 vs. baseline.

studies, has been investigated. The fact that HT and T urinary recoveries are dependent on the phenolic content of the olive oil administered, after doses compatible with dietary habits, confirms the usefulness of these compounds as biomarkers of compliance in clinical trials. With regard to the dose-effect relationship, 24-h urinary T seems to be a better biomarker of sustained and moderate doses of virgin olive oil consumption than HT (Miró-Casas et al., 2003b). This is mainly due to the cross-metabolism between HT and dopamine. Both HT and T urinary concentrations have been used, and are currently in use, in nutritional intervention studies as biomarkers of treatment compliance (Covas et al., 2006a, b; Fitó et al., 2007b).

6.1.5 BINDING OF OLIVE OIL PHENOLIC COMPOUNDS AND THEIR METABOLITES TO HUMAN LIPOPROTEINS

The susceptibility of low density lipoproteins (LDL) to oxidation depends not only on their fatty acid content, but also on LDL antioxidant content (i.e., vitamin E and polyphenols) bound to the LDL (Fuller and Jialal, 1994). Phenolic compounds that could bind LDL would likely perform their peroxyl scavenging activity in the arterial intima, where full LDL oxidation occurs in microdomains sequestered from the richness of antioxidants present in plasma (Steinberg et al., 1989; Witzum et al., 1994).

Several reports converge on the ability of olive oil phenolic compounds to protect lipoproteins against oxidation (Grignaffini et al., 1994; Wiseman et al., 1996; Stupans et al., 2002). Some reports have provided evidence that the incorporation of phenolic compounds and their metabolites in lipoproteins may explain their protective antioxidant effects. In a first study, T and HT were recovered in all lipoprotein fractions, except in very low density lipoproteins (VLDL), with concentrations peaking between 1 and 2 h after olive oil ingestion (Bonanome et al., 2000). In other studies, not only T and HT, but also several metabolites were identified in LDL: HT monoglucuronide, HT monosulfate, T glucuronide, T sulfate, and homovanillic acid sulfate (de la Torre-Carbot et al., 2006, 2007). In addition, the concentration of total phenolic compounds in LDL has been shown to be directly correlated with the phenolic concentration of olive oils and with the resistance of LDL to their *in vitro* oxidation (Gimeno et al., 2007). At postprandial state, after ingestion of a virgin olive oil with high phenolic content (366 mg/kg of olive oil), the phenolic content of LDL directly correlated with the plasma concentrations of T and HT (Covas et al., 2006a). The nature of the bond between LDL and phenolic compounds, including olive oil phenolic compounds and their metabolites, deserves further investigation due to the physiopathological implications involved.

6.2 ANTIOXIDANT EFFECT OF OLIVE OIL PHENOLIC COMPOUNDS IN HUMANS

6.2.1 OXIDATIVE STRESS, OXIDATIVE DAMAGE, AND OLIVE OIL PHENOLIC COMPOUNDS

Oxidative stress is defined as an imbalance between the oxidant and antioxidant systems of the body, in favor of the oxidants (Sies, 1997). The oxidant systems are free radicals, molecules, or molecular fragments containing one or more unpaired electrons (Valko et al., 2007). Radicals derived from oxygen, including the so-called reactive oxygen species (ROS), such as the superoxide anion or the hydroxyl radical, represent the most important class of free radical species, and are produced in normal aerobic metabolism (Gutteridge, 1995; Sies, 1997; Valko et al., 2007). Several situations such as infection, inflammation, ultraviolet radiation, and tobacco smoke can increase free radical production. Free radicals can interact with fatty acids, thus forming peroxyl and alkoxyl radicals, and also with nitric oxide, proteins, and transition metals, such as iron and copper, resulting in new radical molecules (Gutteridge, 1995). Targets for free radicals are lipids, deoxyribonucleic acid (DNA), and proteins (Gutteridge, 1995; Sies, 1997; Valko et al., 2007). If a fatty acid is damaged by free radicals it becomes a free radical itself setting up a chain reaction of lipid peroxidation (Gutteridge, 1995; Valko et al, 2007). Oxidation of the lipid part (Steinberg et al., 1989), or directly of the apolipoprotein (apo) B of the LDL particle (Hazen and Heinecke, 1997), leads to a change in the lipoprotein conformation by which the LDL is better able to enter into the monocyte/macrophage system of the arterial wall, and develop the atherosclerotic process (Witzum, 1994). The modified apoB has immunogenic properties prompting the generation of auto-antibodies against oxidized LDL (Steinberg et al., 1989). In addition, 3-chloro- and nitro-tyrosine generation, via myeloperoxidase activity, in high density lipoproteins (HDL) converts the lipoprotein in a pro-inflammatory HDL, and reduces its capacity to remove cholesterol from cells (Fogelman, 2004). Nucleic acids are also targets for free radicals. Oxidative stress leads to a plethora of mutagenic DNA lesions in purines, pyrimidines, deoxyribose, and DNA single- and double-strand breaks (Poulsen et al., 1998; Whiteman et al., 2002). Accumulation of mutations from oxidative DNA damage is considered to be a crucial step in human carcinogenesis (Poulsen et al., 1998; Evans et al., 2004). Oxidative stress produced by free radicals has been linked to the development of several diseases such as cardiovascular, cancer, and neurodegenerative diseases, and also with the process of ageing (Witzum, 1994; Southom and Powis, 1998).

The biological oxidative effects of free radicals on lipids, DNA, and proteins are controlled by a wide spectrum of enzymatic antioxidants, such as the scavenger enzymes superoxide dismutase and glutathione peroxidase (GSH-Px), and nonenzymatic antioxidants, such as vitamin E and glutathione (Gutteridge, 1995; Valko et al., 2007). Some nonenzymatic antioxidants provided by diet, such as vitamins C and E, and phenolic compounds, may be key factors in the pathogenesis of oxidative stress-related disorders (Southom and Powis, 1998; Valko et al., 2007). As has been referred to in previous chapters, olive oil is the primary source of fat in the Mediterranean diet, and it is a functional food that besides having a high level of monounsaturated fatty acid (MUFA), the oleic acid, contains multiple minor components with biological properties. In most human studies, oleate-rich LDL have been shown to be less susceptible to oxidation than linoleate-rich LDL. Some studies performed from 1991–2004 on this topic are referred to in a recently reported review (Lapointe et al., 2006). In only 2 of the 14 studies referred to (Lapointe et al., 2006) did MUFA-rich diets not promote a higher resistance of LDL to oxidation compared with polyunsaturated fatty acids (PUFA)-rich ones.

Among olive oil minor components, the phenolic compounds have been the focus of intensive research in recent years, and are the best-studied olive oil minor components, particularly their antioxidant properties. In experimental studies, olive oil phenolics have been shown to have antioxidant effects, greater than those of vitamin E, on lipids and DNA oxidation (Visioli et al., 1995; De la Puerta et al., 1999; Fitó et al., 2000; Owen et al., 2000; Masella et al., 2004). Olive oil phenolic compounds have also been shown to be able to prevent endothelial dysfunction by decreasing expression of cell adhesion molecules (Carluccio et al., 2003), increasing nitric oxide (NO) production and inducible nitric oxide synthase (Moreno, 2003), and scavenging vascular endothelium intracellular free radicals (Massaro et al., 2002). Also, olive oil phenolic compounds inhibited platelet-induced aggregation (Petroni et al., 1995) and enhanced the mRNA transcription of the scavenger enzyme GSH-Px. Controversial results, however, have been obtained on this last issue depending on the tissue in which the gene expression was evaluated (Quiles et al., 2002; Masella et al., 2004). Other potential benefits include a chemopreventive activity (Owen et al., 2000). In experimental studies, olive oil phenolic compounds, like other plant-derived polyphenols (Vinson et al., 1995), counteracted the metal-, radical-, and macrophage-mediated oxidation of lipids and LDL (Visioli et al., 1995; Fitó et al., 2000; Masella et al., 2004). In animal models, olive oil phenolics retained their antioxidant properties *in vivo* (Visioli et al., 2000c) and delayed the progression of atherosclerosis (Aviram, 1996). The administration of high doses of HT (10 mg/kg/day) to apoE-deficient mice, however, enhanced the atherosclerotic lesion development (Acín et al., 2006). This fact points out the importance of the matrix and that of the combination of all antioxidants present in natural foods such as olive oil.

A large number of studies, both in experimental models and in humans, have been performed on the antioxidant capacity of olive oil phenolic compounds. However, the precepts of Evidence-Based Medicine require first-level scientific evidence to be provided before nutritional recommendations for the general public are formulated (Wolff et al., 1990). The scientific evidence required is provided by randomized, controlled, double-blind clinical trials (level I of Evidence) and to some extent by large cohort studies (level II of Evidence). Basic research, despite its usefulness in permitting a mechanistic approach to be adopted, does not provide evidence for nutritional recommendations. Of course, the level of evidence of a particular study depends not only on its type of design but also on the quality of the study (external and internal validity, homogeneity of the sample, and statistical power). Finally, evidence is built by agreement of results of several similar studies (Wolff et al., 1990; Goodman, 1993). Here we summarize the state of the art of the body of knowledge and the extent to which we, the scientific community, have evidence of antioxidant benefits of olive oil phenolic compounds in humans.

6.2.2 Postprandial Studies on the Antioxidant Effect in Humans of Olive Oil Phenolic Compounds

After a fatty meal postprandial lipemia occurs (Roche et al., 1998). Postprandial lipemia is recognized as a risk factor for atherosclerosis development as it is, together with postprandial hyperglycemia, associated with oxidative changes (Roche and Gibney, 2000). After an oral load of 50 ml of virgin olive oil an oxidative stress occurs in plasma, reflected in an increase of lipid peroxides and in a decrease of activities of antioxidant scavenger enzymes GSH-Px and glutathione reductase (Fitó et al., 2002). A decrease of antioxidant defenses with an increase of lipid oxidation is a common feature in an increased oxidative status situation (Ruíz et al., 1999). Oxidized chylomicrons and triacylglycerol-rich VLDL produced in the postprandial phase may be a metabolic factor involved in injury of the arterial wall, and may also constitute a potential link between postprandial lipemia and atherogenesis (Cohn, 1998). In our experience, postprandial triacylglycerol–rich VLDL are prone to oxidation after 50 ml of virgin olive oil ingestion in healthy humans (Figure 6.2). Postprandial triglyceride enrichment of VLDL has been shown to correlate with postprandial oxidative stress in type 2 diabetic patients (Evans et al., 2000), and postprandial remnant-like protein particles

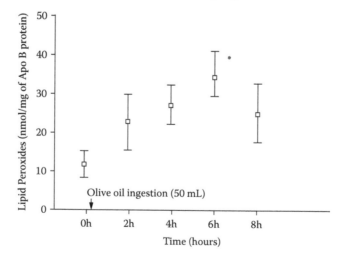

FIGURE 6.2 Time course of lipid peroxides formation in very low density lipoproteins (VLDL) after ingestion of 50 ml of virgin olive oil. P = 0.007 for quadratic trend, general linear model. * = P < 0.05 from baseline. (Adapted from Fitó, M. et al., 2002, *Lipids*, 37, 245–251.)

have been shown to increase intracellular oxidant levels, thus impairing endothelial function (Doi et al., 2000).

Some studies have examined the postprandial effect of olive oil phenolic compounds on biomarkers of oxidative stress. Some of them did not report changes at the postprandial state, neither of the *ex vivo* susceptibility of LDL to oxidation (Nicolaïew et al., 1998; Bonanome et al., 2000; Vissers et al., 2004) nor of the *in vivo* measurements of oxidized LDL and DNA oxidation (Weinbrenner et al., 2004b) after ingestion of olive oils providing from 0–100 mg of phenolic compounds. The ingestion of 50 ml of virgin olive oil enhanced total plasma antioxidant capacity (Bonanome et al., 2000), while ingestion of 25 ml of low phenolic content (10 mg/kg) olive oil reduced the activity of the antioxidant scavenger enzyme GSH-Px (Weinbrenner et al., 2004a). In this last bioavailability study (Weinbrenner et al., 2004a), reduction in GSH-Px activity was not observed after ingestion of 25 ml of olive oil with medium (133 mg/kg) and high (486 mg/kg) phenolic content (Figure 6.3). The reduction of GSH-Px activity after ingestion of olive oil with low phenolic content could reflect consumption of enzyme when counteracting the postprandial lipid oxidation, due to lack of phenolic compounds in olive oil (Weinbrenner et al., 2004a). Visioli et al. (2000a) described a decrease in urinary F2-isoprostanes, considered to be the best systemic markers of oxidative damage, after a 50-ml dose of olive oil enriched with T and HT. After 4 days of sustained consumption (25 ml/day), a decrease in postprandial levels of circulating oxidized LDL and DNA oxidation has been reported after ingestion of a single 25-ml dose of a high phenolic content olive oil (486 mg/kg). This effect was not observed after the same dose of olive oil with medium (133 mg/kg) or low phenolic content (10 mg/kg) (Weinbrenner et al., 2004b).

The results of the postprandial studies performed are difficult to evaluate and compare because some studies do not mention whether postprandial lipemia and/or hyperglycemia occurs (Visioli et al., 2000a; Vissers et al., 2004), while in other studies neither hyperlipemia nor hyperglycemia occurs after olive oil ingestion (Nicolaïew et al., 1998; Bonanome et al., 2000; Weinbrenner et al., 2004a, b). In our experience, ingestion of a 25-ml olive oil dose did not promote postprandial oxidative stress with independence of phenolic content of the olive oil (Weinbrenner et al., 2004a,b), whereas single doses of 40 (Covas et al., 2006a) and 50 ml did (Fitó et al., 2002) (Figure 6.2).

With olive oil doses at which oxidative stress occurs, data from randomized, crossover, controlled studies in humans show: (1) an increase in serum antioxidant capacity after virgin olive oil ingestion, but not after ordinary olive oil, in comparison with corn oil, suggesting a role for phenolic compounds of virgin olive oil (Bogani et al., 2007); and (2) the phenolic content of an olive oil modulates the degree of lipid and LDL oxidation, the lipid oxidative damage being lower after high- than after low-phenolic content olive oil ingestion (Ruano et al., 2005; Covas et al., 2006a).

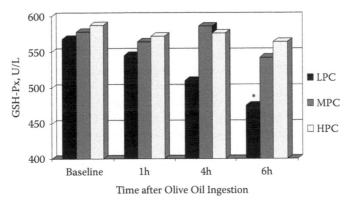

FIGURE 6.3 Activity of glutathione peroxidase (GSH-Px) after ingestion of olive oil with low (10 mg/kg, LPC), medium (133 mg/kg, MPC), and high (486 mg/kg, HPC) phenolic content. * = P < 0.05 vs. baseline.

6.2.3 STUDIES ON ANTIOXIDANT EFFECT IN HUMANS OF SUSTAINED CONSUMPTION OF OLIVE OIL PHENOLIC COMPOUNDS

Considerable differences exist among the randomized, crossover, controlled studies performed in humans to assess the effects of sustained consumption of phenolic compounds provided by olive oil (Covas et al., 2006c). These differences are reflected not only in the length of the intervention periods, from 4 days to 8 weeks, but also in the experimental design, control of diet, sample population, age of participants, sample size, measurement of markers of compliance of the intervention, and in sensitivity and specificity of the oxidative stress biomarkers evaluated (Fitó et al., 2007a). Table 6.1 shows a summary of the randomized, crossover, controlled studies performed to date in healthy volunteers. Concerning lipid oxidative damage, in four studies performed up to 2002 with healthy volunteers, there was no evidence that consumption of phenolic compounds from dietary olive oil accounted for benefits on *ex vivo* susceptibility of LDL to oxidation (Nicolaïew et al., 1998; Bonanome et al., 2000; Vissers et al., 2001; Moschandreas et al., 2002). In two studies *in vivo* biomarkers such as plasma malondialdehyde (MDA), lipid peroxides (LPO), and protein carbonyls (PC) were also evaluated without any effect being identified that could be attributed to the phenolic content of olive oil (Vissers et al., 2001; Moschandreas et al., 2002). Most recently, two further studies (Marrugat et al., 2004; Weinbrenner et al., 2004b) reported protective effects of olive oil phenols on *in vivo* circulating oxidized LDL, MDA in urine, DNA oxidation, plasma GSH-Px (Table 6.1), and also in HDL cholesterol levels in healthy male subjects. No changes in F2-isoprostanes were observed. Despite the differences in length of intervention periods among the two studies, from 4 days (Weinbrenner et al., 2004b) to 3 weeks (Marrugat et al., 2004), there was a similar approach in experimental design. Subjects were subjected to a strict very low-antioxidant diet in both washout and intervention periods (Weinbrenner et al., 2004b), or to a controlled diet in all the study in order to avoid a high antioxidant consumption (Marrugat et al., 2004). Low-phenolic olive oil was used for cooking purposes during intervention periods, and for all purposes during washout periods, in both studies. This fact permitted homogenization of both the main fat ingestion of participants and that of LDL fatty acid content (Marrugat et al., 2004; Weinbrenner et al., 2004b).

Concerning DNA oxidation, the most abundant DNA modification is hydroxylation of guanine in the 8-position to 8-oxo-deoxyguanosine (8-dG) (Kasai, 1997). Urinary excretion of 8-dG is advocated as a biomarker of whole body DNA oxidation (Poulsen, 2005). As has been previously referred to, the protective effects of olive oil phenolics on *in vivo* DNA oxidation, measured as 8-dGuo in mononuclear cells and in urine, were found in healthy male subjects in a short-term study in which participants were submitted to a very low antioxidant diet (Weinbrenner et al., 2004b). A protective effect on DNA oxidation, measured by the comet assay in peripheral blood lymphocytes, has also been reported in postmenopausal women (Salvini et al., 2006). The intake of ω6-PUFA has been associated with an increase of etheno-DNA adducts, another marker of DNA oxidation, in urine (Hanaoka et al., 2002) and in white blood cells (Nair et al., 1997) in female subjects. In contrast, consumption of 25 ml/day of virgin olive oil during 3 weeks did not modify urinary excretion of etheno-DNA adducts in healthy volunteers (Hillestrøm et al., 2006).

As pointed out in the Consensus Report made by the Expert Panel in the International Conference of Olive Oil and Health held in Jaen, Spain, October 2004 (Pérez-Jimenez et al., 2004; Covas et al., 2006c), the protective effects of olive oil phenolic compounds on oxidative damage in humans are better displayed in situations in which participants are submitted to oxidative stress conditions (males, males submitted to a low antioxidant diet, post-menopausal females). In this sense, all randomized, crossover, controlled studies with patients in which an enhanced oxidative stress status has been reported (Moriel et al., 2000; Weinbrenner et al., 2003; Mueller et al., 2004) showed a protective effect of olive oil phenolic compounds on oxidative damage (Table 6.2) (Ramírez-Tortosa et al., 1999; Fitó et al., 2005; Ruano et al., 2005; Visioli et al., 2005). This can be explained by the fact that the balance of pro-oxidant and antioxidant reactions is well regulated in the body. For this reason, an intervention with an antioxidant-rich compound without any oxidative stress involved

TABLE 6.1

Sustained Effects due to Olive Oil Phenolic Compounds Consumption on Oxidative Biomarkers in Randomized, Crossover, Controlled Studies in Healthy Volunteers

Intervention	Subjects (n, sex)	Intervention Period	Washout Period	Baseline Adjustment	Compliance Biomarkers	Oxidative Markers	Effects	Ref.
Virgin olive oil vs. oleic acid-rich sunflower oil[a]	10 (men)	3 weeks	1 week with usual diet	No	No	LDL resistance to oxidation	Decrease of dienes	Nicolaïew et al., 1998
Virgin olive oil (50 g/day)	14 (4 men) 10 (women)	4 weeks	4 weeks[b]	No	No	LDL resistance to oxidation	None	Bonanome et al., 2000
High-phenol vs. low-phenol olive oil (69 g/d)	46 (15 men) 31 women	3 weeks	2 weeks without olives and olive oil	Nc	No	LDL resistance to oxidation MDA, FRAP, LPO, PC	None (all markers)	Vissiers et al., 2001
High-phenol vs. low-phenol olive oil (70 g/d, raw)	25 (11 men) 14 (women)	3 weeks	2 weeks without olives and olive oil	Nc	No	LDL resistance to oxidation MDA, FRAP, LPO, PC	None (all markers)	Moschandreas et al., 2002
Virgin vs. ordinary vs. refined olive oil (25 mL/d, raw)	30 (men)	3 weeks with refined olive oil	2 weeks with refined olive oil for cooking for raw and cooking purposes	Yes	Yes	LDL resistance to oxidation, circulating oxidized LDL OLAB	Increase with olive oil phenolics Decrease with olive oil phenolics None	Marrugat et al., 2004
High vs. medium vs low phenol olive oil (25 mL/d, raw)	12 (men)	4 days with refined olive oil for cooking very low-antioxidant diet	10 days with refined olive oil for all purposes; very low-antioxidant diet	Yes	Yes	In vivo oxidized LDL MDA in urine 8dG in urine and lymphocytes F2 isoprostanes Glutathione peroxidase	Decrease with olive oil phenol content (all markers) None Increase with olive oil phenolics	Weinbrenner et al., 2004b
High vs. low phenol virgin olive oil	10 women, menopause	8 weeks	4 weeks usual diet	Yes	No	Comet assay	Decrease in DNA oxidation with olive oil phenolics	Salvini et al., 2006
Virgin vs. ordinary vs. refined olive oil	200 men[d]	3 weeks	3 weeks without olives and olive oil	Yes	Yes	In vivo oxidized LDL Uninduced dienes Hydroxy fatty acids F2-isoprostans Antioxidant enzymes GSH/GSSG	Decrease with olive oil phenolics None	Covas et al., 2006b

(continued)

TABLE 6.1 (continued)

Sustained Effects due to Olive Oil Phenolic Compounds Consumption on Oxidative Biomarkers in Randomized, Crossover, Controlled Studies in Healthy Volunteers

Intervention	Subjects (n, sex)	Intervention Period	Washout Period	Baseline Adjustment	Compliance Biomarkers	Oxidative Markers	Effects	Ref.
Virgin vs. ordinary vs. refined olive	200 men[d]	3 weeks	3 weeks without olives and olive oil	Yes	Yes	8-dG in urine	Decrease non-related with olive oil phenolics	Machowetz et al., 2007
28 (men)[d]	Virgin vs. common vs. refined olive oil	3 weeks	3 weeks without olives and olive oil	Yes	Yes	8-oxo-guanosine 8-oxo-guanine Etheno-DNA adducts in urine	None None None	Hillestrøm et al., 2006

[a] Nondefined quantity ingested with meals.

[b] Characteristics of the washout period not defined.

[c] Olive oil ingested in sauces and baked products.

[d] The EUROLIVE study.

MDA, malondialdehyde; FRAP, ferric reducing ability of plasma; LPO, lipid peroxides; PC, protein carbonyl; OLAB, antibodies against oxidized LDL; 8-dG, 8-oxo-deoxyguanosine in urine.

TABLE 6.2

Antioxidant Effects of Phenolic Compounds from Olive Oil in Randomized, Crossover, Controlled Studies in Patients with High Oxidative Status

Intervention	Subjects (n, sex)	Intervention Period	Washout Period	Baseline Adjustment	Compliance Markers	Oxidative Markers	Effects	Ref.
Virgin vs. refined olive oil (all purposes)	Peripheral vascular disease patients (24, men)	3 months, usual diet	3 months, usual diet	No	No	Lipid peroxides in LDL Macrophase plasma oxidized LDL uptake	Decrease with olive oil phenol content (all markers)	Ramírez-Tortosa et al., 1999
Virgin vs. refined (raw) (40 mL/day)	Hyperlipemic (22) (12 men; 10 women)	7 weeks usual diet	4 weeks with usual diet	Yes	No	Plasma total antioxidant capacity F2-isoprostanes	Increase with olive oil phenol content None	Visioli et al., 2005
Virgin vs. refined olive oil (50 mL/day, raw)	Coronary heart disease patients (40 men)	3 weeks with refined olive oil for cooking for all purposes	2 weeks with refined olive oil for all purposes	Yes	Yes	Circulating oxidized LDL Lipid peroxides Glutathione peroxidase	Decrease with olive oil phenol content (all markers) Increase with olive oil phenol content	Fitó et al., 2005
Meal with high phenol vs. phenol olive oil	Hyper-cholesterolemic (18 men)	Single dose (postprandial)	1 week	No	No	Lipid peroxides	Decrease with olive oil phenol content	Ruano et al., 2005

may exert only a marginal effect that could not be detected with the current state of the art of the oxidative biomarkers.

The Consensus Report previously referred to (Pérez-Jimenez et al., 2004; Covas et al., 2006c) also pointed out that not only carefully controlled but large sample size trials would be needed in order to assess the *in vivo* antioxidant effect in humans of phenolic compounds from olive oil. The reason is that only modest changes in biomarkers are expected after administration of real-life doses of a single food, which in turn cannot be consumed in great quantities per day such as raw olive oil. The results of the recently delivered EUROLIVE study (Covas et al., 2006b) confirmed this statement. The EUROLIVE (Effect of olive oil consumption on oxidative damage in European populations) study was a large, randomized, crossover, multicenter clinical trial performed in 200 individuals from 5 European countries. Participants were randomly assigned to receive 25 ml/day of three similar olive oils, but with differences in their phenolic content (2.7, 164, and 366 mg/kg of olive oil), in intervention periods of 3 weeks preceded by 2-week washout periods. All olive oils increased the HDL-cholesterol and the ratio between reduced and oxidized forms of glutathione (Table 6.1). The antioxidant activity of HDL on LDL lipid peroxidation is well known (Fogelman et al., 2004), and reduced glutathione is a major mechanism for cellular protection against oxidative stress (Hayes and McLellan, 1999). In the EUROLIVE study, consumption of medium- and high-phenolic content olive oil decreased lipid oxidative damage biomarkers such as plasma-oxidized LDL, uninduced conjugated dienes (a measure of polyunsaturated fatty acid oxidation), and hydroxy fatty acids (a measure of the unsaturated fatty acids oxidation), without changes in F_2-isoprostanes. The increase in HDL cholesterol and the decrease in the lipid oxidative damage were dose-dependently related to phenolic content of olive oil consumed (Table 6.1). The results of the EUROLIVE study have provided evidence of: (1) the *in vivo* protective role of phenolic compounds from olive oil on lipid cardiovascular risk factors, including lipid oxidative damage, in humans at real-life olive oil doses (Covas et al., 2006b); and (2) the fact that olive oil is more than a MUFA fat.

Also, results of the EUROLIVE study showed that consumption of 25 ml of olive oil per day during 3 weeks reduced DNA oxidation in 182 healthy males, as measured by the 24-h urinary excretion of 8dG, irrespective of the olive oil phenolic content (Machowetz et al., 2007). It must be pointed out that the decrease in oxidative damage to DNA after olive oil consumption observed in the EUROLIVE study, in spite of the consistency of the results through three randomized intervention periods, was evaluated on a linear basis due to lack of a placebo group other than the low phenolic olive oil group. From the EUROLIVE results, olive oil phenolic compounds do not contribute in reducing levels of urinary 8dG in healthy males. The role of phenolic compounds from olive oil on DNA oxidative damage remains controversial, and perhaps more sensitive methods would be required to detect differences among types of olive oil consumed. As has been previously mentioned, the protective role of olive oil phenolic compounds on DNA oxidative damage has been displayed in studies, but with low sample size, where DNA oxidative damage was measured in mononuclear cells or lymphocytes from peripheral blood (Weinbrenner et al., 2004b; Salvini et al., 2006). There is still a debate concerning the best method for DNA oxidative damage measurement, steady-state levels of 8dG in lymphocytes being considered at present the best biomarker for oxidative damage to DNA (Thompson, 2004). Unfortunately this method is difficult to apply in large sample size intervention studies. Further studies are required to establish the effect of olive oil and its phenolic compounds on oxidative damage to DNA vs. other types of fat in potential target populations (i.e., smokers, postmenopausal females, diabetic patients, etc.).

6.3 KEY POINTS FOR FUTURE RESEARCH ON THE ANTIOXIDANT EFFECT OF OLIVE OIL PHENOLIC COMPOUNDS IN HUMANS

6.3.1 OXIDATIVE MARKERS

The protective effect of olive oil phenolic compounds on lipid oxidative damage is established. However, further clinical studies with individuals who are prone to oxidative stress are required in order to determine which are the population groups in which ingestion of phenolic compounds from olive oil could provide the greatest benefits. Oxidative damage to DNA also deserves to be explored in both healthy individuals and target populations with high sensitive biomarkers. The human clinical trials to be performed are those capable of providing first-level evidence, the randomized, controlled ones with an appropriate sample size (Wolff et al., 1990; Goodman, 1993). To be crossover in design is not mandatory for a clinical trial in order to provide evidence. However, the crossover design requires a smaller sample size than the parallel design, and also permits the same participants to be included in different interventions with several types of olive oils, thus minimizing interferences with other possible confounder variables (Senn, 2002).

6.3.2 OXIDATIVE STRESS–ASSOCIATED PROCESSES

Besides oxidative damage markers, biomarkers related to oxidative stress–associated processes must be explored. Oxidative stress and lipid oxidation are linked with other atherosclerosis-associated processes such as inflammation and endothelial dysfunction. Oxidized lipids, through NFκB-like transcription factors, initiate an inflammatory response that leads to the development of the fatty streak (Berliner et al., 1995). The anti-inflammatory properties of olive oil as monounsaturated fat, and those of the phenolic compounds from olive oil, have been displayed in several experimental models and in some human studies, and have been reviewed recently (López-Miranda et al., 2006; Covas, 2007). The anti-inflammatory effects of olive oil and its phenolic compounds consumption in humans is a promising field, and further studies are required to obtain full evidence on the topic. Oxidative stress and LDL oxidation are also related with endothelial dysfunction and hypertension (Cai and Harrison, 2000; Guzik et al., 2002). Some data exist concerning possible benefits in humans of phenolic compounds from olive oil on both systolic blood pressure and endothelial dysfunction markers, linked with a concomitant reduction in oxidative lipid damage (Fitó et al., 2005; Ruano et al., 2005), as well as on inflammatory markers (Fitó et al., 2007c). The effect of olive oil phenolic compounds on oxidative stress–associated markers, which in turn are risk factors for disease, deserves to be explored.

6.3.3 NUTRITIONAL INTERVENTIONS

We must underline some key characteristics required for nutritional intervention studies in humans on antioxidant effects of phenolic compounds or other minor components. First, a dietary control of washout and intervention periods, primarily of the type of fat ingested, must be carried out. The type of fat ingested influences oxidative damage to lipids (Reaven et al., 1994) and can be an important confounder in the assessment of effects of phenolic compounds from olive oil. Second, adjustment of the end-point values of the biomarkers for the baseline of each intervention period must be performed. In general, as far as baseline values are concerned, the statistical treatment of the results in crossover trials is limited to an adjustment for values at the beginning of the study that are considered a sole baseline for all intervention periods (Senn, 2002). However, when dealing with dietary components and oxidative damage, from beginning to end of a crossover study, there is a long time span for interferences with other confounding variables. Oxidative stress is a short-term response to several stimuli that influence steady-state balance, and biological variability of oxidative stress markers is high (Sen, 1995; Halliwell and Whiteman, 2004). Third, measurement in urine of phenolic compounds from olive oil, such as T and HT, as compliance markers of intervention, is essential. In our experience in the EUROLIVE (Covas et al., 2006b; Machowetz et al., 2007) and other olive oil sustained consumption studies (Marrugat et al., 2004; Weinbrenner et al., 2004b; Fitó et al., 2005, 2007c; Covas et al., 2006a, b) some participants may identify low phenolic content olive oil or very high phenolic content by the color and taste; if they do not like them, they may fail to observe full compliance with the scheduled protocol.

6.3.4 SELECTION OF BIOMARKERS

Finally, biomarkers for oxidative damage or associated processes as secondary end points for the disease must be selected on the basis of biomarker sensitivity and clinical significance. The sensitivity and specificity of some tests and *ex vivo* measurements for lipid and LDL oxidation are currently questioned (Halliwell and Whiteman, 2004). Markers to be selected are preferentially those that have been shown to be predictors for an oxidative stress–associated disease in large sample size cohort studies (or if not available in case-control studies), such as *in vivo* plasma-oxidized LDL or urinary F_2-isoprostanes (Schwedhelm et al., 2004; Shimada et al., 2004).

REFERENCES

Acín, S., Navarro, M.A., Arbonés-Manar, J.M., Guillén, N., Sarría, A.J., Carnicer, R., et al., 2006, Hydroxytyrosol administration enhances atherosclerotic lesion development in ApoE deficient mice, *J. Biochem. (Tokyo)*, 140, 383–391.

Aviram, M., 1996, Interaction of oxidized low density lipoprotein with macrophages in atherosclerosis, and the antiatherogenicity of antioxidants, *Eur. J. Clin. Chem. Clin. Biochem.*, 34, 599–608.

Bazoti, F.N., Gikas, E., Puel, C., Coxam, V., and Tsarbopoulos, A., 2005, Development of a sensitive and specific solid phase extraction–gas chromatography–tandem mass spectrometry method for the determination of elenolic acid, hydroxytyrosol, and tyrosol in rat urine, *J. Agric. Food Chem.*, 53, 6213–6221.

Berliner, J.A., Navab, M., Fogelman, A.M., Frank, J.S., Demer, L.L., Edwards, P.A., et al., 1995, Atherosclerosis: basic mechanisms. Oxidation, inflammation, and genetics, *Circulation*, 91, 2488–2496.

Bogani, P., Galli, C., Villa, M., and Visioli, F., 2007, Postprandial anti-inflammatory and antioxidant effects of extra virgin olive oil, *Atherosclerosis,* 190, 181–186.

Bonanome, A., Pagnan, A., Caruso, D., Toia, A., Xamin, A., Fedeli, E., et al., 2000, Evidence of postprandial absorption of olive oil in humans, *Nutr. Metab. Cardiovas. Dis.,* 10, 111–120.

Cai, H. and Harrison, D.G., 2000, Endothelial dysfunction in cardiovascular diseases: the role of oxidant stress, *Circ. Res.*, 87, 840–844.

Carluccio, M.A., Siculella, L., Ancora, M.A., Massaro, M., Scoditti, E., Storelli, C., et al., 2003, Olive oil and red wine antioxidant polyphenols inhibit endothelial activation: antiatherogenic properties of the Mediterranean diet phytochemicals, *Arterioscler. Thromb. Vasc. Biol.*, 23, 622–629.

Carrasco-Pancorbo, A., Arraez-Roman, D., Segura-Carretero, A., and Fernández-Gutiérrez, A., 2006, Capillary electrophoresis-electrospray ionization-massspectrometry method to determine the phenolic fraction of extra-virgin olive oil, *Electrophoresis*, 27, 2182–2196.

Cohn, S., 1998, Postprandial lipemia: emerging evidence for atherogenicity of remnant lipoproteins, *Can. J. Cardiol.*, 14(Suppl. B), 18B–27B.

Corona, G., Tzounis, X., Assunta-Dessa, M., Deiana, M., Debnam, E.S., Visioli, F., et al., 2006, The fate of olive oil polyphenols in the gastrointestinal tract: implications of gastric and colonic microflora-dependent biotransformation, *Free Radic. Res.,* 40, 647–658.

Covas, M.I., 2007, Olive oil and the cardiovascular system, *Pharmacol. Rev.,* 55, 175–178.

Covas, M.I., de la Torre, K., Farre-Albaladejo, M., Kaikkonen, J., Fitó, M., López-Sabater, C., et al., 2006a, Postprandial LDL phenolic content and LDL oxidation are modulated by olive oil phenolic compounds in humans, *Free Rad. Biol. Med.,* 40, 608–616.

Covas, M.I., Nyyssonen, K., Poulsen, H.E., Kaikkonen, J., Zunft, H.J., Kiesewetter, H., et al., EUROLIVE Study Group, 2006b, The effect of polyphenols in olive oil on heart disease risk factors: a randomized trial, *Ann. Intern. Med.,* 145, 333–341.

Covas, M.I., Ruiz-Gutiérrez, V., de la Torre, R., Kafatos, A., Lamuela-Raventós, R., Osada, J., et al., 2006c, Minor components of olive oil: evidence to date of health benefits in humans, *Nutr. Rev.,* 64, 20–30.

D'Angelo, S., Manna, C., Migliardi, V., Mazzoni, O., Morrica, P., Capasso, G., et al., 2001, Pharmacokinetics and metabolism of hydroxytyrosol, a natural antioxidant from olive oil, *Drug Metab. Dispos.*, 11, 1492–1498.

De la Puerta, R., Ruiz Gutierrez, V., and Hoult, J.R., 1999, Inhibition of leukocyte 5-lipooxigenase by phenolics from virgin olive oil, *Biochem. Pharmacol.*, 157, 445–449.

de la Torre, R., Covas, M.I., Pujadas, M.A., Fitó, M., Farré, M., et al., 2006, Is dopamine behind the health benefits of red wine? *Eur. J. Nutr.*, 45, 307–310.

De la Torre-Carbot, K., Jauregui, O., Castellote, A.I., Lamuela-Raventós, R.M., Covas, M.I., Casals, I., et al., 2006, Rapid high-performance liquid chromatography–electrospray ionization tandem mass spectrometry method for qualitative and quantitative analysis of virgin olive oil phenolic metabolites in human low-density lipoproteins, *J. Chromatogr. A*, 1116, 69–75.

De la Torre-Carbot, K., Chavez-Servin, J.L., Jáuregui, O., Castellote, A.I., Lamuela-Raventós, R.M., Fitó, M., et al., 2007, Presence of virgin olive oil phenolic metabolites in human low density lipoprotein fraction: determination by high-performance liquid chromatography–electrospray ionization tandem mass spectrometry, *Anal. Chim. Acta*, 583, 402–410.

Del Boccio, P., Di Deo, A., De Curtis, A., Celli, N., Iacoviello, L., and Rotilio, D., 2003, Liquid chromatography–tandem mass spectrometry analysis of oleuropein and its metabolite hydroxytyrosol in rat plasma and urine after oral administration, *J. Chromatogr. B Analyt. Technol. Biomed. Life Sci.*, 785, 47–56.

Doi, H., Kugiyama, K., Oka, H., Sugiyama, S., Ogata, N., Koide, S.I., et al., 2000, Remnant lipoproteins induce proatherothrombotic molecules in endothelial cells through a redox-sensitive mechanism, *Circulation*, 102, 670–676.

Edgecombe, S.C., Stretch, G.L., and Hayball, P.J., 2000, Oleuropein, an antioxidant polyphenol from olive oil, is poorly absorbed from isolated perfused rat intestine, *J. Nutr.*, 130, 2996–3002.

Evans, M., Anderson, R.A., Graham, J.B., Ellis, G.R., Morris, K., Davies, S., et al., 2000, Ciprofibrate therapy improves endothelial function and reduces postprandial lipemia and oxidative stress in type 2 diabetes mellitus, *Circulation*, 101, 1773–1779.

Evans, M.D., Dizdaroglu, M., and Cooke, M.S., 2004, Oxidative DNA damage and disease: induction, repair and significance, *Mutat. Res.*, 567, 1–61.

Fitó, M., Covas, M.I., Lamuela-Raventós, R.M., Vila, J., Torrents, L., de la Torre, C., et al., 2000, Protective effect of olive oil and its phenolic compounds against low density lipoprotein oxidation, *Lipids*, 35, 633–638.

Fitó, M., Gimeno, E., Covas, M.I., Miró, E., López-Sabater, M.C., Farré, M., et al., 2002, Postprandial and short-term effects of dietary virgin olive oil on oxidant/antioxidant status, *Lipids*, 37, 245–251.

Fitó, M., Cladellas, M., de la Torre, R., Martí, J., Alcántara, M., Pujadas-Bastardes, M., et al., 2005, Antioxidant effect of virgin olive oil in patients with stable coronary heart disease: a randomised, crossover, controlled, clinical trial, *Atherosclerosis*, 181, 149–158.

Fitó, M., de la Torre, R., and Covas, M.I., 2007a, Olive oil and oxidative stress, *Mol. Nutr. Food Res.*, 51, 1215–1224.

Fitó, M., Guxens, M., Corella, D., Sáez, G., Estruch, R., de la Torre, R., et al., for the PREDIMED Study Investigators, 2007b, Effect of a traditional Mediterranean diet on lipoprotein oxidation: a randomized controlled trial, *Arch. Intern. Med.*, 67, 1195–1203.

Fitó, M., Cladellas, M., de la Torre, R., Martí, J., Muñoz, D., Schröder, H., et al., 2007c, Anti-inflammatory effect of virgin olive oil in stable coronary disease patients: a randomized, crossover, controlled trial, *Eur. J. Clin. Nutr.*, in press (available on PubMed.).

Fogelman, A.M., 2004, When good cholesterol goes bad, *Nature Med.*, 10, 902–903.

Fuller, C.J. and Jialal, I., 1994, Effects of antioxidants and fatty acids on low density lipoprotein oxidation, *Am. J. Clin. Nutr.*, 60, 1010–1013.

Gimeno, E., de la Torre-Carbot, K., Lamuela-Raventos, R.M., Castellote, A., Fitó, M., de la Torre, R., et al., 2007, Changes in the phenolic content of low density lipoprotein after olive oil consumption in men. A randomized crossover controlled trial, *Br. J. Nutr.*, 98, 1243–1250.

Goodman, C., 1993, Literature Searching and Evidence Interpretation for Assessing Health Care Practices, The Swedish Council of Technology Assessment in Health Care, Stockholm, Sweden.

Grignaffini, P., Roma, P., Galli, C., and Catapano, A.L., 1994, Protection of low-density lipoprotein from oxidation by 3,4-dihydroxyphenylethanol, *Lancet*, 343, 1296–1297.

Gutteridge, J.M., 1995, Lipid peroxidation and antioxidants as biomarkers of tissue damage, *Clin. Chem.*, 41, 1819–1828.

Guzik, T.J., West, N.E., Pillai, R., Taggart, D.P., and Channon, K.M., 2002, Nitric oxide modulates superoxide release and peroxynitrite formation in human blood vessels, *Hypertension*, 39, 1088–1094.

Halliwell, B. and Whiteman, M., 2004, Measuring reactive species and oxidative damage *in vivo* and in cell culture: how should you do it and what do the results mean? *Br. J. Pharmacol.*, 142, 231–255.

Hanaoka, T., Nair, J., Takahashi, Y., Sasaki, S., Bartsch, H., and Tsugane, S., 2002, Urinary level of 1,N-6-ethenodeoxyadenosine, a marker of oxidative stress, is associated with salt excretion and omega 6-polyunsaturated fatty acid intake in postmenopausal Japanese women, *Int. J. Cancer*, 100, 71–75.

Hayes, J.D. and McLellan, L.I., 1999, Glutathione and glutathione-dependent enzymes represent a coordinately regulated defence against oxidative stress, *Free Rad. Res.*, 31, 273–300.

Hazen, S.L. and Heinecke, J.W., 1997, 3-Chlorotyrosine, a specific marker of myeloperoxidase-catalyzed oxidation, is markedly elevated in low density lipoprotein isolated from human atherosclerotic intima, *J. Clin. Invest.*, 99, 2075–2081.

Hillestrøm, P.R., Covas, M.I., and Poulsen, H.E., 2006, Effect of dietary virgin olive oil on urinary excretion of etheno-DNA adducts, *Free Rad. Biol. Med.*, 41, 1133–1138.

Kasai, H., 1997, Analysis of a form of oxidative DNA damage, 8-hydroxy-2′-deoxyguanosine, as a marker of cellular oxidative stress during carcinogenesis, *Mutat. Res.*, 387, 147–163.

Khymenets, O., Joglar, J., Clapes, P., Parella, T., Covas, M.I., and de la Torre, R., 2006, Biocatalyzed synthesis and structural characterization of monoglucuronides of hydroxytyrosol, tyrosol, homovanillic alcohol, and 3-(4′-hydroxyphenyl)propanol, *Adv. Synthesis Catalysis*, 348, 2155–2162.

Lapointe, A., Couillard, C., and Lemieux, S., 2006, Effects of dietary factors on oxidation of low-density lipopropotein particles, *J. Nutr. Biochem.*, 17, 645–658.

López-Miranda, J., Badimon, L., Bonanome, A., Lairon, D., Kris-Etherton, P., Mata, P., et al., 2006, Monounsaturated fat and cardiovascular risk, *Nutr. Rev.*, 64(Suppl. 1), 2–12.

Machowetz, A., Poulsen, H.E., Gruendel, S., Weimann, A., Fitó, M., Marrugat, J., et al., 2007, Effect of olive oils on biomarkers of oxidative DNA stress in North and South Europeans, *FASEB J.*, 137, 84–87.

Manna, C., Galletti, P., Maisto, G., Cucciolla, V., D'Angelo, S., and Zappia, V., 2000, Transport mechanism and metabolism of olive oil hydroxytyrosol in Caco-2 cells, *FEBS Lett.*, 470, 341–344.

Marrugat, J., Covas, M.I., Fitó, M., Schröder, H., Miró-Casas, E., and Gimeno, E., 2004, Effects of differing phenolic content in dietary olive oils on lipids and LDL oxidation. A randomized controlled trial, *Eur. J. Nutr.*, 43, 140–147.

Masella, R., Vari, R., D'Archivio, M., Di Benedetto, R., Matarrese, P., Malorni, W., et al., 2004, Extra virgin olive oil biophenols inhibit cell-mediated oxidation of LDL by increasing the mRNA transcription of glutathione-related enzymes, *J. Nutr.*, 134, 785–791.

Massaro, M., Basta, G., Lazzerini, G., Carluccio, M.A., Bosetti, F., Solaini, G., et al., 2002, Quenching of intracellular ROS generation as a mechanism for oleate-induced reduction of endothelial activation in early atherogenesis, *Thromb. Haemost.*, 88, 335–344.

Mateos, R., Espartero, J.L., Trujillo, M., Ríos, J.J., León-Camacho, M., Alcudia, F., et al., 2001, Determination of phenols, flavones, and lignans in virgin olive oils by solid-phase extraction and high-performance liquid chromatography with diode array ultraviolet detection, *J. Agric. Food Chem.*, 49, 2185–2192.

Mateos, R., Goya, L., and Bravo, L., 2005, Metabolism of the olive oil phenols hydroxytyrosol, tyrosol, and hydroxytyrosyl acetate by human hepatoma HepG2 cells, *J. Agric. Food Chem.*, 53, 9897–9905.

Miró-Casas, E., Farré-Albadalejo, M., Covas, M.I., Fitó Colomer, M., Lamuela Raventós, R.M., et al., 2001, Tyrosol bioavailability in humans after ingestion of virgin olive oil, *Clin. Chem.*, 47, 341–343.

Miró-Casas, E., Covas, M.I., Farré, M., Fito, M., Ortuño, J., Weinbrenner, T., et al., 2003a, Hydroxytyrosol disposition in humans, *Clin. Chem.*, 49, 945–952.

Miró-Casas, E., Covas, M.I., Fitó, M., Farré-Albadalejo, M., Marrugat, J., and de la Torre, R., 2003b, Tyrosol and hydroxytyrosol are absorbed from moderate and sustained doses of virgin olive oil in humans, *Eur. J. Clin. Nutr.*, 57, 186–190.

Moreno, J.J., 2003, Effect of olive oil minor components on oxidative stress and arachidonic acid mobilization and metabolism by macrophages RAW 264.7, *Free Radic. Biol. Med.*, 35, 1073–1081.

Moriel, P., Plavnik, F.L., Zanella, M.T., Bertolami, M.C., and Abdalla, D.S., 2000, Lipid peroxidation and antioxidants in hyperlipidemia and hypertension, *Biol. Res.*, 33, 105–112.

Moschandreas, J., Vissers, M.N., Wiseman, S., van Putte, K.P., and Kafatos, A., 2002, Extra virgin olive oil phenols and markers of oxidation in Greek smokers: a randomized cross-over study, *Eur. J. Clin. Nutr.*, 56, 1024–1029.

Mueller, T., Dieplinger, B., Gegenhuber, A., Haidinger, D., Schmid, N., Roth, N., et al., 2004, Serum total 8-iso-prostaglandin $F_{2\alpha}$: a new and independent predictor of peripheral arterial disease, *J. Vasc. Surg.*, 40, 268–273.

Nair, J., Vaca, C.E., Velic, I., Mutanen, M., Valsta, L.M., and Bartsch, H., 1997, High dietary omega-6 polyunsaturated fatty acids drastically increase the formation of etheno-DNA base adducts in white blood cells of female subjects, *Cancer Epidemiol. Biomarkers Prev.*, 6, 597–601.

Nicolaïew, N., Leniort, N., Adorni, L., Berra, B., Montorfano, G., Rapelli, S., et al., 1998, Comparison between extra virgin olive oil and oleic acid rich sunflower oil: effects on postprandial lipemia and LDL susceptibility to oxidation, *Ann. Nutr. Metab.,* 42, 251–280.

Owen, R.W., Giacosa, A., Hull, W.E., Haubner, R., Spiegelhalder, B., and Bartsch, H., 2000, The antioxidant/anticancer potential of phenolic compounds from olive oil, *Eur. J. Cancer,* 36, 1235–1247.

Pérez-Jimenez, F., Alvarez de Cienfuegos, G., Badimon, L., Barja, G., Battino, M., Blanco, A., et al., 2004, Internacional conference on the healthy effect of virgin olive oil. Consensus Report, Jaen (Spain), *Eur. J. Clin. Invest.,* 35, 421–424.

Petroni, A., Blasevich, M., Salami, M., Papini, N., Montedoro, G.F., and Galli, C., 1995, Inhibition of platelet aggregation and eicosanoid production by phenolic components of olive oil, *Thromb. Res.,* 78, 151–160.

Poulsen, H.E., Prieme, H., and Loft, S., 1998, Role of oxidative DNA damage in cancer initiation and promotion, *Eur. J. Cancer Prev.,* 7, 9–16.

Poulsen, H.E., 2005, Oxidative DNA modifications, *Exp. Toxicol. Pathol.,* 57, 161–169.

Quiles, J.L., Farquharson, A.J., Simpson, D.K., Grant, I., and Wahle, K.W., 2002, Olive oil phenolics: effects on DNA oxidation and redoxenzyme RNA in prostate cells, *Br. J. Nutr.,* 88, 225–234.

Ramírez-Tortosa, M.C., Urbano, G., Lopez-Jurado, M., Nestares, T., Gomez, M.C., Mir, A., et al., 1999, Extra-virgin olive oil increases the resistance of LDL to oxidation more than refined olive oil in free-living men with peripheral vascular disease, *J. Nutr.,* 129, 2177–2183.

Reaven, P.D., Grasse, B.J., and Tribble, D.L., 1994, Effects of linoleate-enriched and oleate-enriched diets in combination with alpha-tocopherol on the susceptibility of LDL and LDL subfractions to oxidative modifications in humans, *Arterioscler. Thromb.,* 14, 557–566.

Roche, H.M., Zampelas, A., Jackson, K.G., Williams, C.M., and Gibney, M.J., 1998, The effect of test meal monounsaturated fatty acid:saturated fatty acid ratio on postprandial lipid metabolism, *Br. J. Nutr.,* 79, 419–424.

Roche, H.M. and Gibney, M.J., 2000, The impact of postprandial lipemia in accelerating atherothrombosis, *J. Cardiovasc. Risk,* 7, 317–324.

Ruano, J., López-Miranda, J., Fuentes, F., Moreno, J.A., Bellido, C., Perez-Martinez, P., et al., 2005, Phenolic content of virgin olive oil improves ischemic reactive hyperemia in hypercholesterolemic patients, *J. Am. Coll. Cardiol.,* 46, 1864–1868.

Ruíz, C., Alegría, A., Barbera, R., Farré, R., and Lagarda, M.J., 1999, Lipid peroxidation and antioxidant enzyme activities in patients with type 1 diabetes mellitus, *Scand. J. Clin. Lab. Invest.,* 59, 99–105.

Sallustio, B.C., Sabordo, L., Evans, A.M., and Nation, R.L., 2000, Hepatic disposition of electrophilic acyl glucuronide conjugates, *Curr. Drug. Metab.,* 1, 163–180.

Salvini, S., Sera, F., Caruso, D., Giovannelli, L., Visioli, F., Saieva, C., et al., 2006, Daily consumption of a high-phenol extra-virgin olive oil reduces oxidative DNA damage in postmenopausal women, *Br. J. Nutr.,* 95, 742–751.

Schwedhelm, E., Bartling, A., and Lenzen, H., 2004, Urinary 8-iso-prostaglandin $F_{2\alpha}$ as a risk marker in patients with coronary heart disease. A matched case-control study, *Circulation,* 109, 843–848.

Sen, C.K., 1995, Oxidants and antioxidants in exercise, *Am. J. Physiol.,* 30, 675–684.

Senn, S., 2002, *Cross-Over Trials in Clinical Research,* 2nd ed., John Wiley & Sons, Chichester, 157–202.

Servili, M., Selvaggini, R., Esposto, S., Taticchi, A., Montedoro, G., and Morozzi, G., 2004, Health and sensory properties of virgin olive oil hydrophilic phenols: agronomic and technological aspects of production that affect their occurrence in the oil, *J. Chromatogr. A,* 1054, 113–127.

Shimada, K., Mokuno, H., Matsunaga, E., Miyazaki, T., Sumiyoshi, K., Miyauchi, K., et al., 2004, Circulating oxidized low-density lipoprotein is an independent predictor for cardiac event in patients with coronary heart disease, *Atherosclerosis,* 174, 343–347.

Sies, H., 1997, Oxidative stress: oxidants and antioxidants, *Exp. Physiol.,* 82, 291–295.

Southom, P.A. and Powis, G., 1998, Free radicals in medicine. II. Involvement in human disease (Review), *Mayo Clin. Proc.,* 63, 390–408.

Sperker, B., Backman, J.T., and Kroemer, H.K., 1997, The role of beta-glucuronidase in drug disposition and drug targeting in humans, *Clin. Pharmacokinet.,* 33, 18–31.

Steinberg, D., Parthasarathy, S., Carew, T.E., Khoo, J.C., and Witztum, J.L., 1989, Beyond cholesterol. Modifications of low-density lipoprotein that increase its atherogenicity, *N. Engl. J. Med.,* 320, 915–924.

Stupans, I., Kirlich, A., Tuck, K.L., and Hayball, P.J., 2002, Comparison of radical scavenging effect, inhibition of microsomal oxygen free radical generation, and serum lipoprotein oxidation of several natural antioxidants, *J. Agric. Food Chem.,* 50, 2464–2469.

Thompson, H.J., 2004, DNA oxidation products, antioxidant status, and cancer prevention, *J. Nutr.*, 134, 3186S–3187S.

Trichopoulou, A., Costacou, T., Bamia, C., and Trichopoulos, D., 2003, Adherence to a Mediterranean diet and survival in a Greek population, *N. Engl. J. Med.*, 348, 2599–2608.

Tsimidou, M., 1998, Polyphenols and quality of virgin olive oil in retrospect, *Ital. J. Food Sci.*, 2, 99–116.

Tuck, K.L., Freeman, M.P., Hayball, P.J., Stretch, G.L., and Stupans, I., 2001, The *in vivo* fate of hydroxytyrosol and tyrosol, antioxidant phenolic constituents of olive oil, after intravenous and oral dosing of labeled compounds to rats, *J. Nutr.*, 131, 1993–1996.

Tuck, K.L., Hayball, P.J., and Stupans, I., 2002, Structural characterization of the metabolites of hydroxytyrosol, the principal phenolic component in olive oil, in rats, *J. Agric. Food Chem.*, 50, 2404–2409.

Valko, M., Leibfritz, D., Moncol, J., Cronin, M.T., Mazur, M., and Telser, J., 2007, Free radicals and antioxidants in normal physiological functions and human disease, *Int. J. Biochem. Cell Biol.*, 39, 44–84.

Vinson, J.A., Jang, J., Dabbagh, Y.A., Liang, X., Serry, M., Proch, J., et al., 1999, Vitamins and especially flavonoids in common beverages are powerful *in vitro* antioxidants which enrich lower density lipoproteins and increase their oxidative resistance after ex vivo spiking in human plasma, *J. Agric. Food Chem.*, 47, 2502–2504.

Visioli, F., Bellomo, G., Montedoro, G., and Galli, C., 1995, Low density lipoprotein oxidation is inhibited in vitro by olive oil constituents, *Atherosclerosis*, 117, 25–32.

Visioli, F., Caruso, D., Galli, C., Viappiani, S., Galli, G., and Sala, A., 2000a, Olive oils rich in natural catecholic phenols decrease isoprostane excretion in humans, *Biochem. Biophys. Res. Commun.*, 278, 797–799.

Visioli, F., Galli, C., Bornet, F., Mattei, A., Patelli, R., Galli, G., et al., 2000b, Olive oil phenolics are dose-dependently absorbed in humans, *FEBS Lett.*, 468, 159–160.

Visioli, F., Galli, C., Plasmati, E., Viappiani, S., Hernandez, A., Colombo, C., et al., 2000c, Olive oil phenol hydroxytyrosol prevents passive smoking-induced oxidative stress, *Circulation*, 102, 2169–2171.

Visioli, F., Caruso, D., Plasmati, E., Patelli, R., Mulinacci, N., and Romani, A., 2001, Hydroxytyrosol, as a component of olive mill waste water, is dose-dependently absorbed and increases the antioxidant capacity of rat plasma, *Free Radic. Res.*, 34, 301–305.

Visioli, F., Galli, C., Grande, S., Colonnelli, K., Patelli, C., Galli, G., et al., 2003, Hydroxytyrosol excretion differs between rats and humans and depends on the vehicle of administration, *J. Nutr.*, 133, 2612–2615.

Visioli, F., Caruso, D., Grande, S., Bosisio, R., Villa, M., Galli, G., et al., 2005, Virgin Olive Oil Study (VOLOS): vasoprotective potential of extra virgin olive oil in mildly dyslipidemic patients, *Eur. J. Nutr.*, 44, 121–127.

Vissers, M.N., Zock, P.L., Wiseman, S.A., Meyboom, S., and Katan, M.B., 2001, Effect of phenol-rich extra virgin olive oil on markers of oxidation in healthy volunteers, *Eur. J. Clin. Nutr.*, 55, 334–341.

Vissers, M.N., Zock, P.L., Roodenburg, A.J., Leenen, R., and Katan, M.B., 2002, Olive oil phenols are absorbed in humans, *J. Nutr.*, 132, 409–417.

Vissers, M.N., Zock, P.L., and Katan, M.B., 2004, Bioavailability and antioxidant effects of olive oil phenols in humans: a review, *Eur. J. Clin. Nutr.*, 58, 955–965.

Weinbrenner, T., Cladellas, M., Covas, M.I., Fitó, M., Tomás, M., and Sentí, M., 2003, High oxidative stress in patients with stable coronary heart disease, *Atherosclerosis*, 168, 99–106.

Weinbrenner, T., Fitó, M., Farré-Albaladejo, M., Saez, G.T., Rijken, P., Tormos, C., et al., 2004a, Bioavailability of olive oil phenolic compounds from olive oil and oxidative/antioxidative status at postprandial state in humans, *Drugs Exp. Clin. Res.*, 5/6, 207–212.

Weinbrenner, T., Fitó, M., de la Torre, R., Saez, G.T., Rijken, P., and Tormos, C., 2004b, Olive oils high in phenolic compounds modulate oxidative/antioxidative status in men, *J. Nutr.*, 134, 2314–2321.

Whiteman, M., Hong, H.S., Jenner, A., and Halliwell, B., 2002, Loss of oxidized and chlorinated bases in DNA treated with reactive oxygen species: implications for assessment of oxidative damage *in vivo*, *Biochem. Biophys. Res. Commun.*, 296, 883–889.

Wiseman, S.A., Mathot, J.N., de Fouw, N.J., and Tijburg, L.B., 1996, Dietary non-tocopherol antioxidants present in extra virgin olive oil increase the resistance of low density lipoproteins to oxidation in rabbits, *Atherosclerosis*, 120, 15–23.

Witzum, J.L., 1994, The oxidation hypothesis of atherosclerosis, *Lancet*, 344, 793–795.

Wolff, SM., Battista, R.N., Anderson, G.M., Logan, A.G., and Wang, E., 1990, Assessing the clinical effectiveness of preventive manoeuvres: analytic principals and systematic methods in reviewing evidence and developing clinical practice recommendations. A report by the Canadian Task Force on the Periodic Health Examination, *J. Clin. Epidemiol.*, 43, 891–905.

7 Olive Oil Phenols, Basic Cell Mechanisms, and Cancer

Marilena Kampa, Vassiliki Pelekanou,
George Notas, and Elias Castanas

CONTENTS

7.1 INTRODUCTION

In the Mediterranean basin, the "Mediterranean diet" has been widely considered to be responsible for a healthy and relatively disease-free population. Epidemiological data show that this diet and way of life have significant protective effects against different types of chronic diseases, including cancer and coronary heart disease. To a certain degree, these effects can be attributed to olive oil consumption, one of the major constituents of the Mediterranean diet. The beneficial role of olive oil is mainly due to a combination of its high oleic acid content (peroxidation-resistant lipid) and its minor components like polar phenolic compounds. More than 40 phenols have been identified in olive oil and a large number have been isolated and used in *in vitro* and *in vivo* studies conducted in order to investigate their actions. The major polar phenolic compounds identified and quantified in olive oil, as already mentioned in previous chapters of the book, belong to four different classes: simple phenols (hydroxytyrosol, tyrosol); secoiridoids (oleuropein, the aglycon of ligstroside, and their respective decarboxylated dialdehyde derivatives); flavonoids (apigenin, luteolin); and lignans [(+)-1-acetoxypinoresinol and pinoresinol]. A limited number of studies deal with cellular or molecular actions of olive oil lignans. However, it is known that pinoresinol can be converted to mammalian lignans, called enterolignans (enterodiol and enterolactone) (Heinonen et al., 2001), formed by the intestinal microflora after the consumption of plant lignans (Milder et al., 2005).

Initially, the antioxidant potential of olive oil phenolics appeared as the main beneficial mechanism of action; however, soon enough researchers realized that this mechanism alone could not explain the whole spectrum of their beneficial properties. Indeed, an accumulating body of evidence reveals a number of pharmacological effects induced by (poly)phenols. Therefore, one has to be cautious with the interpretation of these extraordinary properties. It should be pointed out that the biological properties of these compounds *in vivo* will depend on the extent of their absorption and metabolism. It is essential to decipher the chemical form of circulating olive oil polyphenols, after their absorption and possible primary (bio)transformation, and to find in which chemical form they ultimately reach their target tissues. Presently, the majority of information in the literature is based on analysis of blood and urine samples from animals and humans. Oleuropein, for example, is not absorbed in its parental form in the small intestine and is not degraded under acidic conditions. Consequently, it is likely to reach the large intestine, where it is subjected to rapid biotransformation by the colonic microflora to yield hydroxytyrosol (Corona et al., 2006). On the other hand, hydroxytyrosol was reported to diffuse passively across a colon carcinoma cell line Caco-2 monolayer (Manna et al., 2000).

In the following sections, we review in brief the effects of olive oil phenols and their cellular actions, linked to the generation and/or progression of cancer.

7.2   OLIVE OIL PHENOLS AND CANCER

Cancer, a noncontrolled proliferation of a given cellular population, is a multistep disease that:

1. Initiates with transformation of the genetic content of a cell
2. Proceeds to a preneoplastic stage, that
3. Leads to tumor formation and finally
4. Metastasis

Olive oil polyphenols, as will be presented below, can exert an inhibitory action on cancer, acting as blocking and/or suppressive agents at several stages of cancer progression.

7.2.1   EPIDEMIOLOGICAL STUDIES

A large number of epidemiological studies point out the beneficial role of olive oil against cancer (see, for example, Gallus et al., 2004; La Vecchia, 2004). Indeed, studies conducted in countries around the Mediterranean basin (especially Greece, Italy, and Spain) demonstrate a clear association between olive oil consumption and a reduced cancer risk. In fact, a protective role for olive oil has been shown against different malignancies such as breast (La Vecchia et al., 1995; Trichopoulou et al., 1995; Lipworth et al., 1997; Franceschi and Favero, 1999; Sieri et al., 2004), ovarian (Bosetti et al., 2002b), endometrial (Tzonou et al., 1996), colorectal (Franceschi and Favero, 1999; Rouillier et al., 2005), laryngeal (Bosetti et al., 2002a; Petridou et al., 2002; Gallus et al., 2003), esophageal (Bosetti et al., 2000), lung (Fortes et al., 2003), and pancreatic cancer (Soler et al., 1998). Based on these data, a lot of research has been performed in order to find the components responsible for olive oil effects and elucidate their mechanisms of action that remain largely unknown.

7.2.2 ANIMAL MODELS

Epidemiological evidence, demonstrating cancer protective activity of olive oil, was supported by numerous experimental animal studies. Indeed the effect of olive oil and/or its different components has been studied in different cancer models. The majority of studies focused on the presence of unsaturated fats in olive oil and to a lesser extent on its phenolic content. For example, it was reported that in 7,12-dimethylbenz(a)anthracene (DMBA)-induced rat mammary tumorigenesis, rats fed with high fat diets, rich in oleic acid, had lower tumor incidence, fewer tumors per rat, and longer tumor-free time (Lasekan et al., 1990). In addition, 9,10-dimethyl-1,2-benzanthracene-induced rat mammary gland cancer showed a significantly reduced tumor incidence when 15% olive oil was included in the diet (Zusman, 1998). Dietary olive oil prevented the development of aberrant crypt foci and colon carcinomas in rats, suggesting that olive oil may have chemopreventive activity against colon carcinogenesis (Bartoli et al., 2000; Schwartz et al., 2004). Similarly, dietary olive oil was found to effectively inhibit 4-(methylnitrosamino)-1-(3-pyridyl)-1-butanone–induced lung tumorigenesis (Smith et al., 1998). Moreover, in studies using the N-nitrosomethylurea mammary tumor model, the level of oleic acid was a key determinant of olive oil protective effects, mainly affecting the histological type of formed tumors (Cohen et al., 2000).

Additionally, a number of studies investigated the antitumor action of different olive oil phenolic constituents. In a mouse model of developing spontaneous tumors, orally administered oleuropein regressed tumors in 9–12 days (Hamdi and Castellon, 2005). Apigenin was found to block colon carcinogenesis in two mouse models: azoxymethane (AOM)-induced CF-1 mice and Min mice with a mutant adenomatous polyposis coli (APC) gene (Au et al., 2006). The same compound was also shown to inhibit skin tumorigenesis (Baliga and Katiyar, 2006) initiated by DMBA and promoted by 12-O-tetradecanoylphorbol-13-acetate (TPA) in the SENCAR mouse model; it prolonged the latency period of tumor appearance by 3 weeks and significantly inhibited the incidence of carcinoma and number of tumors (Wei et al., 1990). Similarly, apigenin inhibited ultraviolet light-induced skin carcinogenesis in SKH-1 mice (Birt et al., 1997). A tumor inhibitory effect of apigenin has been also observed in a prostate cancer 22Rv1 xenograft (Shukla et al., 2005). Moreover, a significant, dose-dependent delay of tumor growth was reported in syngeneic C57BL/6N mice inoculated with B16-BL6 melanoma cells and treated with apigenin (Caltagirone et al., 2000). In addition, luteolin-treated rats showed a decreased incidence of colon tumors induced by 1,2-dimethylhydrazine (Manju and Nalini, 2005, 2007). A strong chemopreventive activity against the genesis of 7,12-dimethylbenz(a)anthracene-induced mammary tumors was suggested, since luteolin, combined with cyclophosphamide, inhibited the incidence rate of tumors and decreased tumor volume (Samy et al., 2006).

7.2.3 IN VITRO STUDIES

The majority of data supporting an inhibitory role of olive oil phenols against cancer derives from the examination of their effects on different cancer cell lines. In several studies, a crude olive oil extract was preferentially tested, since it was believed that it initiates a synergistic effect not achievable by single compounds or limited combinations of olive oil constituents. For example, a virgin olive oil phenol extract decreased the proliferation of the human promyelocytic cell line HL-60. Similar properties were attributed, at least in part, to two compounds isolated from olive oil, the dialdehydic form of elenoic acid, linked to hydroxytyrosol (3,4-DHPEA-EDA) or to tyrosol (pHPEA-EDA) (Fabiani et al., 2006)

Oleuropein has been reported to exhibit an inhibitory effect on the proliferation rate of several different cancer cell lines: LN-18, poorly differentiated glioblastoma; TF-1a, erythroleukemia; 786-O, renal cell adenocarcinoma; T47D, infiltrating ductal carcinoma of the breast; MCF-7, mammary gland adenocarcinoma; RPMI-7951, malignant melanoma; LoVo, colorectal adenocarcinoma (Hamdi and Castellon, 2005). Oleuropein, as well as tyrosol and hydroxytyrosol, decreased breast cancer cell viability, as described by Menendez and co-workers (Menendez et al., 2007). Minimal growth inhibition of McCoys cells, induced by tyrosol, was also observed, as compared to the action of oleuropein (Saenz et al., 1998)

Phenolic acids, such as caffeic, syringic, sinapic, protocatechuic, ferulic, and 3,4-dihydroxy-phenylacetic acid (PAA), were also found to inhibit T47D human breast cancer cells (Kampa et al., 2004). Cinnamic, p-coumaric, ferulic, and sinapic acids were also effective against MK-1 human gastric adenocarcinoma cells, HeLa human uterine carcinoma, and B16F10 murine melanoma (Nagao et al., 2001).

The flavonoids apigenin and luteolin, found among olive and olive oil phenolic compounds, are the most extensively studied due to their presence in a variety of other plants, also. Apigenin resulted in a dose-dependent reduction in the cell number of human colon carcinoma cell lines SW480, HT-29, and Caco-2 (Richter et al., 1999; Wang et al., 2000). A growth inhibitory effect of apigenin was also observed on MCF-7 and MDA-MB-231 breast carcinoma cells (Lindenmeyer et al., 2001; Yin et al., 2001; Vargo et al., 2006) and human thyroid carcinoma cell lines, UCLA NPA-87-1 (NPA) (papillary carcinoma), UCLA RO-82W-1 (WRO) (follicular carcinoma), and UCLA RO-81A-1 (ARO) (anaplastic carcinoma) (Yin et al., 1999a). Similarly, apigenin exhibited a potent cell growth inhibition of prostate (LNCaP, DU-145, PC3) (Shenouda et al., 2004; Morrissey et al., 2005), gastric (SGC-7901) (Wu et al., 2005), lung (A549) (Liu et al., 2005; Vargo et al., 2006), and pancreatic cancer (AsPC-1, CD18, MIA PaCa2, and S2-013) (Ujiki et al., 2006); neuroblastoma (NUB-7, LAN-5, and SK-N-BE) (Torkin et al., 2005); and monocytic and lymphocytic leukemia cells (monocytic leukemia THP-1 and U937 lines, promyelocytic HL60, acute T cell leukemia Jur-kat, K562 chronic myelogenous leukemia, and the NIH-3T3 fibroblast cell line) (Vargo et al., 2006). Equally, luteolin significantly inhibited the proliferation of human myeloid leukemia HL-60 (Ko et al., 2002), pancreatic cancer MiaPaCa-2 (Lee, L.T. et al., 2002), NK/Ly ascites tumor (Molnar et al., 1981), and melanoma B16F10 and SK-MEL-1 cells (Rodriguez et al., 2002; Yanez et al., 2004).

Olive oil-contained lignans (mainly 1-acetoxypinoresinol, hydroxypinoresinol, and pinoresinol) were examined in a few studies. They exhibited cytotoxicity against human colon (HCT-116) and hepatocellular carcinoma (HepG2) cell lines *in vitro* (Lee, D.Y. et al., 2007). However, pinoresinol can be converted to mammalian enterolignans (enterodiol and enterolactone) (Heinonen et al., 2001) by intestinal microflora (Milder et al., 2005). Enterolignans have been shown to inhibit skin, lung, breast, colon, and prostate carcinoma (Lin et al., 2001; Owen et al., 2000).

Finally, the response of oral cavity-derived cells (i.e., the initial site of exposure upon ingestion of olive oil) upon olive oil phenols was studied. This is an important factor, in view of the potential cytotoxicity of phenolic molecules at high concentrations. Indeed, high concentrations of oleuro-pein aglycon, oleuropein glycoside, caffeic acid, *o*-coumaric acid, and cinnamic acid exhibited a cytotoxic effect on normal GN61 gingival fibroblasts, immortalized nontumorigenic S-G gingival epithelial cells, and malignant HSG$_1$ cells derived from the salivary gland (Babich and Visioli, 2003).

7.3 MODE OF ACTION OF OLIVE OIL CONSTITUENTS

7.3.1 MODIFICATION OF THE REDOX STATUS

Human cells, in order to sustain optimal physiological conditions, should retain a balance between oxidants (endogenously produced or externally supplied) and antioxidants. In cases of an oxidant imbalance, oxidative stress occurs, damaging different cell macromolecules (lipid proteins and DNA), increasing the risk of carcinogenesis and tumor promotion. Reactive oxygen species can act as fine regulators of cell replication (Ames et al., 1993) and exert important signal transduction activities (Poli et al., 2004). Therefore, the inhibitory action of phenolic compounds in cancer can be in part attributed to their ability to scavenge or reduce the generation of free radicals. Olive oil per se and the contained phenolic compounds possess potent antioxidant properties. Ichihashi and co-workers reported that when olive oil was used immediately after UVB radiation (known to produce reactive oxygen species and damage DNA leading to gene mutation and abnormal cell proliferation in skin), it significantly delayed the onset and reduced the number of skin cancers (Ichihashi et al., 2000). Oleuropein, acting as free radical scavenger and inhibiting free radical production (Kruk et al., 2005), decreased the intracellular levels of reactive oxygen species (ROS), and reduced the amount of oxidized proteins in human embryonic fibroblasts (Katsiki et al., 2007). Pretreatment of HepG2 with hydroxytyrosol prevented cell damage, evoked by t-BOOH, by reducing oxygen species generation (Goya et al., 2007). In J774 murine macrophages, hydroxytyrosol completely inhibited ROS production (Maiuri et al. 2005; Di Benedetto et al., 2007), while it prevented oxidative stress in human melanoma M13 UVA-irradiated cells (D'Angelo et al., 2005). Furthermore it blocked DNA damage *in vitro*, induced by peroxynitrite (Deiana et al., 1999), and decreased hydrogen peroxide–induced formation of single-strand breaks in nuclear DNA (Nousis et al., 2005). Apigenin reduced the damage of hepatocytes *in vitro* by inhibiting ROS in a concentration-dependent manner (Zheng, Q.S. et al., 2005). Luteolin was also protective against oxidative DNA damage in HepG2 cells (Kanazawa et al., 2006; Lima et al., 2006), human lymphocyte, myelogenous leukemia (K562), and L1210 murine leukemia cells; apigenin was less potent in the latter condition (Noroozi et al., 1998; Horvathova et al., 2003; Horvathova et al., 2004), while luteolin had no effect on bleomycin-Fe complex–induced DNA damage (Ng et al., 2000). Finally, both enterodiol and enterolactone inhibited oxidative stress–induced DNA scissions, in a concentration-dependent manner (Kitts et al., 1999).

In addition to their antioxidant activity, a polyphenol pro-oxidant nature also has been demonstrated, suggesting an alternative *in vitro* mechanism of action (Matsuo et al., 2005). The pro-oxidant property is due to the generation of free radicals, at high polyphenol concentrations. Oxidative digestive gland cell-protein modification was increased in a concentration-dependent manner in cells incubated with phenolic acids (Labieniec and Gabryelak, 2007). Equally, caffeic- and ferulic acid-evoked dose-related elevation of intracellular ROS in HepG2 human hepatoma cells reduced cell viability and induced apoptotic cell death (Lee, Y.S., 2005). Ferulic acid has been reported to exert a pro-oxidant action, accelerating DNA damage, in the presence of a bleomycin-iron complex (Scott et al., 1993) or copper (Li and Trush, 1994). Luteolin and apigenin intensified cell death after exposure to H_2O_2 and were unable to protect HUVEC cells from oxidant-induced apoptosis and DNA damage (Choi et al., 2003).

7.3.2 Interference with Basic Cell Functions

7.3.2.1 Cell Cycle and Apoptosis

Cell cycle is an ordered set of events, culminating in cell growth and division into two daughter cells. A defective cell cycle regulation can lead to uncontrolled cell proliferation and tumor formation. The cell cycle consists of four distinct phases: G1, S, G2 (collectively known as interphase), and M (mitotic) phase. The relay of a cell from one phase to another is governed by a cascade of enzyme-protein phosphorylations that involve cyclical activation of the cyclin/cyclin-dependent kinase (cdks) complexes and cyclin-dependent kinase inhibitors (CKIs). In addition a set of checkpoints exists, monitoring completion of critical events and regulating progression to the next stage. Important cell cycle regulators are the retinoblastoma protein (pRb) and the p53 protein. Their phosphorylation is also controlled by cyclin/cdk complexes, while in cancer mutations in pRb and/or p53 proteins and cyclin/cdk, overexpression is found.

Cell cycle arrest can occur either at G_1/S or G_2/M phase. Arrest of cells at G_1 is mainly due to activation of p53, detecting aberrant DNA lesions. Since the majority of cancer cells has a mutated p53 gene unable to arrest G_1 phase, consequently, a G_2 arrest may occur. In both cases, any agent downregulating cyclins or cdks (like endogenous cdk inhibitors) will result in cell cycle arrest, an irreversible process that ultimately will lead to cell apoptosis. The latter is the most potent defense against cancer, activated by the host immune system (Lee, E.J. et al., 2004; Rigolio et al., 2005) and several chemotherapeutic agents (Mansour et al., 2004; Shenouda et al., 2004). Two main pathways regulate this process. The first is initiated at the cell surface by activation of death receptors (e.g., TNF or Fas receptor), recruiting caspase 8 and pro-apoptotic Bcl-2 family member Bid. The second pathway involves direct permeabilization of the mitochondrial membrane, due to the disturbance of pro-apoptotic (Bax, Bad, and Bak) to antiapoptotic family members (Bcl-2 and Bcl-X_L) ratio. In both cases, mitochondrial protein release induces caspase activation, leading to DNA and protein degradation, resulting in apoptosis.

In rats exposed to DMBA but fed with a 15% olive oil–rich diet, a high expression of FasL and p53 proteins (inducers of apoptosis) and a decreased production of Bcl-2 protein (inhibitor of apoptosis) were observed in mammary tumors (Kossoy et al., 2001). A decreased Bcl-2 expression and apoptosis were also found in colorectal cancer cells (Caco-2 and HT-29) that were supplemented with olive oil (Llor et al., 2003). Virgin olive oil phenol extract has been found to accumulate HL60 promyelocytic cells in the G_0/G_1 phase and to induce apoptosis (Fabiani et al., 2006). This effect was (partially) attributed to the dialdehydic forms of elenoic acid, linked to hydroxytyrosol and tyrosol. It should be noted that hydroxytyrosol did not induce apoptosis on freshly isolated human lymphocytes and polymorphonuclear, or HL60, cells (Ragione et al., 2000), while it led colon adenocarcinoma cells HT-29 to apoptosis (Fabiani et al., 2002; Guichard et al., 2006).

Apigenin has been reported to arrest at G_2/M the cell cycle of B104 rat neuronal cells (Sato et al., 1994), MCF7, and MDA-MB-468 breast carcinoma cells (Ford et al., 2000; Yin et al. 2001) due to a significant decrease in cyclin B1, D1, and A and inhibition of cdk1 and cdk4 (Way et al., 2005). Additionally, G_2/M cell cycle arrest and induction of apoptosis were also observed in apigenin-treated human prostate adenocarcinoma (CA-HPV-10, PC3, and LNCaP) (Gupta et al., 2001; Shenouda et al., 2004) and HeLa cells (Czyz et al., 2004). In the latter, an additional G_1 phase arrest was also reported (Zheng, P.W. et al., 2005) with induction of Fas/APO-1, caspase-3, and apoptosis. Work by Shukla and co-workers also showed a G_1 arrest in apigenin-treated PC3 and LNCaP cells, accompanied by a decrease in total and phosphorylated Rb protein (Shukla and Gupta, 2007). G_2/M cycle arrest was also induced by apigenin and several of its analogs in SW480, HT-29, and Caco-2 colon carcinoma cells (Wang et al., 2000; Wang et al., 2004) with inhibited activity of p34 (cdc2) kinase and reduced accumulation of p34 (cdc2) and cyclin B1 proteins. Reduced phosphorylated forms of cdks cdc2 and cdc25 and cyclin A, cyclin B, responsible for G_2/M phase cell cycle arrest, were found in pancreatic cancer cells (Ujiki et al., 2006). Furthermore, in the p53-mutant cancer cell lines HT-29 and MG63, treatment with apigenin resulted in G_2/M phase arrest, associated with marked increase in protein expression of the cdk inhibitor p21/WAF1 (Takagaki et al., 2005). On the other hand, in DU-145 prostate carcinoma a G_1 phase arrest was also induced by apigenin, related to a marked decrease in protein expression of cyclin D1, D2, and E and cdk2, 4, and 6, with concomitant upregulation of the cdk inhibitors p21/WAF1, p27/KIP1, p16/INK4a, and p18/INK4c. In addition, apigenin treatment also resulted in alteration in Bax/Bcl2 ratio in favor of apoptosis that was associated with the release of cytochrome c and induction of apoptotic protease-activating factor-1 (Apaf-1) (Shukla and Gupta, 2004a). This effect was found to result in a significant increase in cleaved fragments of caspase-9, -3, and poly(ADP-ribose) polymerase (PARP). Furthermore, apigenin-induced apoptosis also has been detected in a number of different cancer cell types, such as leukemic (Lee, W.R. et al., 2002; Chen et al., 2005; Vargo et al., 2006), human anaplastic thyroid (ARO) (Yin et al., 1999a), breast (Way et al., 2004), neuroblastoma (NUB-7, LAN-5, SK-N-BE, and SH-SY5Y) (Torkin et al., 2005; Das et al., 2006), gastric (SGC-7901) (Wu et al., 2005), or prostate carcinoma (PWR-1E, LNCaP, PC-3, and DU145) (Morrissey et al., 2005).

In a similar manner luteolin induced cell cycle arrest and apoptosis. Several studies demonstrated a G_1 phase arrest of human melanoma (OCM-1) (Casagrande and Darbon, 2001), gastric (HGC-27) (Matsukawa et al., 1993) or prostate carcinoma (LNCaP, through a p53-independent pathway) (Kobayashi et al., 2002), and hepatoma cells (HepG2, SK-Hep-1, PLC/PRF/5, Hep3B, and HA22T/VGH) (Yee et al., 2003). In the latter, cycle arrest was correlated to downregulated expression of CDK4 and increase of p53 and the cdk inhibitor p21. Apoptosis was also observed as the result of an increased Bax/Bcl-XL ratio and activated caspase-3 (Yee et al., 2003). In OCM-1 melanoma cells, in parallel to the G_1 arrest, cdk2 activity inhibition was observed, attributed to the presence of a hydroxyl group at the 3′-position of ring B (Casagrande and Darbon, 2001). In HT-29 colon cancer cells, a 2-h treatment with luteolin inhibited cdks (2 and 4) and decreased cyclin D1, resulting in G_1 cell cycle arrest and a concomitant decrease of phosphorylation of retinoblastoma protein (pRb). In contrast, after 24 h, it promoted G_2/M arrest and apoptosis with increased activation of caspases 3, 7, and 9 (Lim do et al., 2007). In addition, luteolin induced apoptosis in HL-60 human myeloid leukemia (Yamashita and Kawanishi, 2000; Lee, W.R. et al., 2002), MiaPaCa-2 pancreatic tumor (Lee, L.T. et al., 2002), HeLa cervical cancer, CH27 human lung carcinoma (Leung et al., 2005), HLF hepatoma (Selvendiran et al., 2006), and colorectal cancer cells (Shi et al., 2004). Recently, it has been shown that luteolin-induced apoptosis is mediated through death receptor 5 (DR5) upregulation, since it markedly induced the expression of DR5, in parallel with caspases 8, 10, 9, and 3 activation (Horinaka et al., 2005)

Finally, certain phenolic acids and cinnamic acid present in olive oil have been tested for their effect on cell cycle and apoptosis of different cancer cells. More specifically, cinnamic acid and its derivative TPY-835 induced G_1 cell cycle arrest in human lung cancer cells (A549 and SBC-5) (Jin et al., 2002; Aoyagi et al., 2005) by suppressing cdk2 activity and phosphorylation of pRb. Similarly, hydroxycinnamic acid induced apoptosis and G_1 phase arrest in human cervix epithelial carcinoma (HeLa) cells, by increasing the expression of p53, caspase-3, Bax, and cyclin B (Chuang et al., 2005). G_1 phase accumulation and apoptosis have also been observed in human chronic mycloid leukemia blast crisis (CML-BC) K562 and in acute leukemia MV4-11 cells by the cinnamic-hydroxamic acid analog LBH589 (George et al., 2005). A study by our group demonstrated that caffeic acid and 3,4-dihydroxy-phenylacetic acid induced apoptosis in T47D cells via the Fas/FasL system (Kampa et al., 2004). In addition, apoptotic cell death was also shown in HepG2 human hepatoma cells treated with caffeic and ferulic acid (Lee, Y.S., 2005). Moreover, ferulic acid and para-coumaric acid increased the proportion of colonic endothelial tumor Caco-2 cells in S and G_2 phases (Janicke et al., 2005).

7.3.2.2 Angiogenesis

Angiogenesis is a normal process in growth, development, and wound healing. However, it is also a fundamental step in tumor progression. Tumors induce angiogenesis by secreting various growth factors that cause capillary growth into the tumor. These new vessels assist the supply of oxygen and nutrients to the cancer cells, allowing tumor expansion, and provide the pathways for metastasis. Important regulators of angiogenesis (among numerous others) are shear stress, vascular endothelial (VEGF) and fibroblast growth factor (FGF), angiopoietins (Ang1 and Ang2), endothelins (ETs), matrix metalloproteinases (MMPs), MMP inhibitors (TIMPs), nitric oxide (NO), and nitric oxide synthases (NOS). Angiogenesis is a target of intense study of new antitumor mechanisms and therapies in the last few years and a number of antiangiogenetic compounds are currently in clinical trial.

Several phenolic compounds included in olive oil (especially apigenin and luteolin) interact with the process of tumor angiogenesis (Owen et al., 2003). Both have been reported to decrease the proliferation of normal and tumor cells, as well as *in vitro* bFGF-stimulated proliferation of human umbilical vein endothelial cells (HUVEC) and other endothelial cell lines (Fotsis et al., 1997). In a series of elegant experiments Trochon et al. report that apigenin inhibited the proliferation and, to a lesser degree, the migration of CPAE (calf pulmonary-artery endothelial) and HMEC-1 (human microvascular endothelial) cells, while stimulating the proliferation of human artery smooth-muscle cells (HUASMC). Endothelial derived cells were blocked in the G_2/M phase as a result of the accumulation of the hyperphosphorylated form of pRb, while smooth-muscle cell stimulation was attributed to the reduced expression of cyclin-dependent kinase inhibitors, p21 and p27, which negatively regulate the G_1 phase cyclin-dependent kinase (Trochon et al., 2000). In another report pretreatment of HUVEC cells with apigenin completely inhibited the VEGF/bFGF-stimulated increase in MMP-1 expression and pro-MMP-2 activation, decreased TIMP-1, and completely abolished TIMP-2 and urokinase-type plasminogen activator (uPA) expression (Kim, M.H., 2003). Apigenin also inhibited hypoxia-induced levels of VEGF mRNA in HUVEC cells, via degradation of hypoxia-inducible factor 1 alpha (HIF-1alpha) through PI3K/AKT/p70S6K1 and HDM2/p53 pathways and interference with the function of heat shock protein 90 (Hsp90) (Osada et al., 2004; Fang et al., 2005). This result was further verified in the chicken chorioallantoic membrane and Matrigel plug assays (Fang et al., 2007a). A similar effect of inhibition of both VEGF and HIF-1 alpha by apigenin was found in A549 lung cancer cells (Liu et al., 2005), while in MDA human breast cancer, U-343 and U-118 glioma cells, it inhibited VEGF release (Schindler and Mentlein, 2006). Apigenin has also been shown to be effective in inhibiting laser-induced choroidal neovascularization by inhibiting endothelial cell proliferation (Zou and Chiou, 2006). Luteolin inhibited VEGF-induced *in vivo* angiogenesis in rabbit corneal assay and blocked VEGF-induced survival and proliferation of HUVEC via a PI3K/Akt dependent pathway (Bagli et al., 2004). The antiangiogenic effect of luteolin might be related to its ability to inhibit the hypoxia-response element (HRE) of several genes including VEGF (Hasebe et al., 2003). Like apigenin, topical application of luteolin can inhibit bFGF-induced corneal neovascularization in rabbits (Joussen et al., 2000). Sodium caffeate (SC), the sodium salt of caffeic acid, was found to inhibit lung carcinoma pulmonary metastasis and angiogenesis in animal models. It also inhibited proliferation of transformed HUVEC (ECV304) by inducing apoptosis and inhibited secretion of MMP-2 and MMP-9 (Xu et al., 2004). Another olive oil phenolic acid, protocatechuic acid, inhibited the angiogenetic effect of Cu^{2+} by blocking Cu^{2+}/H_2O_2-dependent induction of VEGF expression (Sen et al., 2002).

Oleanolic acid (a triterpenic acid found in olive oil) also inhibited angiogenesis in the chick embryo chorioallantoic membrane (CAM) assay and inhibited the proliferation of bovine aortic endothelial cells in a dose-dependent manner (Sohn et al., 1995). Furthermore, it has been reported to cause a dose- and time-dependent inhibition of HUVEC viability, although it did not have an effect on matrigel-induced angiogenesis at micromolar concentrations (Barthomeuf et al., 2004). Finally several oleanolic acid derivatives also have significant antiangiogenic effects (Ovesna et al., 2004; Shishodia et al., 2006).

Incubation of embryoid bodies with acteoside (verbascoside), one of the major constituents of olives, also significantly inhibited angiogenesis (Wartenberg et al., 2003). Enterodiol and enterolactone were able to block estradiol-induced growth and angiogenesis induction of MCF-7 breast cancer solid tumors in mice, possibly via inhibition of estradiol-induced VEGF secretion (Bergman et al., 2007).

Finally, secoiridoids, a secondary class of metabolites found in a wide variety of plants and in some animals, are believed to possess antioxidant potential. The only olive-derived secoiridoid that has been referred to as having antiangiogenic effects is oleuropein (Hamdi and Castellon, 2005), while only a few studies about the role of secoiridoids from other sources in angiogenesis exist. Both geniposide and its derivative genipin were shown to contain potent antiangiogenic activity in a dose-dependent manner, which was detected by chick embryo chorioallantoic membrane assay (Koo et al., 2004a,b). However, in another study, ginsenoside induced dose-dependent proliferation, migration, and tube formation of HUVEC cells (Huang et al., 2005). It is therefore obvious that further studies are needed to decipher the role of secoiridoids in angiogenesis.

7.3.2.3 Invasion and Metastasis

The progressing of a tumor from *in situ* to invasive is a prerequisite for cancer metastasis, a major cause of morbidity and mortality. It involves increased cell migration, loss of cell–cell adhesion along with a gain of cell–matrix adhesion, and increased expression and activation of extracellular proteases to degrade the extracellular matrix (ECM). The process of metastasis follows a series of sequential steps that include invasion, intravasation, and survival in circulation, as well as adhesion, extravasation, proliferation, and angiogenesis. Malignant cells are released from the primary tumor and disseminate to distant sites via lymphatic and/or circulatory systems, and halt in distant lymph nodes or in the microvasculatures of secondary sites. The emergence of metastasis in organs distant from the primary tumor is the most devastating aspect of cancer. In light of the above, several secreted proteins and adhesion molecules, as well as their downstream kinases and transcription factors, are determinant of these complicated processes.

Phenolic compounds represent the cornerstone of scientific investigation on olive oil's pleiotropic effects. They have been found to control tumor cell migration, invasion, and metastasis. Below we discuss their role in a critical step of cell motility, directly related to their metastatic potential, namely, their role in modulation of the cytoskeleton. It is of special interest that all actions of olive oil compounds described below are exerted without important cytotoxicity. This property offers new insights in the use of natural pharmaceutical agents in anticancer therapy.

7.3.2.4 Action on Adhesion Molecules and Cytoskeleton

Cell motility, a requirement for tumor invasion, is a coordinated balance between cell adhesion receptors, predominately integrins, and the ECM. Olive oil flavonoids have been found to inhibit the expression of cellular adhesion molecules. Apigenin and luteolin inhibit the expression of ICAM-1 (intercellular adhesion molecule-1) in TNF-stimulated A549 alveolar epithelial cancer cells. The attenuation of this inflammatory response by flavonoids was mediated via mitogen-activated protein kinase (MAPK) activity, c-fos and c-jun mRNA expressions, and transcriptional activity of AP-1 and NF-κB. All three MAPK were inhibited, including extracellular signal-regulated kinase (ERK), p38 and c-Jun NH2-terminal kinase (JNK) (Chen et al., 2004). In a more recent study, hydroxytyrosol and oleuropein aglycon were found to downregulate the expression of ICAM-1 and VCAM-1 (vascular adhesion molecule) mRNA in HUVEC cells, while homovanillyl alcohol induced a reduction of expression of these same molecules, without important modifications of their transcriptional level (Dell'Agli et al., 2006). Lotito and co-workers investigated whether the inhibitory potency of olive oil flavonoids on cellular adhesion molecules correlates with their structural features. They suggested that only flavones, such as apigenin, were able to inhibit adhesion molecules and this property was attributed to 5,7-dihydroxyl substitution of a flavonoid A-ring and 2,3-double bond and 4-keto group of the C-ring. On the other hand, hydroxyl substitutions of the B- and C-rings confer antioxidant activity. In addition, active flavonoids triggered significant attenuation of E-selectin and ICAM-1, but not of VCAM-1. Moreover, using a hepatocyte model mimicking first pass metabolism, they showed that this inhibitory effect was attenuated; they concluded that the effect of dietary flavonoids on endothelial adhesion molecule expression depends on their molecular structure, concentration, and metabolic transformation but not on their antioxidant activity (Lotito and Frei, 2006).

In another study, Gill et al., using virgin olive oil phenolic extract (rich in oleuropein aglycon, lignans, ligstroside aglycon, 3,4 DHPEA-EDA, and p-HPEA-EDA), showed that it inhibited the invasiveness of colon cancer cell lines (HT29, HT115, CACO2, and MRC5) (Gill et al., 2005). Olive oil phenols increased barrier function by 25% compared to untreated cells. Barrier function arises from epithelial cells and tight junctions (TJ), which govern the paracellular permeability, acting as cell-cell adhesion structures, and their aberration is closely associated with metastasis (Martin and Jiang, 2001). Note that in HT115 cells, the inhibition of invasion seems independent of matrix metalloproteinases (MMP). Olive oil extract diminished the attachment of cells in culture flasks and this antiattachment effect was more pronounced when cells were cultured on an ECM-like surface (matrigel). This finding led Gill et al. (2005) to assume that olive oil phenolic compounds interfere with integrin-mediated attachment. Integrins are the primary ECM receptors mediating ECM remodeling and tumor-associated desmoplasia (stromatogenesis). They are responsible not only for cellular attachment with collagens, laminins, and fibronectin, but also for signal transduction, which induces cytoskeletal modifications among other things (for recent reviews, see Hood and Cheresh, 2002; Del Pozo and Schwartz, 2007; Hehlgans et al., 2007). Moreover, ellagic acid, caffeic acid, and luteolin inhibited invasion of PC-3 prostate cancer cells across matrigel, both individually and in combination, where they exerted a supra-additive inhibition (Lansky et al., 2005). However, in another study conducted by Magee et al., lignans failed to exert significant reduction of invasion in the breast cancer cell-line MDA-MB-231, through matrigel (Magee et al., 2004).

It is also known that gap-junction proteins such as connexins are mediators of heterocellular interactions and functional cell coupling. Czyz et al. showed that apigenin inhibits connexin signaling. Apigenin treatment of both HeLa-connexin 43 transfectants and their normal counterparts resulted in a significant inhibition of translocation. In addition, highly invasive HeLa-connexin 43 cells, in the presence of apigenin, failed to invade and engulf chick heart tissue fragments in a co-culture system (Czyz et al., 2005). These findings are in accordance with older studies in animal models, suggesting that apigenin enhances gap junctional communication, in a dose-dependent manner, and counteracts tumor-induced inhibition of this communication in rat liver epithelial cells (Chaumontet et al., 1994; Chaumontet et al., 1997). Furthermore, it was shown that apigenin inhibited ras oncogene, reversing, in consequence, the malignant phenotype of HCT116 cells, appearing to counteract downregulation of gelsolin, an actin-binding protein, absent or with diminished expression in colorectal cancer cell lines (Apc-) and primary tumors (Klampfer et al., 2004).

Oleuropein has been found to disrupt actin cytoskeleton, triggering in this way inhibition of cell growth, motility, and invasiveness, *in vitro* in a series of cancer cell lines (LN-18, TF-1a, 786-O, T-47D, MCF-7, RPMI-7951, and LoVo) and *in vivo* (Hamdi and Castellon, 2005). However, in normal fibroblasts, this effect of oleuropein on actin cytoskeleton was transient. Another interesting finding of this study was that tumor regression was achieved more rapidly than with any established chemotherapeutic agents (complete regression of tumors within 9–12 days) and that oleuropein mainly targeted tumor cells and not tumor vasculature. The authors suggest that oleuropein attacks nascent tumor cells before the latter obtain a more aggressive phenotype, induced by hypoxic stimuli. This assumption could give new insights in anticancer pharmaceutical research (Hamdi and Castellon, 2005). Furthermore, luteolin exerted its inhibitory effect on hepatocyte growth factor (HGF)-induced invasion and migration in HepG2 cells, in a dose-dependent manner and independently of its cellular cytotoxicity (Lee, W.J. et al., 2006). In addition, luteolin induced potent actin cytoskeleton reorganization and inhibited the HGF-induced formation of filopodia and lamellipodia, by promoting a more peripheral redistribution of actin microfilaments, while pretreatment with luteolin was partially effective on HGF-induced cell scattering. This inhibitory effect on HGF signaling is attributed to suppression of c-Met phosphorylation (HGF cognitive receptor) and of both MAPK/ERK and PI3-AKT pathways, as confirmed by specific inhibitors such as PD98059 and wortmanin (Lee, W.J. et al., 2006).

Olive oil phenolic acids (caffeic, vanillic, coumaric, ferulic, syringic) have also been studied for their effect on tumor invasion and possible antimetastatic activity. All have revealed an antimetastatic effect, but in the majority of reports, this action was attributed to alteration of MMP secretion and/or expression (see below). There are only few studies on the inhibitory effect on cell adhesion and ECM. Caffeic acid phenethyl ester (CAPE), at relatively low concentrations (2.5–7.5 μg/ml), induced an impressive reorganization of the cytoskeleton and loss of actin stress fibers, in a dose-dependent manner, in human colon carcinoma DLD-1 cells. In addition, CAPE significantly reduced migration of NIH3T3 cells in the matrigel assay. The dramatic effect of CAPE on cell-adhesion and integrin-mediated signaling pathways was due to reduction of phosphorylation of focal adhesion kinase (FAK) (Weyant et al., 2000). FAK is a nonreceptor tyrosine kinase. Its phosphorylation is a crucial event after integrin activation and displays a key regulator role in processes involved in tumorigenesis and cancer promotion (van Nimwegen and van de Water, 2007). On the other hand, cinnamic acid treatment did not alter adhesion of colon adenocarcinoma cells (Caco2) on collagen type I (Ekmekcioglu et al., 1998). However, the authors suggest that this effect is not mandatory for cinnamic acid on other matrix substances, such as laminin.

Lignans are phytoestrogens; their effect on tumor malignant behavior is linked to both estrogen- and nonestrogen-related mechanisms, interfering with the expression of molecules that promote a more aggressive phenotype, such as Her2/neu, EGFR, IGF-1, VEGF, and HIF-1. Another special characteristic of lignans (or their metabolites) is that they exert their effect directly on the colonic epithelium, possibly meditated by gut microflora, without intervention of first pass metabolism. Lignan metabolites enterodiol (EDL) and enterolactone (ENL) are called mammalian lignans and are thought to be in part responsible for the lignan anticancer effect, since they appear as the major lignan representatives found in serum, urine, bile urine, and plasma seminal fluids of humans and animals (Wang, 2002). A series of studies reveals the multiple effects of lignans in tumor invasion and metastasis. In a nude mouse animal model, Dabrosin et al. (2002) showed that dietary supplementation with lignans was able to counteract the high metastatic ability of MDA-MB-435 estrogen receptor-negative human breast carcinoma cells, and diminish distant metastases. This effect was attributed to slow tumor growth, in parallel with attenuated VEGF expression, and limited angiogenesis. In another murine study, Chen et al. (2002), using the same cancer cell line, reported significant reduction in lymph node and lung metastases in mice fed with lignans, partly due to downregulation of IGF-1and EGFR expression. In a more recent report, ovariectomized mice with MCF-7 (estrogen receptor-positive) tumors receiving a continuous treatment of estradiol (E2) were fed with flaxseed (a plant rich in lignans), ED, or ENL. All three compounds were able to subvert E_2-induced secretion of VEGF and limit angiogenesis and metastatic ability (Bergman et al., 2007). However, it should be noted that the plasma concentrations of both EDL and ENL do not strictly correlate to lignan dietary intake, but also depend on a number of other parameters, like age, smoking history, use of antibiotics (Milder et al., 2007), as well as gut bacterial activity and host conjugating enzyme activity (Clavel et al., 2006). So far, the knowledge in this field indicates that elucidating the sources of variation and measuring the relevant panel of compounds are important in order to use these measures effectively in evaluating the impact of lignans and their derivatives on human health (Lampe et al., 2006).

7.3.3 Mechanism of Action

7.3.3.1 Interaction with Steroid and Growth Factor Receptor–Mediated Functions

Steroid hormones and their receptors are important factors for the growth and function of hormone responsive tissues and play a crucial role in the development and progression of different types of cancer. Several phenolic compounds, due to their structural similarity to estrogens, are able to interact with steroid receptors and/or modulate their expression and function. The so-called "phytoestrogens" can exert both estrogenic and antiestrogenic properties (Griffiths et al., 1999). In breast cancer cells apigenin and luteolin and the lignan enterolactone can interact with the estrogen receptor, exhibiting a biphasic effect on DNA synthesis in a concentration-dependent manner (Wang and Kurzer, 1997; Harris et al., 2005). In addition, apigenin and syringic acid exhibited weak progestational activity, while ferrulic, coumaric, and syringic acids express significant antiprogestational and/or antiandrogenic activity (Rosenberg et al., 1998).

A number of investigators have demonstrated that polyphenols modulate growth factors. The latter are major growth-regulatory molecules for both normal and neoplastic cells. Decreased requirement for specific growth factors is a common occurrence in neoplastically transformed cells and may lead to a growth advantage over their normal counterparts. Tumor cells are characterized by overexpression of growth factors, such as epidermal growth factor (EGF), platelet-derived growth factor (PDGF), insulin-like growth factor I (IGF-I), and vascular endothelial growth factor (VEGF) and their cognitive receptors (see Spencer-Cisek [2002] for a review). Any agent that interferes with growth factor actions, either by ligand-competition or inhibition of growth factor receptor expression, activity, homo- or hetero-dimerization, and/or downstream signaling, has been shown to inhibit cell growth and induce apoptosis.

It has been reported that a high olive oil diet decreased EGFR and ERB-B2/neu signal transduction pathway (Moral et al., 2003). Moreover, olive oil phenolics such as verbascoside, apigenin, and luteolin inhibit EGFR-tyrosine autophosphorylation and its downstream signaling (Huang et al. 1999; Kunvari et al., 1999; Yin et al., 1999b; Lee, L.T. et al., 2002). In addition, enterodiol and enterolactone inhibit EGF receptor-linked protein tyrosine kinase in MDA-MB-468 cells (Schultze-Mosgau et al., 1998). Caffeic acid phenethyl ester also inhibited EGF receptor-mediated effects in a concentration- and time-dependent manner in SV40 transformed keratinocytes (Z114) (Zheng et al., 1995). Apigenin was also reported to inhibit FGF receptor and pp60v-src protein tyrosine kinases in a mouse mutagenesis model (Huang et al., 1996), or VEGF expression and transcriptional activation in human ovarian and lung cancer cells (Fang et al., 2005; Liu et al., 2005). Luteolin inhibited insulin-like growth factor 1 (IGF-1)-induced activation of IGF-1R and Akt in prostate cancer PC-3 and DU145 cells (Fang et al., 2007b). Inhibition of phosphorylation has been also reported for PDGRF-beta by luteolin (Kim, J.H. et al., 2005), that further inhibited the angiogenesis-promoting effect of VEGF, by interacting with downstream molecules like phosphatidylinositol 3'-kinase (PI3K) (Bagli et al., 2004). Furthermore, in prostate cancer cells, apigenin increased accumulation of IGFBP-3, leading to subsequent reduction in IGF-I secretion, and growth inhibition and apoptosis (Shukla et al., 2005). In contrast, there are reports indicating that apigenin and luteolin either increased or had no effect on EGF receptor tyrosine kinase activity (Agullo et al., 1997; Schlupper et al., 2006).

7.3.3.2 Interaction with Specific Protein Kinases and Oncogenes/Oncoproteins

Protein kinases modify proteins by chemically adding phosphate groups to them. As they have profound effects on cell function, their activity is highly regulated. Dysfunctional kinase activity is a frequent cause of disease, particularly cancer, since kinases regulate many aspects of cell growth, movement, and death. *Oncogenes*, on the other hand, are genes whose activation can contribute to the development of cancer. Several genes have been reported to be activated in human cancer and their experimental activation in cell cultures or animal models can induce specific malignancies. Oncogene products are usually growth factor receptors, kinases, and transcription factors. *Tumor suppressor genes*, in contrast, are genes whose loss of function results in the promotion of malignancy. They are usually negative regulators of growth or other functions that affect invasive or metastatic potential. Recent work has presented evidence that olive oil polyphenols might have numerous anticancer effects, via interactions with kinases, oncogenes, and tumor suppressor genes. This work will be reviewed in this section.

7.3.3.2.1 Protein Kinases A and C

Caffeic acid has been reported to inhibit *in vitro* the activity of phosphorylase kinase, protein kinase C, and protein kinase A (Nardini et al., 2000). However, in another study, rat brain protein kinase C activity was not affected by the same agent (Huang et al., 1991). Caffeic acid phenethyl ester was also found to interfere with collagen binding to platelet membranes, via activation of protein kinase C (Hsiao et al., 2007), a result not confirmed in cultured HepG2 human hepatoma cells (Jaiswal et al., 1997). *In vitro* rat brain protein kinase C activity was not affected by ferulic acid (Huang et al., 1991). Oleanolic acid (a triterpenic acid) was reported to inhibit rat liver cyclic AMP-dependent protein kinase (protein kinase A) and rat brain Ca^{2+}- and phospholipid-dependent protein kinase C (PKC) (Wang and Polya, 1996).

Acteoside (verbascoside) has been found to inhibit PKC by interacting with the catalytic domain of PKC, explaining its antitumor activity (Herbert et al., 1991; Zhou et al., 1998; Daels-Rakotoarison et al., 2000). However, it has also been reported that acteoside did not affect PKC in PMA-activated peripheral human neutrophils (PMNs) and mononuclear cells (Lin et al., 2006). In a mouse skin tumor-promoting model protocatechuic acid moderately inhibited TPA-stimulated PKC activity, mainly by affecting the translocation of PKCalpha (Szaefer et al., 2007). Similarly, luteolin was found to exert its inhibition on lipopolysaccharide (LPS)-stimulated NF-κB transcriptional activity in Rat-1 fibroblasts via PKA (Kim, S.H. et al., 2003). Luteolin and apigenin were also inhibitors of PKC, competing with ATP (Huang et al., 1996; Lee and Lin, 1997; Lin et al., 1997; Cesen-Cummings et al., 1998; Kimata et al., 2000), while apigenin was reported to block mast cell phosphorylation of Ca^{2+}-dependent PKC alpha/beta II activity (Kim, J.Y. et al., 2005). However, in A431 cells, luteolin but not apigenin was found to inhibit PKC activity (Agullo et al., 1997). Although PKCdelta activity inhibition was found to be a key step in the effect of apigenin on TPA-induced skin carcinogenesis (Balasubramanian et al., 2006), its activation was also found to be important in apigenin-induced apoptosis in monocytic and lymphocytic leukemia cells (THP-1, U937, HL60, Jurkat, K562, A549) (Vargo et al., 2006).

7.3.3.2.2 Protein Tyrosine Kinases

Caffeic acid inhibits ceramide-induced apoptosis in U937 cells by interfering with its signal transduction pathway, through blocking tyrosine protein kinase activity and NF-κB (Nardini et al., 2001). Caffeic acid esters also inhibit the activity of tyrosine protein kinase in HT-29 cells (Rao et al., 1992), as well as in rat liver and colon (Rao et al., 1993). Furthermore, caffeic acid phenethyl ester blocks tyrosine phosphorylation of focal adhesion kinase in human colon carcinoma cells DLD-1, HT-29, and NIH3T3, a signaling mediator for the integrin-mediated cell-matrix contact, regulating cellular proliferation, migration, and apoptosis (Weyant et al., 2000). Hydroxytyrosol, too, amplifies peroxynitrite-dependent upregulation of Band 3, the anion channel and the major intrinsic membrane protein of the human erythrocyte, tyrosine phosphorylation through the activation of lyn, a src-family kinase (Maccaglia et al., 2003).

7.3.3.2.3 Mitogen-Activated Protein Kinases Family (MAPKs)

Hydroxytyrosol upregulates Erk1/2 and c-Jun N-terminal kinase (JNK) in HL-60 cells, activating apoptosis (Della Ragione et al., 2002). Phosphorylation of ERK was also induced in HUVEC cells by oleanolic acid, an action that is not related to its antiproliferative effect (Barthomeuf et al., 2004). In WI-38 cells, caffeic acid prevented H_2O_2-induced cell damage via the activation of Erc (Kang et al., 2006). In a rat model caffeic acid was reported to abolish the tyrosine phosphorylation of JAK2 and STAT1 and attenuate the proliferation of vascular smooth muscle cells under Angiotensin-II treatment, by partially blocking the JAK/STAT and Ras/Raf-1/ERK1/2 signaling cascade (Li et al., 2005). It should be noted that caffeic acid phenethyl ester has been reported to be a potent inhibitor of NF-κB (Natarajan et al., 1996) and has been used in several studies for this purpose (Lee, H.W. et al., 2002; Mendez-Samperio et al., 2002; Menschikowski et al., 2004). Caffeic acid phenethyl ester was also found to interfere with collagen binding to platelet membranes, via activation of mitogen-activated protein kinases (ERK2, JNK, and p38 MAPK) and Akt phosphorylation (Hsiao et al., 2007). Chlorogenic acid, caffeic acid ester with quinic acid, inhibited the proliferation of A549 human cancer cells by blocking UVB-induced transactivation of AP-1 and NF-κB and by decreasing the phosphorylation of c-Jun NH2-terminal kinases, p38 kinase, and MAPK kinase 4, induced by UVB or TPA (Feng et al., 2005). The antiproliferative mechanism of ferulic acid on serum-induced ECV304 cells, a human umbilical vein endothelial line, was found to be mediated by a nitric oxide-regulated inactivation of extracellular signal-regulated kinase (ERK1/2) mechanism (Hou et al., 2004a) and inactivation of the c-Jun N-terminal kinases (JNK) (Hou et al., 2004a). However, the sodium salt of ferulic acid (sodium ferulate) prevented amyloid-beta-induced neurotoxicity, through suppression of p38 MAPK and upregulation of ERK-1/2 and Akt/protein kinase B, in rat hippocampus (Jin, Y. et al., 2005). Ferulic acid also promotes cellular proliferation of MCF7, BT474, MDA-MB-231, and SKBR3 cells, at least partially via increased phosphorylation of ERK1/2 (Chang et al., 2006a, b). Protocatechuic acid induced apoptosis in human gastric adenocarcinoma (AGS) cells, via a sustained phosphorylation and activation of JNK and p38 MAPK, but not ERK. This effect was also prominent in MKN45, HT29, and HepG2 cells (Yip et al., 2006; Lin et al., 2007).

In MCF-7 and MDA-MB-468 breast cancer cells MAPK inhibition by apigenin blocked PMA-induced apoptosis (Yin et al., 2001; Weldon et al., 2005). The ability of apigenin to inhibit MAPK phosphorylation was also related to its antimetastatic effect in bombesin-enhanced peritoneal metastasis from intestinal adenocarcinomas, induced by azoxymethane in male Wistar rats (Tatsuta et al., 2000). In a well-documented study, both apigenin and luteolin blocked ERK2, p38, and c-Jun NH2-terminal kinase (JNK) (the complete MAPK system) and inhibited TNF-alpha-induced upregulation of intercellular adhesion molecule-1 (ICAM-1) in respiratory epithelial cells (Chen et al., 2004). Luteolin was also found to block the activation of ERKs and JNK in human basophils and murine mast cells (Kimata et al., 2000), while in murine macrophages RAW 264.7, pretreatment with luteolin inhibited LPS-induced ERK1/2 and p38, but not JNK1/2 phosphorylation, and blocked LPS-induced TNF-alpha release from these cells (Xagorari et al., 2002). Luteolin treatment of HepG2 cells was found to induce c-Jun NH2-terminal kinase (JNK) activation and through this and Bax/Bak it induced apoptosis (Lee, H.J. et al., 2005). Luteolin also inhibited TNF-alpha-induced phosphorylation of p38 MAPK and ERK in HT29 colon cancer cells (Kim, J.A. et al., 2005), HGF-induced ERK1/2 and Akt, but not JNK1/2 phosphorylation in HepG2 cells (Lee, W.J. et al., 2006) and LPS-induced ERK1/2 phosphorylation in human gingival fibroblasts (Gutierrez-Venegas et al., 2006). However, the effect of luteolin on JNK seems to be cell line-dependent. Indeed, luteolin can induce JNK and sensitize cells to the anticancer effect of cisplatin, via p53 phosphorylation and stabilization, both *in vivo* and *in vitro* (Shi et al., 2007). The inhibitory effect of apigenin on MAP kinases and especially of ERK via inhibition of its phosphorylation has been found in several other studies (Kuo and Yang, 1995; Grewal et al., 1999; Yano et al., 2005) and therefore apigenin has been used in several other studies as a MAPK inhibitor (Carrillo et al., 1998; Kanda et al., 1998; Niisato et al., 1999; Zhang et al., 2000; Garnovskaya et al., 2004). However, pre-treatment with apigenin of PC12 rat pheochromocytoma cells prolonged EGF-stimulated extracellular signal-regulated protein kinases1/2 (ERK1/2) phosphorylation (Llorens et al., 2002), a result equally found in the HepG2 cell line (Miro et al., 2002). Induction of phospho-JNK and phospho-ERK activity was also observed after incubation of AP1-transfected PC3 cells with apigenin (Gopalakrishnan et al., 2006). Finally, in HeLa cells, apigenin induced cytotoxicity via a marked and unbalanced increase in ERK1/2 but not MEK1/2 phosphorylation, and this effect did not involve p38-MAPK or JNK1/2, PI3kinases, or protein kinase CK2 (Llorens et al., 2004). Apigenin also interacts with the downstream MAPKK kinases and has been reported to block PMA-stimulated AP-1 activity, inhibiting in this way PMA-induced MCF-7 breast carcinoma apoptosis (Weldon et al., 2005).

7.3.3.2.4   Other Kinases

Caffeic acid has been reported to selectively inhibit a G-type casein kinase (CKG) (Cochet et al., 1982). Apigenin has also been reported to inhibit IκB alpha degradation and IκB alpha phosphorylation by significantly decreasing IKKalpha kinase activity in PC-3 prostate cancer cells, interacting in this way with the NFk-beta pathway (Shukla and Gupta, 2004b).

7.3.3.2.5   HER-2/neu Oncogene

The Her-2/neu (or c-erbB-2) oncogene, which is the second member of the EGFR family (EGFR-2), encodes a transmembrane tyrosine receptor kinase. In contrast, however, to other members of the family, it lacks an extracellular binding domain. Overexpression of Her-2/neu was reported in breast cancer and found to be associated with poor overall survival (Hortobagyi et al., 1999), increased metastatic potential, and resistance to chemotherapeutic agents. Transgenic mice overexpressing Her-2/neu develop focal mammary tumors (Guy et al., 1992). Apigenin exhibited potent growth-inhibitory activity in MDA-MB-453, BT-474, and SKBr-3 breast cancer cell lines, all of which overexpress HER2/neu, and MCF-7, which expresses the basal level of HER2/neu, through loss of HER2/neu protein and inhibition of PI3K/Akt pathway, cytochrome c release, or caspase-3 activation (Way et al., 2004, 2005). On the other hand, ferulic acid not only promoted cellular proliferation of MCF7, BT474, MDAMB231, and SKBR3 breast cancer cells, but also increased the phosphorylation and induced overexpression of HER-2/neu on MCF7 cells (Chang et al., 2006a, b).

7.3.3.2.6 Phosphatidylinositol 3-Kinase (PI3K) and Akt Protein Kinase

Several reports show an interaction of polyphenols with PI3 kinase, an important factor in carcinogenesis. In an extensive study of flavonoids/kinases interactions, luteolin and apigenin were reported as potent inhibitors of PI 3-kinase activity in A431 cells (Agullo et al., 1997), a result equally verified in breast cancer cells (Way et al., 2004). Therefore, apigenin has been used as a PI 3-kinase inhibitor (Mounho and Thrall, 1999). In another study luteolin inhibited VEGF-induced PI3K activity in HUVEC cells, an action critical for the antisurvival and antimitotic effects of the compound. Furthermore, luteolin abolished VEGF-induced activation of Akt, a downstream target of PI3K, conveying both survival and mitotic downstream signals (Bagli et al., 2004). Caffeic acid phenethyl ester was found to suppress the motility of lung adenocarcinoma cells, promoted by TGF-beta through Akt inhibition (Shigeoka et al., 2004), while it interfered with collagen binding to platelet membranes via Akt phosphorylation (Hsiao et al., 2007). Sodium ferulate prevented amyloid-beta-induced neurotoxicity, at least partially, via upregulation of Akt/protein kinase B in rat hippocampus (Jin, Y. et al., 2005) and promoted cellular proliferation of MCF7, BT474, MDAMB231, and SKBR3 cells via increased AKT phosphorylation (Chang et al., 2006a, b). Both apigenin and luteolin selectively blocked Akt phosphorylation/activity in the murine intestinal epithelial cell (IEC) line Mode-K (Ruiz and Haller, 2006). Apigenin also inhibits Akt function in breast cancer tumor cells by inhibiting Akt kinase activity and blocking HER-2 autophosphorylation (Way et al., 2004).

7.3.3.2.7 The Retinoblastoma Pathway, Cyclins, Cyclin-Dependent Kinases, and Cyclin-Dependent Kinase Inhibitors

As previously mentioned, entrance into cell cycling and active proliferation is a tightly regulated process. Cyclins regulate cyclin-dependent kinases (CDKs) and cyclin-dependent kinase inhibitors (CKIs), thus controlling the phosphorylation of retinoblastoma protein (pRb), a primary gatekeeper, allowing cells to transit from a resting G_0 state into active cycling and mitosis (Bartek et al., 1997). Polyphenols have been reported to interact with pRb/cyclin-dependent mechanisms in many ways.

Caffeic acid phenethyl ester (CAPE) inhibited the growth of C6 glioma cells in a dose- and time-dependent manner, by decreasing the protein level of hyperphosphorylated pRb, and upregulation of cyclin-dependent kinase inhibitors p21, p27, and p16 (Kuo et al., 2006). In serum-induced ECV304 cells (a human umbilical vein endothelial line), ferulic acid inhibited cellular proliferation, elevated the protein content of p21 (waf1/cip1), decreased expression of cyclin D1, and inhibited phosphorylation of retinoblastoma protein, suggesting that ferulic acid inhibited VSMC proliferation by regulating the cell progression from G_1 to S phase (Hou et al., 2004a, b). Ferulic acid also effectively decreased the iron-induced activation of caspase 3, as well as the expression of p53 and p21 and attenuated iron-induced oxidative damage and apoptosis, in primary cultures of rat cerebellar granule cells (Zhang et al., 2003). In premalignant and malignant (but not normal) human oral epithelial cell lines, ferulic acid treatment led to increased levels of cyclin B1 and cdc2 and p21 (Han et al., 2005). Protocatechuic acid was found to inhibit the survival of human promyelocytic leukemia HL-60 cells in a concentration- and time-dependent manner and caused an increase in the level of hypophosphorylated pRb and a decline in hyperphosphorylated Rb and a rapid loss of pRb, when the treatment period was extended (Tseng et al., 2000).

In an ultraviolet-induced mouse skin tumorigenesis model, apigenin caused a dose-dependent cell-cycle arrest, at both the G_0/G_1 and G_2/M phases, via increase in cyclin D1 expression, dose-dependent inhibition of cdk2, accumulation of the hypophosphorylated form of pRb, and induction of the cdk inhibitor p21/WAF1 (Lepley and Pelling, 1997). In MCF-7 and MDA-MB-468 breast carcinoma cells, apigenin was reported to induce a significant decrease in cyclin B1 and CDK1 protein levels, resulting in a marked inhibition of CDK1 kinase activity. Apigenin also reduced the protein levels of CDK4 and cyclins D1 and A, but did not affect cyclin E, CDK2, and CDK6 protein expression (Yin et al., 2001). Apigenin treatment of LNCaP and PC-3 prostate cancer cells resulted in G_1 arrest, which was associated with a marked decrease in the protein expression of cyclin D1, D2, and E and their activating partner cdk2, 4, and 6, with a concomitant induction of WAF1/p21 and KIP1/p27 and inhibition of the hyperphosphorylation of the pRb protein (Gupta et al., 2002; Shukla and Gupta, 2007). In a model of human prostate tumors implanted in athymic nude mice, oral intake of apigenin resulted in: (1) increased protein expression of WAF1/p21, KIP1/p27, INK4a/p16, and INK4c/p18; (2) reduced expression of cyclins D1, D2, and E and cyclin-dependent kinases cdk2, cdk4, and cdk6; (3) decrease in pRb phosphorylation, with a concurrent increase in the binding of cyclin D1 toward WAF1/p21 and KIP1/p27; and (4) decrease in the binding of cyclin E to cdk2 (Shukla and Gupta, 2006). Apigenin also inhibited the proliferation and, to a lesser degree, the migration of endothelial cells, and capillary formation *in vitro* and stimulated vascular smooth-muscle-cell proliferation. Endothelial-cell inhibition was a result of the accumulation of the hyperphosphorylated pRb, while stimulation of smooth-muscle cells was attributed to the reduced expression of cyclin-dependent kinase inhibitors p21 and p27, which negatively regulate the G_1 phase cyclin-dependent kinase (Trochon et al., 2000). In human LNCaP prostate cancer cells, apigenin and luteolin increased p21 levels through a p53-dependent and -independent manner, respectively (Kobayashi et al., 2002). Furthermore, in HepG2 human hepatocellular carcinoma cells, luteolin and apigenin downregulated CDK4 and increased CDK inhibitor p21/WAF1/CIP1 (Yee et al., 2003). In the HT-29 human colon cancer cell line, luteolin inhibited CDK4 and CDK2 activity, resulting in G1 arrest with a concomitant decrease of phosphorylation of retinoblastoma protein. Luteolin also decreased cyclin D1 levels, although no changes in expression of cyclin A, cyclin E, CDK4, or CDK2 were detected, downregulated cyclin B1 expression and decreased expression of p21 (Lim do et al., 2007). Finally, the enterolignans enterodiol and enterolactone decreased the cyclin A protein levels in human colonic cancer SW480 cells (Qu et al., 2005).

7.3.3.2.8   p53

p53 is probably the most studied tumor suppressor gene. Under normal conditions, it acts as a regulating mechanism for cell division. A number of studies have focused on the effect of olive oil polyphenols on p53 in several cancer models. Caffeic acid had no effect on p53 expression in the breast cancer cell lines T47D and MDA-MB-486, but increased p53 content of MCF-7 breast cancer cells (Soleas et al., 2001). In rat cerebellar granule cells, ferulic acid decreased iron-induced activation of p53 expression (Zhang et al., 2003). Protocatechuic acid induced apoptosis in human gastric adenocarcinoma (AGS) cells and increased phosphorylation and expression of p53 (Lin et al., 2007). Apigenin and luteolin induced p53 accumulation and apoptosis in the nontumor cell line C3H10T1/2CL8, but not in p53-knockout fibroblasts (Plaumann et al., 1996). In HepG2 cells both agents inhibited cell proliferation and increased p53 protein (Yee et al., 2003). Apigenin increased the levels of p53 and the p53-induced p21 and Bax and induced apoptosis in human neuroblastoma cell lines NUB-7, LAN-5, while it had no effect on p53-mutant SK-N-BE(2) cells (Torkin et al., 2005). In human cervical carcinoma cells (HeLa) and in HepG2 cells, apigenin inhibited growth through an apoptotic pathway that involved p53-dependent induction G_1 phase arrest, which was associated with a marked increment of the expression of p21/WAF1 protein (Zheng, P.W. et al., 2005; Chiang et al., 2006). Luteolin also sensitized cells to the anticancer effect of cisplatin, via c-Jun NH_2-terminal kinase-mediated p53 phosphorylation and stabilization (Shi et al., 2007). Apigenin also induced p53 protein accumulation in the mouse keratinocyte 308 cell line and LNCAP prostate cancer cells, where it increased p53 DNA-binding activity and transcriptional activation (McVean et al., 2000; Gupta et al., 2002; Kobayashi et al., 2002).

7.3.3.2.9   Other Oncogenes (Ras, c-myc, c-fos)

Apigenin, acting as inhibitor of the MAPK pathway, is an effective inhibitor of ras-mediated functions. However, apigenin also exhibited a reverting effect on the transformed phenotypes of v-H-ras-transformed NIH 3T3 cells and significantly inhibited their proliferation, suggesting that the flavonoid is capable of reverting the properties of v-H-ras transformed cells (Kuo and Yang, 1995; Lin et al., 1997). Furthermore, in wild-type NIH 3T3 cells apigenin inhibited TPA-induced c-jun and c-fos expression (Huang et al., 1996). Interestingly, in HeLa cells, where apigenin is cytotoxic, activation of the Ras pathway conferred cellular protection (Llorens et al., 2004). Apigenin also suppressed TPA-mediated tumor promotion of mouse skin, by reducing the level of TPA-stimulated phosphorylation of cellular proteins and induction of c-jun and c-fos expression (Lin et al., 1997), while in human keratinocytes, it caused a dramatic loss of c-myc (Segaert et al., 2000). The latter is an expected secondary event, since phosphorylated c-Myc is a nuclear substrate for MAPK and apigenin is a potent inhibitor of MAPKs (Yin et al., 1999b). Apigenin has also been reported to inhibit c-fos expression in LNCaP and PC-3 prostate cancer (Shukla and Gupta, 2007), C6 glioma cells (Zhang et al., 2000), and platelet-derived growth factor-BB (PDGF-BB)-induced expression of c-fos mRNA in primary cultured rat VSMCs (Kim, T.J. et al., 2002). It has also been reported that the inhibitory effects of apigenin and luteolin on TNF-induced ICAM-1 expression in U937 cells are mediated by attenuation of the c-fos and c-jun mRNA expressions (Chen et al., 2004). Luteolin also inhibited PDGF-induced c-fos gene expression in rat aortic VSMCs (Kim, J.H. et al., 2005). Oleanolic acid has been shown to inhibit mouse skin tumor promotion by TPA and also prevented c-fos gene expression (Oguro et al., 1998). Enterolactone and enterodiol were the only lignans with a weak inhibitory effect on TPA-mediated c-fos transcription in human breast cancer-derived MDA-MB-468 cells (Schultze-Mosgau et al., 1998).

7.3.3.3 Inhibition of Enzymes Related to Tumor Promotion and Metastasis

Tumor promotion is an essential process in multistage cellular (and cancer) development, providing the conditions for clonal expansion and genetic instability of preneoplastic and premalignant cells. It is caused by a continuous dysfunction of cellular signal transduction, resulting in an overstimulation of metabolic pathways, along which mediators of cell proliferation and inflammation, as well as genotoxic by-products, are generated. Polyphenols' beneficial effects also have been attributed to their competitive inhibition of enzymes, such as proteasome, matrix metalloproteinases, nitric oxide synthases, and cytochromes P450 enzymes.

7.3.3.3.1 Proteasome

The ubiquitin-proteasome pathway represents the main proteolytic system in eukaryotic cells and has a pivotal role in the control of protein and cellular function. Proteasome proteolysis involves the conjugation of ubiquitin molecules to protein substrates, followed by degradation of the latter by proteasome. There are three major proteasomal activities: chymotrypsin-like, trypsin-like, and peptidyl-glutamyl peptide hydrolyzing activity. The chymotrypsin-like is associated with tumor cell survival. Many cell cycle and cell death regulators have been identified as targets of the ubiquitin-proteasome-mediated degradation pathways, including p53, p21, p27Kip1, IκB-α, and Bax. In recent years, proteasome inhibition has emerged as a promising target in novel anticancer therapy for hemopoietic malignancies and solid tumors, such as androgen-independent prostate and ovarian cancer (Dou and Goldfarb, 2002; Richardson et al., 2005; Landis-Piwowar et al., 2006). Proteasomes have been found to control metastatic potency through inhibition of angiogenesis and induction of tumor cell death (Daniel et al., 2005). Apart from established proteasome inhibitors in anticancer therapy, such as Bortezomib, a plethora of studies focus on new low toxicity molecules, including polyphenols (for a recent review, see Kampa et al. [2007]). The emerging structure-activity of green-tea polyphenols triggered the production and evaluation of several synthetic analogs (Kuhn et al., 2005).

Olive oil compounds can inhibit chymotrypsin-like activity. Apigenin, as reported by Way et al., induced apoptosis in HER2/neu overexpressing breast cancer cells (MDA-MB-453, BT-474, and SKBr-3) via the PI3/Akt pathway (Way et al., 2004). This proteasomal degradation of HER2/neu involves cytochrome c release and rapid caspase-3 activation (Way et al., 2005). According to the authors, this polyubiquitination of HER2/neu, and the subsequent degradation, can be attributed to the position of B ring; and the existence of the 3′, 4′-hydroxyl group on the 2-phenyl group of apigenin. These findings gave new insight to the structure-activity relationship of flavonoids. More recent studies provide new evidence on the structure-proteasome-inhibitory effect and apoptosis potency of apigenin and luteolin (Chen et al., 2007), as well as HER2/neu depletion by oleuropein (Menendez et al., 2007). Apigenin inhibited the chymotrypsin-like activity of purified 20S and 26S proteasomes in intact leukemia Jurkat T cells, leading to the accumulation of Bax and IκB-α (Chen et al., 2005), and subsequently to apoptosis. In addition, apigenin appeared to interfere with HIF-1 (hypoxia inducible factor) degradation, through regulation of CK-2 (casein kinase 2), an ubiquitous serine/threonine kinase (Mottet et al., 2005). Moreover, luteolin was reported to inhibit HIF-1 activity in Chinese hamster ovary (CHO) A4-4 cells by promoting proteasome and p53 activity (Hasebe et al., 2003). In another study, Shi et al. reported that luteolin inhibits PKC (protein kinase C) by caspase-8 induction and caspase-3 enhanced maturation. As a result, downregulation of XIAP (X-linked inhibitor of apoptosis protein) was observed and that enhanced TRAIL (TNF-related apoptosis-inducing ligand) induced apoptosis (Shi et al., 2005). Oleuropein has been found to enhance proteasome activity through conformational changes (Katsiki et al., 2007). As regards phenolic acids, caffeic and cinnamic esters have been shown to inhibit proteasome activity, but this inhibitory effect has not been observed for caffeic or cinnamic acid per se (Arbiser et al., 2005). Hence, CAPE was reported to selectively inhibit NF-κB and partially attenuate peroxisome activity in alveolar epithelial cells (Haddad and Fahlman, 2002). Gallic acid, another phenolic compound of olive oil, affects 20S proteasome functionality, depending on the complex subunit composition, and, in cell extracts, behaves both as antioxidant and proteasome effectors, as reported by Pettinari et al. (Pettinari et al., 2006).

7.3.3.3.2   Matrix Metalloproteinases

The matrix metalloproteinases (MMPs) are a family of Zn^{2+}- and Ca^{2+}-dependent endopeptidases that are key mediators of ECM remodeling. They are secreted in a nonactive form and become activated by partial proteolytic cleavage. They are grouped by their substrate preferences and domain structures: collagenases degrading fibrillar collagen (MMP-1, MMP-8, and MMP-13), gelatinases (MMP-2 and MMP-9) are potent in nonfibrillar and denatured collagen degradation, stromelysins (MMP-3, MMP-10, and MMP-11) preferring proteoglycans and glycoproteins as substrates, and membrane-type MMPs (MT1-, MT2-, MT3-, MT4-, and MT5-MMP) containing C-terminal transmembrane anchorage domain (Nagase and Woessner, 1999). MT1-MMP plays an essential role in basement membrane degradation by activating pro-MMP-2. The activity of MMPs can be inhibited by interaction with their endogenous inhibitors, tissue inhibitors of MMPs (TIMPs) (Chirco et al., 2006; Nagase et al., 2006). MMPs are associated with tumor cell invasion of the basement membrane and stroma, blood vessel penetration, and metastasis, and they have more recently been implicated in primary and metastatic growth and angiogenesis. In particular, gelatinases (MMP-2 and -9) are abundantly expressed in various malignant tumors.

Polyphenols have been shown *in vitro* to profoundly affect ECM turnover by regulating gelatinases expression and activity, acting at both the pre- and post-transcriptional level (Dell'Agli et al., 2005). According to Kim, in a HUVEC model, apigenin inhibited *in vitro* angiogenesis, in part via preventing VEGF/bFGF-induced MMP-1 and uPA (urokinase-type plasminogen activator) expression, as well as the activation of pro-MMP-2. The above actions are achieved by modulation of distinct MMP inhibitors, TIMP-1 and -2, and PAI-1. uPA is a serine protease that is highly specific for the transformation and subsequent activation of plasminogen to plasmin, which, in turn, can cleave matrix components such as fibrin and fibronectin and activate several MMPs (Kim, M.H., 2003). In a more recent study Lee and co-workers reported that apigenin, as well as other phenolic compounds, inhibits both collagenase activity and MMP expression in a dose- and structure-dependent manner (Sim et al., 2007). However, findings on apigenin effects on MMP secretion remain inconsistent. In a series of studies, apigenin seemed not to directly affect MMP-9 expression (Tatsuta et al., 2000; Zhu et al., 2003). Moreover, both luteolin and apigenin appeared as MMP-1 inhibitors (Kim, J.H. et al., 2004). Emerging data on luteolin demostrate an inhibitory effect on MMP-9 and MMP-2 and according to Huang et al. this is due to the double bond between C2 and C3 in ring C and the OH groups on C3' and C4' in ring B (Huang et al., 1999). The inhibitory effect of luteolin on MMP secretion and in parallel of FAK phosphorylation in MiaPaCa-2 cells provided new evidence on the regulation of MMP secretion (Lee, L.T. et al., 2004).

Phenolic acids equally exert a modulatory effect on MMPs. Caffeic acid, one of olive oil's "minor" components, displays a "major" inhibitory role on MMP-9 expression and/or activity as shown in the majority of published data. Caffeic acid is a selective inhibitor of MMP-2 and MMP-9 *in vivo* and *in vitro*, in fibrosarcome-derived cell lines (Hwang et al., 2006), hepatocarcinoma (Chung et al., 2004; Jin, U.H. et al., 2005), human high metastatic giant cell carcinoma of the lung (PG) (Xu et al., 2004), and CT26 colon adenocarcinoma (Liao et al., 2003). However, in HaCaT cells (normal immortalized keratinocytes), caffeic acid-induced modification in MMP-9 expression was moderate (Holvoet et al., 2003). Caffeic acid modifies MMP levels in multiple ways, acting on secretion, transcription, or regulation of the MMP inhibitor TIMP1-2 (Hwang et al., 2006). The inhibitory effect of caffeic acid on MMP levels and the dramatic effect on invasion and metastasis were achieved at low concentrations, while no cytotoxicity was found against normal cells (Jin, U.H. et al., 2005). On the other hand, Liu and co-workers suggested that cinnamic acid (a nonphenolic acid found in olive oil) altered MMP and TIMP-2 expression in glioblastoma, melanoma, prostate, and lung carcinoma cells (Liu et al., 1995). In contrast, vanillic acid did not exert important activity on mouse breast cancer cells (Lirdprapamongkol et al., 2005).

7.3.3.3.3   Cycloxygenase-Lipoxygenase

Although inflammation has long been considered as a localized protective reaction of tissue to irritation, injury, or infection, there has been a new realization about its role in a wide variety of diseases, including cancer. While acute inflammation is part of the defense response, chronic inflammation can lead, among other diseases, to cancer. Several pro-inflammatory gene products have been identified as critical mediators of suppression of apoptosis, proliferation, angiogenesis, invasion, and metastasis. They include TNF and members of its superfamily, cycloxygenase-2 (COX-2), and lipoxygenase-5 (5-LOX). The expression of their genes is mainly regulated by the transcription factor NF-κB, which is constitutively active in most tumors and is induced by carcinogens (Aggarwal et al., 2006). Cyclooxygenase (COX) catalyzes the formation of prostaglandins (PG) from arachidonic acid. COX has two isoforms: COX-1 and COX-2. The former is expressed constitutively in a variety of cells and tissues, whereas COX-2 is inducible by cytokines, growth factors, and tumor promoters. The aberrant overexpression of COX-2 is a characteristic feature of more than two-thirds of all human neoplasias (such as colon, lung, breast, esophagus, prostate, and melanoma) and the specific inhibition of this enzyme gains increasing interest in a targeted anticancer strategy (Marks et al., 2007). COX-2 induced prostaglandins, which in turn promote tumor cell growth by stimulating cell proliferation and angiogenesis and by suppressing apoptosis and immune defense. Lipoxygenases (LOXs) are nonheme iron dioxygenases that insert molecular oxygen into polyunsaturated fatty acids, resulting in the formation of hydroperoxyeicosatetraenoic acid molecules. Their oxidation products have also been reported to be important regulators of the proliferation and apoptosis of cancer cell lines, as well as promoters of tumor angiogenesis (Tang et al., 1996; Ye et al., 2004). Three lipoxygenases (LOXs: 5-LOX, 12-LOX, and 15-LOX) have been reported to be present in human tissues. The above data suggest that the regulation of arachidonic acid metabolism is important in the prevention and evolution of different types of cancer, and especially those of the digestive tract. A great body of studies has been inspired by the effects of natural antioxidants on the COX pathway. Flavonoids and flavonoid-containing foods have been investigated as potential selective COX-2 inhibitors. However, we should note at this point that data on olive oil are limited if compared to other plant sources of (poly)phenols.

Several mechanisms of inhibition appear to be implicated in COX-2 regulation by flavonoids. In the majority of studies, it was suggested that the main regulatory effect of flavonoids on COX-2 was at the transcriptional level (O'Leary et al., 2004; Ziyan et al., 2007). One model of action involves the peroxisome proliferator activated factor gamma (PPARγ). PPARs bind to specific response elements as a heterodimer with the retinoid X factor, activating transcription in response to a variety of different exogenous or endogenous ligands such as NSAIDS, arachidonic acid metabolites, and some drugs. Apigenin and luteolin can bind to PPARγ *in vitro*, acting as possible PPARγ allosteric ligands, and reduce COX-2 promoter activity. PPARγ activation seems structure-dependent (Liang et al., 2001). Moreover, flavonoids were shown to downregulate COX-2 expression through NO regulation. Apigenin decreased iNOS and COX expression, as well as prostaglandin E_2 (PGE_2) release in a dose-dependent manner, in the macrophage cell line J774A (Raso et al., 2001). Similar findings were reported for luteolin in bacterial lipopolysaccharide (LPS)-activated mouse macrophages RAW264 (Hu and Kitts, 2004). Another mechanism proposed for inhibition of COX-2 gene expression is through the NF-κB pathway (Liang et al., 1999). Apigenin-induced NF-κB inhibition in prostate cancer cells triggers prostate cancer suppression by transcriptional repression of NF-κB-responsive genes, as well as through selective sensitization of prostate carcinoma cells to TNF-alpha-induced apoptosis (Shukla and Gupta, 2004b). Al-Fayez et al. reported that apigenin has no effect on COX-2 activity, but exerted a strong inhibitory effect on COX-2 expression (Al-Fayez et al., 2006). More recent data, however, revealed that this compound has a coupled inhibitory effect on COX-2 by stabilizing mRNA and suppressing, at the same time, translation through TIAR (T-cell-restricted intracellular antigen 1-related protein) and USF (upstream stimulatory factor) in UVB-exposed mouse 308 keratinocytes (Tong et al., 2007; Van Dross et al., 2007). In addition, flavonoids can suppress COX-2 transcriptional activity by inhibition of phosphorylation of signal transduction molecules. Structurally, the number of hydroxyl groups on the B ring may be related to the molecular conformation that influences the interactions between flavonoids and enzymes such as tyrosine kinase and protein kinase C, which are involved in COX-2 transcriptional activity. In human keratinocytes, apigenin inhibited COX-2 through downregulation of Akt signal transduction and limitation of arachidonic acid release (Van Dross et al., 2005). In another study, however, both apigenin and luteolin induced p38 stress kinase activity, but not JNK (O'Prey et al., 2003). In mouse bone marrow-derived mast cells, both apigenin and luteolin exerted a dual inhibitory effect on COX-2/5-LOX (Kim, J.S. et al., 2006).

Tyrosol and hydroxytyrosol, olive oil's most characteristic minor components, exert an inhibitory effect on COX-2, especially through suppression of the NF-κB pathway (Moreno, 2003; Maiuri et al., 2005; De Stefano et al., 2007). In addition, other molecules seem to interfere in this process, such as STAT-1α (signal transducer and activator of transcription-1alpha) and IRF-1 (interferon regulated factor). Moreover, hydroxytyrosol seems more effective in inhibiting 5-LOX than tyrosol and oleuropein (Kohyama et al., 1997; de la Puerta et al., 1999). Surprisingly, data on the relation of COX/LOX and lignans, which represent one of the most well-studied phenolic compounds due to their phytoestrogenic activities, are very few, and we are still in need of further investigation. There is evidence for the inhibitory effect of lignans on COX-1 and COX-2 in colon tumor models (Bommareddy et al., 2006).

Data on phenolic acid effects on cycloxygenase and lipoxygenase remain contradictory. Rossi et al. reported that neither caffeic acid nor ferulic acid inhibited COX activity in J747 macrophages and rat lung (Rossi et al., 2002). In more recent studies, however, ferulic, caffeic, and cinnamic acid and their esters significantly inhibited both COX-1 and COX-2 enzymes in a dose-dependent manner, in COX enzyme inhibitory assays (Shin et al., 2004; Abdel-Latif et al., 2005; Al-Anati et al., 2005; Hirata et al., 2005; Karlsson et al., 2005; Jayaprakasam et al., 2006; Sang et al., 2006; Manju and Nalini, 2007). The mechanism suggested for the above actions also involves inhibition of the NF-κB pathway.

7.3.3.3.4 Nitric Oxide Synthases

Nitric oxide (NO) is a multifaceted gaseous signaling agent and regulator, influential in many biological systems. As regards cancer, the role of NO and the enzymes that produce it (nitric oxide synthases [NOSs], iNOS inducible, eNOS endothelial, and nNOS neuronal) remain inconsistent. The advantageous or deleterious profile of NO in malignancies appears as two faces of the same coin and displays organ- and cell-specificity. The NO/NOS system provides to phenolic compounds an alternative multiplexing mechanism of action and cross-talk between inflammation and tumor promotion (Williams and Djamgoz, 2005).

Tyrosol and hydroxytyrosol have been reported to downregulate iNOS and COX-2 gene expression in RAW 264.7 macrophages, by attenuation of NF-κB, STAT-1α, and IRF-1 activation mediated through LPS-induced ROS generation (Moreno, 2003; Maiuri et al., 2005; De Stefano et al., 2007). On the other hand, Schmitt et al. concluded that hydroxytyrosol is unlikely to have a direct effect on eNOS in human endothelial EA.hy926cells (Schmitt et al., 2007). With regard to oleuropein, in a study conducted on mouse macrophages by Visioli et al. (1998), it was suggested that under endotoxin stimulation, leuropein triggered NO release through iNOS potentiation.

There is a growing body of evidence on the interrelation of flavonoids and NOS. Both apigenin and luteolin have been found to exert an inhibitory effect on iNOS transcription and activity (Comalada et al., 2006). This regulatory effect appeared to be mediated mainly through downregulation of NF-κB. Indeed, pretreatment with luteolin diminished LPS-induced NF-κB translocation, phosphorylation of Akt and MAPK members, as well as iNOS expression and NO synthesis, in human gingival fibroblasts (Gutierrez-Venegas et al., 2006). Moreover, luteolin was reported to inhibit iNOS expression and degradation of I-κB-alpha in a dose-dependent manner, in LPS-activated BV-2 microglia (Kim, J.S. et al., 2006). It was also reported, that luteolin inhibits both iNOS and COX-2 protein expression, but not enzymatic activity, in RAW264.7 cells (Hu and Kitts, 2004). Apigenin, on the other hand, appeared as a strong inhibitor of iNOS and COX-2 transcription in activated macrophages (Liang et al., 2001; Olszanecki et al., 2002), through stimulation of PPARgamma transcriptional activity. Additionally, it suppressed prostate cancer cells via inhibition of NF-κB, which resulted in a decreased expression of NF-κB-dependent reporter gene and suppressed expression of NF-κB-regulated genes, including iNOS (Shukla and Gupta, 2004b). Conversely, apigenin may upregulate eNOS expression and activity, acting as an inhibitor of MAPK and Akt (Jiang et al., 2007). All the above-mentioned effects mediated by luteolin and apigenin are exerted at low, noncytotoxic levels.

Concerning phenolic acids, a number of conflicting studies exist; most of them focus on their metabolites and not on phehenolic acid per se, with caffeic acid being the most studied compound. Nevertheless, the emerging data remain controversial. In a former study of our group, caffeic acid exerted no effect on NOS-isoenzymes activity in T47D breast cancer cells (Kampa et al., 2004). However, caffeic acid derivatives inhibited iNOS expression and enzyme activity *in vivo* and *in vitro* (da Cunha et al., 2004; Chiang et al., 2005). Inhibition of NOS was associated with suppression of COX-2 and 5-LOX (Chiang et al., 2005; Jatana et al., 2006), mediated through downregulation of the NF-κB pathway (Song et al., 2002; Khan et al., 2007). In addition, caffeic acid, p-coumaric acid, and vanillic acid enhanced eNOS expression moderately, while cinnamic acid appeared as a strong potentiator and ferulic acid had no effect in EA.hy 926 endothelial cells (Wallerath et al., 2005). In a human umbilical vein endothelial line, treatment with ferulic acid enhanced NO secretion (Hou et al., 2004a). In the hippocampus, ferulic acid induced transient increase of eNOS, while pretreatment with ferulic acid derivatives resulted in iNOS inhibition (Cho et al., 2005; Sultana et al., 2005). Moreover, in NCX 20275 macrophages, an NO-releasing derivative of ferulic acid induced iNOS inhibition on both the transcriptional and translational level, while ferulic acid was inactive. This action was mediated by attenuation of LPS-induced NF-κB translocation (Ronchetti et al., 2006).

7.3.3.3.5   Cytochromes P450

Cytochromes P450 (CYPs) constitute a superfamily of heme-thiolate isoenzymes involved in the metabolism of several chemicals (such as drugs, dietary chemicals, or environmental pollutants). In this respect, they play an important role in the bioactivation of several pro-carcinogens and in the activation and inactivation of several anticancer drugs. Metabolic activation of chemical carcinogens is mediated by a limited number of human CYP species, namely, CYP1A1, CYP1A2, CYP1B1, CYP2A6, CYP2B6, CYP2E1, and CYP3A4 (Code et al., 1997). These CYPs are mainly expressed in the liver, except CYP1A1 and CYP1B1, which are extrahepatic isoenzymes in humans. The major olive and olive oil phenolic compounds oleuropein and its two major metabolites, hydroxytyrosol and tyrosol (Zhou et al., 2004), have been shown to inhibit CYPs. Indeed *in vitro* studies indicated that oleuropein inactivated androstenedione 6β-hydroxylase (CYP3A4) activity in human liver microsomes (Stupans et al., 2001). The reactive metabolites of oleuropein remain undetermined, but oleuropein might undergo CYP3A-mediated oxidation to a number of metabolite(s) capable of binding and inactivating CYP3A4. In addition, hydroxytyrosol and tyrosol and/or their metabolites may be involved in this inactivation. Metabolic studies indicated that hydroxytyosol was excreted into the urine unchanged and as its glucuronide and sulfate conjugates. Hydroxytyrosol can also be sequentially oxidized to 3,4-dihydroxyphenylacetic acid and 3,4-dihydroxyphenylacetaldehyde by alcohol and aldehyde dehydrogenase, or methylated by catechol–O-methyltransferase to homovanillic alcohol and then oxidized to homovanillic acid (D'Angelo et al., 2001). Oleuropein was found to be a relatively weak inhibitor of CYP1A2-mediated 7-methoxyresorufin-O-deethylation (24% inhibition at 100 μM), but not CYP2E1-mediated chlorzoxazone 6-hydroxylation. In contrast, CYP1A2 did not undergo mechanism-based inactivation by oleuropein (Stupans et al, 2001). Finally, administration of olive oil in Sprague-Dawley rats resulted in a 31% reduction of CYP2C11 protein levels (Brunner and Bai, 2000).

Flavone aglycons, apigenin, and luteolin exhibited a mixed-type inhibition of CYPs in *vitro*. Kim, H.J. et al. (2005) suggested that these compounds exert a differential inhibitory effect on CYP1A, related to the number and the position of hydroxyl groups. However, the inhibition of CYP1B1 enzyme seemed structure-independent. In HepG2 cells, apigenin increased CYP1A1-induced luciferase activity (Allen et al., 2001). As regards CYP1B1 (which metabolizes estradiol and polycyclic aromatic hydrocarbons to potential carcinogens), apigenin exerted a competitive inhibition in a dose-dependent manner (Chaudhary and Willett, 2006). In addition, apigenin inhibited CYP1A2 and CYP3A with an IC_{50} lower than 10 μg/l (von Moltke et al., 2004). Furthermore, apigenin downregulated CYP19 activity (Moon et al., 2006). However, as flavonoids are metabolized mainly by CYP1A2, leading to formation of metabolites with different properties than those of the parent compounds, as well as the differential expression of CYPs among individuals, questions on flavonoid bioavailability and on their advantageous and health-promoting properties are raised (Breinholt et al., 2002). Data on phenolic acids and their interrelation with CYPs remain controversial. Administration of caffeic acid had no effect on xenobiotic-metabolizing enzymes in rat liver (Debersac et al., 2001). Nevertheless, in a previous study by our group, incubation of T47D breast cancer cells with caffeic acid resulted in a reduction of CYP1A1 by 70% (Kampa et al., 2004). Additionally, gallic acid diminished CYP3A activity in human liver microsomes (Stupans et al., 2002).

7.3.3.4   Direct Effect on Nucleic Acids and Nucleoproteins

DNA damage is a key element of carcinogenesis and cancer progression. DNA function and repair are regulated by a number of proteins inside the nucleus. Nucleoproteins are proteins structurally associated with DNA (and RNA) that play important structural and enzymatic roles in DNA processes. Disruption of the actions of these proteins may lead to dysfunction of nucleic acids or impaired DNA repair leading to cell death or carcinogenesis. The DNA interacting proteins that might be involved are topoisomerases, polymerases, and acetylases. The majority of studies links olive oil polyphenols and their effect on DNA indirectly, via the production of reactive oxygen species that induce oxidative damage of DNA. Moreover, it should be pointed out that this effect usually occurs at relatively high concentrations. Only a few reports demonstrate a direct effect of olive oil microconstituents on DNA and nucleoproteins.

Caffeic acid has been shown to be a potent inhibitor of topoisomerase I (Stagos et al., 2005). A similar topoisomerase I inhibition was also the effect of protocatechuic acid (Stagos et al., 2005), which could also directly inhibit topoisomerase II in Chinese hamster V79 cells (De Graff et al., 2003) and cause a dose-dependent decrease in andriamycin-induced DNA double-strand breaks. Oleanolic acid, a triterpene acid present in olive oil, also inhibits topoisomerases I and II-alpha through a reported mechanism that does not involve stabilization of the cleavable complex or the intercalation of DNA (Syrovets et al., 2000) as well as DNA polymerase beta (Deng et al., 1999; Prakash Chaturvedula et al., 2003). Topoisomerase inhibition was also reported for luteolin, inducing DNA cleavage with subsequent DNA ladder formation, in promyelocytic HL-60, promyelocytic HP-100, and hamster ovary AA8 cells, via formation of a luteolin-topoisomerase II-DNA ternary complex (Yamashita and Kawanishi, 2000; Cantero et al., 2006). However, in another study it was found that the same compound possesses cytotoxic and DNA topoisomerase I poisoning activity (Galvez et al., 2003). Moreover, luteolin has also been found to bind to histones H3 and H4, controlling in this way histone-dependent gene transcription and cellular proliferation, via binding and modulation of core histone/nucleosome functions (Shoulars et al., 2002; Shoulars et al., 2005; Shoulars et al., 2006). Apigenin also interacts with topoisomerases I and II, stabilizing the topoisomerase II-DNA complex (Constantinou et al., 1995; Boege et al., 1996; Snyder and Gillies, 2002). In Reuber H35 hepatoma and CTLL-2 cells this enhanced cytotoxicity, due to topoisomerase II inhibition, was observed when apigenin was applied following an irradiation treatment, leading to decreased repair of DNA (Azuma et al., 1995; van Rijn and van den Berg, 1997). Verbascoside (acteoside), an olive oil phenylpropanoid glycoside, has been reported to induce cell death in promyelocytic leukemia HL-60 cells by internucleosomal breakdown of chromatin DNA (Inoue et al., 1998) and to reduce oxidative stress–induced DNA damage in a Fenton reaction on plasmid model by forming complexes with iron molecules (Zhao et al., 2005). Verbascoside was also reported to inhibit telomerase activity leading human gastric carcinoma cells MKN45 to cell cycle arrest (Zhang et al., 2002). Finally, cinnamic hydroxamic acid (NVP-LAQ824) was found to inhibit histone deacetylase enzymatic activities *in vitro* (Atadja et al., 2004)

7.4 OTHER PENTACYCLIC TRITERPENES

In addition to oleanolic and maslinic acid previously discussed, other biologically active terpenes in olive and olive pomace oil are ursolic acid, betulinic acid, erythrodiol, and uvaol (see Chapter 4). Among them, betulinic and ursolic acids are the agents that have been studied extensively due to their high cytotoxicity toward tumor cells and lack of toxicity against normal cells. Betulinic acid was characterized as melanoma selective cytotoxic agent since it completely inhibited cultured human melanoma cell growth as well as tumor growth in athymic mice carrying human melanomas (Yasukawa et al., 1991; Pisha et al., 1995). Later on betulinic acid was tested in different cancer cells such as breast, colon (Basu et al., 2004), head and neck (Thurnher et al., 2003), prostate (Chintharlapalli et al., 2007), ovary, lung, thyroid, neuroblastoma (Rzeski et al., 2006), glioma (Wick et al., 1999), neuroblastoma (Fulda et al., 1997; Fulda and Debatin, 2000), and leukemia cells (Noda et al., 1997; Raghuvar Gopal et al., 2005). Apart from betulinic acid several derivatives have been produced by simple modifications of the parent structure in order to improve their selective antitumor activity (Kim, D.S. et al., 1998; Kim, J.Y. et al., 2001). The action of betulinic acid and its derivatives as antitumor agents was mainly mediated by the induction of apoptosis that functions in a p53- and CD95-independent fashion through a mitochondrial-mediated pathway (Eiznhamer and Xu, 2004). It involved the activation of caspases that cleaves poly(ADP ribose) polymerase (Wick et al., 1999), while a decreased bcl2 and an increased bax expression were observed (Rzeski et al., 2006). Moreover, it has been shown that betulinic acid induced NFk-B activation (Kasperczyk et al., 2005), induced reactive oxygen species generation, inhibited topoisomerase I, and activated the MAP kinase cascade. In addition, it has been reported to inhibit angiogenesis and cell migration (Rzeski et al., 2006; Chintharlapalli et al., 2007). Similarly, ursolic acid is capable of inducing apoptosis and cell cycle arrest mainly at G_0/G_1 phase in different tumor cells (melanoma, endometrial, multiple myeloma, leukemia, lung, breast, and prostate) (Hsu et al., 2004; Achiwa et al., 2005; Harmand et al., 2005; Zhang et al., 2006; Lai et al., 2007; Liu and Jiang, 2007; Nangia-Makker et al., 2007; Pathak et al., 2007). This apoptotic effect is dependent on the mitochondrial intrinsic pathway, characterized by caspase 3 activation and alteration of the Bax-Bcl-2 balance (Harmand et al., 2005) as well as inhibition of both the PI3K-Akt pathway and the MAPK pathway (Achiwa et al., 2007).

7.5 EFFECTS OF OLEIC ACID

Taking into consideration the large body of evidence indicating the beneficial role of olive oil in cancer, we have to keep in mind its unique characteristics, namely, the presence of the ω-9 mono-unsaturated fatty acid, oleic acid, in high abundance (56–84%). At first, a strong association of a high fat diet and cancer risk (especially colorectal cancer) had been established, but now it becomes widely accepted that the type of dietary fat is the most important element. Indeed, many epidemiological studies revealed that intake of oleic acid is protective against several carcinomas (Bartsch et al., 1999; Wahle et al., 2004; Binukumar and Mathew, 2005). A number of *in vitro* and *in vivo* studies revealed that oleic acid and its derivatives could have effects similar to those reported for polyphenols. Indeed, oleic acid restrained cancer cell growth (breast, colon, lung) (Zhu et al., 1989; Llor et al., 2003; Menendez et al., 2005) by inducing apoptosis and cell cycle arrest (Martinez et al., 2005a). Moreover, it was found that it inhibited angiogenesis (Kimura, 2002) and metastasis (Suzuki et al., 1997). Its mechanism of action also involved activation of certain kinases, such as PKC, increase in cdk inhibitors (CKIs), and decrease of cyclins' concentration (Martinez et al., 2005b). In addition, it was reported to reduce the expression of HER2/neu (erbB-2) oncogene (Nelson, 2005) and to synergistically enhance the growth inhibitory effects of trastuzumab (Herceptin, anti-Her-2/neu immunotherapy) in breast cancer cells (Menendez et al., 2005).

7.6 CONCLUSIONS

From the data presented in this chapter it becomes evident that the beneficial anticancer effect of olive oil is a combination of the specific action of oleic acid and of its minor constituents. Both exhibit a wide spectrum of biological properties, influencing major structural and functional cellular components. Their effects (interaction with key elements of cell function: cell cycle, growth, progression, signaling, apoptosis, etc.) provide the biological background of the beneficial actions of olive oil, a major element of the Mediterranean type of nutrition. They further present data for new, targeted therapeutic interventions in a great spectrum of chronic diseases, including cancer.

REFERENCES

Abdel-Latif, M.M., Windle, H.J., Homasany, B.S., Sabra, K., and Kelleher, D., 2005, Caffeic acid phenethyl ester modulates Helicobacter pylori-induced nuclear factor-kappa B and activator protein-1 expression in gastric epithelial cells, *Br. J. Pharmacol.,* 146, 1139–1147.

Achiwa, Y., Hasegawa, K., Komiya, T., and Udagawa, Y., 2005, Ursolic acid induces Bax-dependent apoptosis through the caspase-3 pathway in endometrial cancer SNG-II cells, *Oncol. Rep.,* 13, 51–57.

Achiwa, Y., Hasegawa, K., and Udagawa, Y., 2007, Regulation of the phosphatidylinositol 3-kinase-Akt and the mitogen-activated protein kinase pathways by ursolic acid in human endometrial cancer cells, *Biosci. Biotechnol. Biochem.,* 71, 31–37.

Aggarwal, B.B., Shishodia, S., Sandur, S.K., Pandey, M.K., and Sethi, G., 2006, Inflammation and cancer: how hot is the link? *Biochem. Pharmacol.*, 72, 1605–1621.

Agullo, G., Gamet-Payrastre, L., Manenti, S., Viala, C., Remesy, C., Chap, H., and Payrastre, B., 1997, Relationship between flavonoid structure and inhibition of phosphatidylinositol 3-kinase: a comparison with tyrosine kinase and protein kinase C inhibition, *Biochem. Pharmacol.*, 53, 1649–1657.

Al-Anati, L., Katz, N., and Petzinger, E., 2005, Interference of arachidonic acid and its metabolites with TNF-alpha release by ochratoxin A from rat liver, *Toxicology,* 208, 335–346.

Al-Fayez, M., Cai, H., Tunstall, R., Steward, W.P., and Gescher, A.J., 2006, Differential modulation of cyclo-oxygenase-mediated prostaglandin production by the putative cancer chemopreventive flavonoids tricin, apigenin and quercetin, *Cancer Chemother. Pharmacol.*, 58, 816–825.

Allen, S.W., Mueller, L., Williams, S.N., Quattrochi, L.C., and Raucy, J., 2001, The use of a high-volume screening procedure to assess the effects of dietary flavonoids on human cyp1a1 expression, *Drug Metab. Dispos.*, 29, 1074–1079.

Ames, B.N., Shigenaga, M.K., and Hagen, T.M., 1993, Oxidants, antioxidants, and the degenerative diseases of aging, *Proc. Natl. Acad. Sci. U.S.A.*, 90, 7915–7922.

Aoyagi, Y., Masuko, N., Ohkubo, S., Kitade, M., Nagai, K., Okazaki, S., Wierzba, K., Terada, T., Sugimoto, Y., and Yamada, Y., 2005, A novel cinnamic acid derivative that inhibits Cdc25 dual-specificity phosphatase activity, *Cancer Sci.*, 96, 614–619.

Arbiser, J.L., Li, X.C., Hossain, C.F., Nagle, D.G., Smith, D.M., Miller, P., Govindarajan, B., DiCarlo, J., Landis-Piwowar, K.R., and Dou, Q.P., 2005, Naturally occurring proteasome inhibitors from mate tea (*Ilex paraguayensis*) serve as models for topical proteasome inhibitors, *J. Invest. Dermatol.*, 125, 207–212.

Atadja, P., Gao, L., Kwon, P., Trogani, N., Walker, H., Hsu, M., Yeleswarapu, L., Chandramouli, N., Perez, L., Versace, R., Wu, A., Sambucetti, L., Lassota, P., Cohen, D., Bair, K., Wood, A., and Remiszewski, S., 2004, Selective growth inhibition of tumor cells by a novel histone deacetylase inhibitor, NVP-LAQ824, *Cancer Res.*, 64, 689–695.

Au, A., Li, B., Wang, W., Roy, H., Koehler, K., and Birt, D., 2006, Effect of dietary apigenin on colonic ornithine decarboxylase activity, aberrant crypt foci formation, and tumorigenesis in different experimental models, *Nutr. Cancer,* 54, 243–551.

Azuma, Y., Onishi, Y., Sato, Y., and Kizaki, H., 1995, Effects of protein tyrosine kinase inhibitors with different modes of action on topoisomerase activity and death of IL-2-dependent CTLL-2 cells, *J. Biochem.* (Tokyo), 118, 312–318.

Babich, H. and Visioli, F., 2003, *In vitro* cytotoxicity to human cells in culture of some phenolics from olive oil, *Farmaco,* 58, 403–407.

Bagli, E., Stefaniotou, M., Morbidelli, L., Ziche, M., Psillas, K., Murphy, C., and Fotsis, T., 2004, Luteolin inhibits vascular endothelial growth factor-induced angiogenesis; inhibition of endothelial cell survival and proliferation by targeting phosphatidylinositol 3′-kinase activity, *Cancer Res,* 64, 7936–7946.

Balasubramanian, S., Zhu, L., and Eckert, R.L., 2006, Apigenin inhibition of involucrin gene expression is associated with a specific reduction in phosphorylation of protein kinase C delta Tyr311, *J. Biol. Chem.*, 281, 36162–36172.

Baliga, M. S. and Katiyar, S.K., 2006, Chemoprevention of photocarcinogenesis by selected dietary botanicals, *Photochem. Photobiol. Sci.*, 5, 243–253.

Bartek, J., Bartkova, J., and Lukas, J., 1997, The retinoblastoma protein pathway in cell cycle control and cancer, *Exp. Cell Res.*, 237(1), 1–6.

Barthomeuf, C., Boivin, D., and Beliveau, R., 2004, Inhibition of HUVEC tubulogenesis by hederacolchiside-A1 is associated with plasma membrane cholesterol sequestration and activation of the Ha-Ras/MEK/ERK cascade, *Cancer Chemother. Pharmacol.*, 54, 432–440.

Bartoli, R., Fernandez-Banares, F., Navarro, E., Castella, E., Mane, J., Alvarez, M., Pastor, C., Cabre, E., and Gassull, M.A., 2000, Effect of olive oil on early and late events of colon carcinogenesis in rats: modulation of arachidonic acid metabolism and local prostaglandin E(2) synthesis, *Gut,* 46, 191–199.

Bartsch, H., Nair, J., and Owen, R.W., 1999, Dietary polyunsaturated fatty acids and cancers of the breast and colorectum: emerging evidence for their role as risk modifiers, *Carcinogenesis,* 20, 2209–2218.

Basu, S., Ma, R., Boyle, P.J., Mikulla, B., Bradley, M., Smith, B., Basu, M., and Banerjee, S., 2004, Apoptosis of human carcinoma cells in the presence of potential anti-cancer drugs. III. Treatment of Colo-205 and SKBR3 cells with: cis-platin, Tamoxifen, Melphalan, Betulinic acid, L-PDMP, L-PPMP, and GD3 ganglioside, *Glycoconj. J.,* 20, 563–577.

Bergman Jungestrom, M., Thompson, L.U., and Dabrosin, C., 2007, Flaxseed and its lignans inhibit estra-diol-induced growth, angiogenesis, and secretion of vascular endothelial growth factor in human breast cancer xenografts in vivo, *Clin. Cancer Res.,* 13, 1061–1067.

Binukumar, B. and Mathew, A., 2005, Dietary fat and risk of breast cancer, *World J. Surg. Oncol.,* 3, 45.

Birt, D.F., Mitchell, D., Gold, B., Pour, P., and Pinch, H.C., 1997, Inhibition of ultraviolet light induced skin carcinogenesis in SKH-1 mice by apigenin, a plant flavonoid, *Anticancer Res.,* 17(1A), 85–91.

Boege, F., Straub, T., Kehr, A., Boesenberg, C., Christiansen, K., Andersen, A., Jakob, F., and Kohrle, J., 1996, Selected novel flavones inhibit the DNA binding or the DNA religation step of eukaryotic topoisomerase I, *J. Biol. Chem.,* 271, 2262–2270.

Bommareddy, A., Arasada, B.L., Mathees, D.P., and Dwivedi, C., 2006, Chemopreventive effects of dietary flaxseed on colon tumor development, *Nutr. Cancer,* 54, 216–222.

Bosetti, C., La Vecchia, C., Talamini, R., Simonato, L., Zambon, P., Negri, E., Trichopoulos, D., Lagiou, P., Bardini, R., and Franceschi, S., 2000, Food groups and risk of squamous cell esophageal cancer in northern Italy, *Int. J. Cancer,* 87, 289–294.

Bosetti, C., La Vecchia, C., Talamini, R., Negri, E., Levi, F., Dal Maso, L., and Franceschi, S., 2002a, Food groups and laryngeal cancer risk: a case-control study from Italy and Switzerland, *Int. J. Cancer,* 100, 355–360.

Bosetti, C., Negri, E., Franceschi, S., Talamini, R., Montella, M., Conti, E., Lagiou, P., Parazzini, F., and La Vecchia, C., 2002b, Olive oil, seed oils and other added fats in relation to ovarian cancer (Italy), *Cancer Causes Control,* 13, 465–470.

Breinholt, V. M., Offord, E.A., Brouwer, C., Nielsen, S.E., Brosen, K., and Friedberg, T., 2002, *In vitro* investigation of cytochrome P450-mediated metabolism of dietary flavonoids, *Food Chem. Toxicol.,* 40, 609–616.

Brunner, L.J. and Bai, S., 2000, Effect of dietary oil intake on hepatic cytochrome P450 activity in the rat, *J. Pharm. Sci.,* 89, 1022–1027.

Caltagirone, S., Rossi, C., Poggi, A., Ranelletti, F.O., Natali, P.G., Brunetti, M., Aiello, F.B., and Piantelli, M., 2000, Flavonoids apigenin and quercetin inhibit melanoma growth and metastatic potential, *Int. J. Cancer,* 8, 595–600.

Cantero, G., Campanella, C., Mateos, S., and Cortes, F., 2006, Topoisomerase II inhibition and high yield of endoreduplication induced by the flavonoids luteolin and quercetin, *Mutagenesis,* 21, 321–325.

Carrillo, C., Cafferata, E.G., Genovese, J., O'Reilly, M., Roberts, A.B., and Santa-Coloma, T.A., 1998, TGF-beta1 up-regulates the mRNA for the Na+/Ca2+ exchanger in neonatal rat cardiac myocytes, *Cell Mol. Biol.* (Noisy-le-grand), 44, 543–551.

Casagrande, F. and Darbon, J.M., 2001, Effects of structurally related flavonoids on cell cycle progression of human melanoma cells: regulation of cyclin-dependent kinases CDK2 and CDK1, *Biochem. Pharmacol.,* 61, 1205–1215.

Cesen-Cummings, K., Warner, K.A., and Ruch, R.J., 1998, Role of protein kinase C in the deficient gap junctional intercellular communication of K-ras-transformed murine lung epithelial cells, *Anticancer Res.,* 18(6A), 4343–4346.

Chang, C.J., Chiu, J.H., Tseng, L.M., Chang, C.H., Chien, T.M., Chen, C.C., Wu, C.W., and Lui, W.Y., 2006a, Si-Wu-Tang and its constituents promote mammary duct cell proliferation by up-regulation of HER-2 signaling, *Menopause,* 13, 967–976.

Chang, C.J., Chiu, J.H., Tseng, L.M., Chang, C.H., Chien, T.M., Wu, C.W., and Lui, W.Y., 2006b, Modulation of HER2 expression by ferulic acid on human breast cancer MCF7 cells, *Eur. J. Clin. Invest.,* 36, 588–596.

Chaudhary, A. and Willett, K.L., 2006, Inhibition of human cytochrome CYP 1 enzymes by flavonoids of St. John's wort, *Toxicology,* 217, 194–205.

Chaumontet, C., Bex, V., Gaillard-Sanchez, I., Seillan-Heberden, C., Suschetet, M., and Martel, P., 1994, Apigenin and tangeretin enhance gap junctional intercellular communication in rat liver epithelial cells, *Carcinogenesis,* 15, 2325–2330.

Chaumontet, C., Droumaguet, C., Bex, V., Heberden, C., Gaillard-Sanchez, I., and Martel, P., 1997, Flavonoids (apigenin, tangeretin) counteract tumor promoter-induced inhibition of intercellular communication of rat liver epithelial cells, *Cancer Lett.,* 114, 207–210.

Chen, C.C., Chow, M.P., Huang, W.C., Lin, Y.C., and Chang, Y.J., 2004, Flavonoids inhibit tumor necrosis factor-alpha-induced up-regulation of intercellular adhesion molecule-1 (ICAM-1) in respiratory epithelial cells through activator protein-1 and nuclear factor-kappaB: structure-activity relationships, *Mol. Pharmacol.,* 66, 683–693.

Chen, D., Daniel, K.G., Chen, M.S., Kuhn, D.J., Landis-Piwowar, K.R., and Dou, Q.P., 2005, Dietary flavonoids as proteasome inhibitors and apoptosis inducers in human leukemia cells, *Biochem. Pharmacol.*, 69, 1421–1432.

Chen, D., Chen, M.S., Cui, Q.C., Yang, H., and Dou, Q.P., 2007, Structure-proteasome-inhibitory activity relationships of dietary flavonoids in human cancer cells, *Front Biosci.*, 12, 1935–1945.

Chen, J., Stavro, P.M., and Thompson, L.U., 2002, Dietary flaxseed inhibits human breast cancer growth and metastasis and downregulates expression of insulin-like growth factor and epidermal growth factor receptor, *Nutr. Cancer*, 43, 187–192.

Chiang, L.C., Ng, L.T., Lin, I.C., Kuo, P.L., and Lin, C.C., 2006, Anti-proliferative effect of apigenin and its apoptotic induction in human Hep G2 cells, *Cancer Lett.*, 237, 207–214.

Chiang, Y.M., Lo, C.P., Chen, Y.P., Wang, S.Y., Yang, N.S., Kuo, Y.H., and Shyur, L.F., 2005, Ethyl caffeate suppresses NF-$_\kappa$B activation and its downstream inflammatory mediators, iNOS, COX-2, and PGE$_2$ *in vitro* or in mouse skin, *Br. J. Pharmacol.*, 146, 352–363.

Chintharlapalli, S., Papineni, S., Ramaiah, S.K., and Safe, S., 2007, Betulinic acid inhibits prostate cancer growth through inhibition of specificity protein transcription factors, *Cancer Res.*, 67, 2816–2823.

Chirco, R., Liu, X.W., Jung, K.K., and Kim, H.R., 2006, Novel functions of TIMPs in cell signaling, *Cancer Metastasis Rev.*, 25, 99–113.

Cho, J.Y., Kim, H.S., Kim, D.H., Yan, J.J., Suh, H.W., and Song, D.K., 2005, Inhibitory effects of long-term administration of ferulic acid on astrocyte activation induced by intracerebroventricular injection of beta-amyloid peptide (1-42) in mice, *Prog. Neuropsychopharmacol. Biol. Psychiatry*, 29, 901–907.

Choi, Y.J., Kang, J.S., Park, J.H., Lee, Y.J., Choi, J.S., and Kang, Y.H., 2003, Polyphenolic flavonoids differ in their antiapoptotic efficacy in hydrogen peroxide-treated human vascular endothelial cells, *J. Nutr.*, 133, 985–991.

Chuang, J.Y., Tsai, Y.Y., Chen, S.C., Hsieh, T.J., and Chung, J.G., 2005, Induction of G0/G1 arrest and apoptosis by 3-hydroxycinnamic acid in human cervix epithelial carcinoma (HeLa) cells, *In Vivo*, 19, 683–688.

Chung, T.W., Moon, S.K., Chang, Y.C., Ko, J.H., Lee, Y.C., Cho, G., Kim, S.H., Kim, J.G., and Kim, C.H., 2004, Novel and therapeutic effect of caffeic acid and caffeic acid phenyl ester on hepatocarcinoma cells: complete regression of hepatoma growth and metastasis by dual mechanism, *FASEB J.*, 18, 1670–1681.

Clavel, T., Borrmann, D., Braune, A., Dore, J., and Blaut, M., 2006, Occurrence and activity of human intestinal bacteria involved in the conversion of dietary lignans, *Anaerobe*, 12, 140–147.

Cochet, C., Feige, J.J., Pirollet, F., Keramidas, M., and Chambaz, E.M., 1982, Selective inhibition of a cyclic nucleotide independent protein kinase (G type casein kinase) by quercetin and related polyphenols, *Biochem. Pharmacol.*, 31, 1357–1361.

Code, E.L., Crespi, C.L., Penman, B.W., Gonzalez, F.J., Chang, T.K., and Waxman, D.J., 1997, Human cytochrome P4502B6: interindividual hepatic expression, substrate specificity, and role in procarcinogen activation, *Drug Metab. Dispos.*, 25, 985–993.

Cohen, L.A., Epstein, M., Pittman, B., and Rivenson, A., 2000, The influence of different varieties of olive oil on N-methylnitrosourea (NMU)-induced mammary tumorigenesis, *Anticancer Res.*, 20, 2307–2312.

Comalada, M., Ballester, L., Bailon, E., Sierra, S., Xaus, J., Galvez, J., de Medina, F.S., and Zarzuelo, A., 2006, Inhibition of pro-inflammatory markers in primary bone marrow-derived mouse macrophages by naturally occurring flavonoids: analysis of the structure-activity relationship, *Biochem. Pharmacol.*, 72, 1010–1021.

Constantinou, A., Mehta, R., Runyan, C., Rao, K., Vaughan, A., and Moon, R., 1995, Flavonoids as DNA topoisomerase antagonists and poisons: structure-activity relationships, *J. Nat. Prod.*, 58, 217–225.

Corona, G., Tzounis, X., Assunta Dessi, M., Deiana, M., Debnam, E.S., Visioli, F., and Spencer, J.P., 2006, The fate of olive oil polyphenols in the gastrointestinal tract: implications of gastric and colonic microflora-dependent biotransformation, *Free Radic. Res.*, 40, 647–658.

Czyz, J., Irmer, U., Zappe, C., Mauz, M., and Hulser, D.F., 2004, Hierarchy of carcinoma cell responses to apigenin: gap junctional coupling versus proliferation, *Oncol. Rep.*, 11, 739–744.

Czyz, J., Madeja, Z., Irmer, U., Korohoda, W., and Hulser, D.F., 2005, Flavonoid apigenin inhibits motility and invasiveness of carcinoma cells in vitro, *Int. J. Cancer*, 114, 12–18.

D'Angelo, S., Manna, C., Migliardi, V., Mazzoni, O., Morrica, P., Capasso, G., Pontoni, G., Galletti, P., and Zappia, V., 2001, Pharmacokinetics and metabolism of hydroxytyrosol, a natural antioxidant from olive oil, *Drug Metab. Dispos.*, 29, 1492–1498.

D'Angelo, S., Ingrosso, D., Migliardi, V., Sorrentino, A., Donnarumma, G., Baroni, A., Masella, L., Tufano, M.A., Zappia, M., and Galletti, P., 2005, Hydroxytyrosol, a natural antioxidant from olive oil, prevents protein damage induced by long-wave ultraviolet radiation in melanoma cells, *Free Radic. Biol. Med.*, 38, 908–919.

da Cunha, F.M., Duma, D., Assreuy, J., Buzzi, F.C., Niero, R., Campos, M.M., and Calixto, J.B., 2004, Caffeic acid derivatives: in vitro and in vivo anti-inflammatory properties, *Free Radic. Res.*, 38, 1241–1253.

Dabrosin, C., Chen, J., Wang, L., and Thompson, L.U., 2002, Flaxseed inhibits metastasis and decreases extracellular vascular endothelial growth factor in human breast cancer xenografts, *Cancer Lett.*, 185, 31–37.

Daels-Rakotoarison, D.A., Seidel, V., Gressier, B., Brunet, C., Tillequin, F., Bailleul, F., Luyckx, M., Dine, T., Cazin, M., and Cazin, J.C., 2000, Neurosedative and antioxidant activities of phenylpropanoids from ballota nigra, *Arzneimittelforschung*, 50, 16–23.

Daniel, K.G., Kuhn, D.J., Kazi, A., and Dou, Q.P., 2005, Anti-angiogenic and anti-tumor properties of proteasome inhibitors, *Curr. Cancer Drug Targets*, 5, 529–541.

Das, A., Banik, N.L., and Ray, S.K., 2006, Mechanism of apoptosis with the involvement of calpain and caspase cascades in human malignant neuroblastoma SH-SY5Y cells exposed to flavonoids, *Int. J. Cancer*, 119, 2575–2585.

De Graff, W.G., Myers, L.S., Jr., Mitchell, J.B., and Hahn, S.M., 2003, Protection against Adriamycin cytotoxicity and inhibition of DNA topoisomerase II activity by 3,4-dihydroxybenzoic acid, *Int. J. Oncol.*, 23, 159–163.

de la Puerta, R., Ruiz Gutierrez, V., and Hoult, J.R., 1999, Inhibition of leukocyte 5-lipoxygenase by phenolics from virgin olive oil, *Biochem. Pharmacol.*, 57, 445–449.

De Stefano, D., Maiuri, M.C., Simeon, V., Grassia, G., Soscia, A., Cinelli, M.P., and Carnuccio, R., 2007, Lycopene, quercetin and tyrosol prevent macrophage activation induced by gliadin and IFN-gamma, *Eur. J. Pharmacol.*, 566(1–3), 192–199.

Debersac, P., Vernevaut, M.F., Amiot, M.J., Suschetet, M., and Siess, M.H., 2001, Effects of a water-soluble extract of rosemary and its purified component rosmarinic acid on xenobiotic-metabolizing enzymes in rat liver, *Food Chem. Toxicol.*, 39, 109–117.

Deiana, M., Aruoma, O.I., Bianchi, M.L., Spencer, J.P., Kaur, H., Halliwell, B., Aeschbach, R., Banni, S., Dessi, M.A., and Corongiu, F.P., 1999, Inhibition of peroxynitrite dependent DNA base modification and tyrosine nitration by the extra virgin olive oil-derived antioxidant hydroxytyrosol, *Free Radic. Biol. Med.*, 26, 762–769.

Del Pozo, M.A. and Schwartz, M.A., 2007, Rac, membrane heterogeneity, caveolin and regulation of growth by integrins, *Trends Cell Biol.*, 17, 246–250.

Dell'Agli, M., Canavesi, M., Galli, G., and Bellosta, S., 2005, Dietary polyphenols and regulation of gelatinase expression and activity, *Thromb. Haemost.*, 93, 751–760.

Dell'Agli, M., Fagnani, R., Mitro, N., Scurati, S., Masciadri, M., Mussoni, L., Galli, G.V., Bosisio, E., Crestani, M., De Fabiani, E., Tremoli, E., and Caruso, D., 2006, Minor components of olive oil modulate proatherogenic adhesion molecules involved in endothelial activation, *J. Agric. Food Chem.*, 54, 3259–3264.

Della Ragione, F., Cucciolla, V., Criniti, V., Indaco, S., Borriello, A., and Zappia, V., 2002, Antioxidants induce different phenotypes by a distinct modulation of signal transduction, *FEBS Lett.*, 532, 289–294.

Deng, J.Z., Starck, S.R., and Hecht, S.M., 1999, DNA polymerase beta inhibitors from Baeckea gunniana, *J. Nat. Prod.*, 62, 1624–1626.

Di Benedetto, R., Vari, R., Scazzocchio, B., Filesi, C., Santangelo, C., Giovannini, C., et al., 2007, Tyrosol, the major extra virgin olive oil compound, restored intracellular antioxidant defences in spite of its weak antioxidative effectiveness, *Nutr. Metab. Cardiovasc. Dis.*, 17, 535–545.

Dou, Q.P. and Goldfarb, R.H., 2002, Bortezomib (millennium pharmaceuticals), *IDrugs*, 5, 828–834.

Eiznhamer, D.A. and Xu, Z.Q., 2004, Betulinic acid: a promising anticancer candidate, *Idrugs*, 7, 359–373.

Ekmekcioglu, C., Feyertag, J., and Marktl, W., 1998, Cinnamic acid inhibits proliferation and modulates brush border membrane enzyme activities in Caco-2 cells, *Cancer Lett.*, 128, 137–144.

Fabiani, R., De Bartolomeo, A., Rosignoli, P., Servili, M., Montedoro, G.F., and Morozzi, G., 2002, Cancer chemoprevention by hydroxytyrosol isolated from virgin olive oil through G1 cell cycle arrest and apoptosis, *Eur. J. Cancer Prev.*, 11, 351–358.

Fabiani, R., De Bartolomeo, A., Rosignoli, P., Servili, M., Selvaggini, R., Montedoro, G.F., Di Saverio, C., and Morozzi, G., 2006, Virgin olive oil phenols inhibit proliferation of human promyelocytic leukemia cells (HL60) by inducing apoptosis and differentiation, *J. Nutr.*, 136, 614–619.

Fang, J., Xia, C., Cao, Z., Zheng, J.Z., Reed, E., and Jiang, B.H., 2005, Apigenin inhibits VEGF and HIF-1 expression via PI3K/AKT/p70S6K1 and HDM2/p53 pathways, *FASEB J.*, 19, 342–353.

Fang, J., Zhou, Q., Liu, L.Z., Xia, C., Hu, X., Shi, X., and Jiang, B.H., 2007a, Apigenin inhibits tumor angiogenesis through decreasing HIF-1alpha and VEGF expression, *Carcinogenesis*, 28, 858–864.

Fang, J., Zhou, Q., Shi, X.L., and Jiang, B.H., 2007b, Luteolin inhibits insulin-like growth factor 1 receptor signaling in prostate cancer cells, *Carcinogenesis*, 28, 713–723.

Feng, R., Lu, Y., Bowman, L.L., Qian, Y., Castranova, V., and Ding, M., 2005, Inhibition of activator protein-1, NF-kappaB, and MAPKs and induction of phase 2 detoxifying enzyme activity by chlorogenic acid, *J. Biol. Chem.*, 280, 27888–27895.

Ford, H.L., Landesman-Bollag, E., Dacwag, C.S., Stukenberg, P.T., Pardee, A.B., and Seldin, D.C., 2000, Cell cycle-regulated phosphorylation of the human SIX1 homeodomain protein, *J. Biol. Chem.*, 275, 22245–22254.

Fortes, C., Forastiere, F., Farchi, S., Mallone, S., Trequattrinni, T., Anatra, F., Schmid, G., and Perucci, C.A., 2003, The protective effect of the Mediterranean diet on lung cancer, *Nutr. Cancer*, 46, 30–37.

Fotsis, T., Pepper, M.S., Aktas, E., Breit, S., Rasku, S., Adlercreutz, H., Wahala, K., Montesano, R., and Schweigerer, L., 1997, Flavonoids, dietary-derived inhibitors of cell proliferation and *in vitro* angiogenesis, *Cancer Res.*, 57, 2916–2921.

Franceschi, S. and Favero, A., 1999, The role of energy and fat in cancers of the breast and colon-rectum in a southern European population, *Ann. Oncol.*, 10(Suppl. 6), 61–63.

Fulda, S., Friesen, C., Los, M., Scaffidi, C., Mier, W., Benedict, M., Nunez, G., Krammer, P.H., Peter, M.E., and Debatin, K.M., 1997, Betulinic acid triggers CD95 (APO-1/Fas)- and p53-independent apoptosis via activation of caspases in neuroectodermal tumors, *Cancer Res.*, 57, 4956–4964.

Fulda, S. and Debatin, K.M., 2000, Betulinic acid induces apoptosis through a direct effect on mitochondria in neuroectodermal tumors, *Med. Pediatr. Oncol.*, 35, 616–618.

Gallus, S., Bosetti, C., Franceschi, S., Levi, F., Negri, E., and La Vecchia, C., 2003, Laryngeal cancer in women: tobacco, alcohol, nutritional, and hormonal factors, *Cancer Epidemiol. Biomarkers Prev.*, 12, 514–517.

Gallus, S., Bosetti, C., and La Vecchia, C., 2004, Mediterranean diet and cancer risk, *Eur. J. Cancer Prev.*, 13, 447–452.

Galvez, M., Martin-Cordero, C., Lopez-Lazaro, M., Cortes, F., and Ayuso, M.J., 2003, Cytotoxic effect of *Plantago* spp. on cancer cell lines, *J. Ethnopharmacol.*, 88, 125–130.

Garnovskaya, M.N., Mukhin, Y.V., Vlasova, T.M., Grewal, J.S., Ullian, M.E., Tholanikunnel, B.G., and Raymond, J.R., 2004, Mitogen-induced rapid phosphorylation of serine 795 of the retinoblastoma gene product in vascular smooth muscle cells involves ERK activation,. *J. Biol. Chem.*, 279, 24899–24905.

George, P., Bali, P., Annavarapu, S., Scuto, A., Fiskus, W., Guo, F., Sigua, C., Sondarva, G., Moscinski, L., Atadja, P., and Bhalla, K., 2005, Combination of the histone deacetylase inhibitor LBH589 and the hsp90 inhibitor 17-AAG is highly active against human CML-BC cells and AML cells with activating mutation of FLT-3, *Blood*, 105, 1768–1776.

Gill, C.I., Boyd, A., McDermott, E., McCann, M., Servili, M., Selvaggini, R., Taticchi, A., Esposto, S., Montedoro, G., McGlynn, H., and Rowland, I., 2005, Potential anti-cancer effects of virgin olive oil phenols on colorectal carcinogenesis models in vitro, *Int. J. Cancer*, 117, 1–7.

Gopalakrishnan, A., Xu, C.J., Nair, S.S., Chen, C., Hebbar, V., and Kong, A.N., 2006, Modulation of activator protein-1 (AP-1) and MAPK pathway by flavonoids in human prostate cancer PC3 cells, *Arch. Pharm. Res.*, 29, 633–644.

Goya, L., Mateos, R., and Bravo, L., 2007, Effect of the olive oil phenol hydroxytyrosol on human hepatoma HepG2 cells. Protection against oxidative stress induced by tert-butylhydroperoxide, *Eur. J. Nutr.*, 46, 70–78.

Grewal, J.S., Mukhin, Y.V., Garnovskaya, M.N., Raymond, J.R., and Greene, E.L., 1999, Serotonin 5-HT2A receptor induces TGF-beta1 expression in mesangial cells via ERK: proliferative and fibrotic signals, *Am. J. Physiol.*, 276(6 Pt 2), F922–F930.

Griffiths, K., Morton, M.S., and Denis, L., 1999, Certain aspects of molecular endocrinology that relate to the influence of dietary factors on the pathogenesis of prostate cancer, *Eur. Urol.*, 35, 443–455.

Guichard, C., Pedruzzi, E., Fay, M., Marie, J.C., Braut-Boucher, F., Daniel, F., Grodet, A., Gougerot-Pocidalo, M.A., Chastre, E., Kotelevets, L., Lizard, G., Vandewalle, A., Driss, F., and Ogier-Denis, E., 2006, Dihydroxyphenylethanol induces apoptosis by activating serine/threonine protein phosphatase PP2A and promotes the endoplasmic reticulum stress response in human colon carcinoma cells, *Carcinogenesis*, 27, 1812–1827.

Gupta, S., Afaq, F., and Mukhtar, H., 2001, Selective growth-inhibitory, cell-cycle deregulatory and apoptotic response of apigenin in normal versus human prostate carcinoma cells, *Biochem. Biophys. Res. Commun., 287,* 914–920.

Gupta, S., Afaq, F., and Mukhtar, H., 2002, Involvement of nuclear factor-kappa B, Bax and Bcl-2 in induction of cell cycle arrest and apoptosis by apigenin in human prostate carcinoma cells, *Oncogene,* 21, 3727–3738.

Gutierrez-Venegas, G., Kawasaki-Cardenas, P., Arroyo-Cruz, S.R., and Maldonado-Frias, S., 2006, Luteolin inhibits lipopolysaccharide actions on human gingival fibroblasts, *Eur. J. Pharmacol.,* 541, 95–105.

Guy, C.T., Webster, M.A., Schaller, M., Parsons, T.J., Cardiff, R.D., and Muller, W.J., 1992, Expression of the neu protooncogene in the mammary epithelium of transgenic mice induces metastatic disease, *Proc. Natl. Acad. Sci. U.S.A.,* 89, 10578–10582.

Haddad, J.J. and Fahlman, C.S., 2002, Nuclear factor-kappa B-independent regulation of lipopolysaccharide-mediated interleukin-6 biosynthesis, *Biochem. Biophys. Res. Commun.,* 291, 1045–1051.

Hamdi, H.K. and Castellon, R., 2005, Oleuropein, a non-toxic olive iridoid, is an anti-tumor agent and cytoskeleton disruptor, *Biochem. Biophys. Res. Commun.,* 334, 769–778.

Han, C., Ding, H., Casto, B., Stoner, G.D., and D'Ambrosio, S.M., 2005, Inhibition of the growth of premalignant and malignant human oral cell lines by extracts and components of black raspberries, *Nutr. Cancer,* 51, 207–217.

Harmand, P.O., Duval, R., Delage, C., and Simon, A., 2005, Ursolic acid induces apoptosis through mitochondrial intrinsic pathway and caspase-3 activation in M4Beu melanoma cells, *Int. J. Cancer,* 114, 1–11.

Harris, D.M., Besselink, E., Henning, S.M., Go, V.L., and Heber, D., 2005, Phytoestrogens induce differential estrogen receptor alpha- or beta-mediated responses in transfected breast cancer cells, *Exp. Biol. Med. (Maywood),* 230, 558–568.

Hasebe, Y., Egawa, K., Yamazaki, Y., Kunimoto, S., Hirai, Y., Ida, Y., and Nose, K., 2003, Specific inhibition of hypoxia-inducible factor (HIF)-1 alpha activation and of vascular endothelial growth factor (VEGF) production by flavonoids, *Biol. Pharm. Bull.,* 26, 1379–1383.

Hehlgans, S., Haase, M., and Cordes, N., 2007, Signalling via integrins: implications for cell survival and anticancer strategies, *Biochim. Biophys. Acta,* 1775, 163–180.

Heinonen, S., Nurmi, T., Liukkonen, K., Poutanen, K., Wahala, K., Deyama, T., Nishibe, S., and Adlercreutz, H., 2001, In vitro metabolism of plant lignans: new precursors of mammalian lignans enterolactone and enterodiol, *J. Agric. Food Chem.,* 49, 3178–3186.

Herbert, J.M., Maffrand, J.P., Taoubi, K., Augereau, J.M., Fouraste, I., and Gleye, J., 1991, Verbascoside isolated from Lantana camara, an inhibitor of protein kinase C, *J. Nat. Prod.,* 54, 1595–6000.

Hirata, A., Murakami, Y., Atsumi, T., Shoji, M., Ogiwara, T., Shibuya, K., Ito, S., Yokoe, I., and Fujisawa, S., 2005, Ferulic acid dimer inhibits lipopolysaccharide-stimulated cyclooxygenase-2 expression in macrophages, *In Vivo,* 19, 849–853.

Holvoet, S., Vincent, C., Schmitt, D., and Serres, M., 2003, The inhibition of MAPK pathway is correlated with down-regulation of MMP-9 secretion induced by TNF-alpha in human keratinocytes, *Exp. Cell Res.,* 290, 108–119.

Hood, J.D. and Cheresh, D.A., 2002, Role of integrins in cell invasion and migration, *Nat. Rev. Cancer,* 2, 91–100.

Horinaka, M., Yoshida, T., Shiraishi, T., Nakata, S., Wakada, M., Nakanishi, R., Nishino, H., Matsui, H., and Sakai, T., 2005, Luteolin induces apoptosis via death receptor 5 upregulation in human malignant tumor cells, *Oncogene,* 24, 7180–7189.

Hortobagyi, G.N., Hung, M.C., and Buzdar, A.U., 1999, Recent developments in breast cancer therapy, *Semin. Oncol.,* 26(4 Suppl. 12), 11–20.

Horvathova, K., Novotny, L., and Vachalkova. A., 2003, The free radical scavenging activity of four flavonoids determined by the comet assay, *Neoplasma,* 50, 291–295.

Horvathova, K., Novotny, L., Tothova, D., and Vachalkova, A., 2004, Determination of free radical scavenging activity of quercetin, rutin, luteolin and apigenin in H_2O_2-treated human ML cells K562, *Neoplasma,* 51, 395–399.

Hou, Y., Yang, J., Zhao, G., and Yuan, Y., 2004a, Ferulic acid inhibits endothelial cell proliferation through NO down-regulating ERK1/2 pathway, *J. Cell Biochem.,* 93, 1203–1209.

Hou, Y.Z., Yang, J., Zhao, G.R., and Yuan, Y.J., 2004b, Ferulic acid inhibits vascular smooth muscle cell proliferation induced by angiotensin II, *Eur. J. Pharmacol.,* 499, 85–90.

Hsiao, G., Lee, J.J., Lin, K.H., Shen, C.H., Fong, T.H., Chou, D.S., and Sheu, J.R., 2007, Characterization of a novel and potent collagen antagonist, caffeic acid phenethyl ester, in human platelets: *in vitro* and *in vivo* studies, *Cardiovasc. Res.*, 75, 782–792.

Hsu, Y.L., Kuo, P.L., and Lin, C.C., 2004, Proliferative inhibition, cell-cycle dysregulation, and induction of apoptosis by ursolic acid in human non-small cell lung cancer A549 cells, *Life Sci.*, 75, 2303–2316.

Hu, C. and Kitts, D.D., 2004, Luteolin and luteolin-7-O-glucoside from dandelion flower suppress iNOS and COX-2 in RAW264.7 cells, *Mol. Cell. Biochem.*, 265, 107–113.

Huang, M.T., Lysz, T., Ferraro, T., Abidi, T.F., Laskin, J.D., and Conney, A.H., 1991, Inhibitory effects of curcumin on in vitro lipoxygenase and cyclooxygenase activities in mouse epidermis, *Cancer Res.*, 51, 813–819.

Huang, Y.C., Chen, C.T., Chen, S.C., Lai, P.H., Liang, H.C., Chang, Y., Yu, L.C., and Sung, H.W., 2005, A natural compound (ginsenoside Re) isolated from Panax ginseng as a novel angiogenic agent for tissue regeneration, *Pharm. Res.*, 22, 636–646.

Huang, Y.T., Kuo, M.L., Liu, J.Y., Huang, S.Y., and Lin, J.K., 1996, Inhibitions of protein kinase C and proto-oncogene expressions in NIH 3T3 cells by apigenin, *Eur. J. Cancer*, 32A, 146–151.

Huang, Y.T., Hwang, J.J., Lee, P.P., Ke, F.C., Huang, J.H., Huang, C.J., Kandaswami, C., Middleton, E., Jr., and Lee, M.T., 1999, Effects of luteolin and quercetin, inhibitors of tyrosine kinase, on cell growth and metastasis-associated properties in A431 cells overexpressing epidermal growth factor receptor, *Br. J. Pharmacol.*, 128, 999–1010.

Hwang, H.J., Park, H.J., Chung, H.J., Min, H.Y., Park, E.J., Hong, J.Y., and Lee, S.K., 2006, Inhibitory effects of caffeic acid phenethyl ester on cancer cell metastasis mediated by the down-regulation of matrix metalloproteinase expression in human HT1080 fibrosarcoma cells, *J. Nutr. Biochem.*, 17, 356–362.

Ichihashi, M., Ahmed, N.U., Budiyanto, A., Wu, A., Bito, T., Ueda, M., and Osawa, T., 2000, Preventive effect of antioxidant on ultraviolet-induced skin cancer in mice, *J. Dermatol. Sci.*, 23(Suppl. 1), S45–S50.

Inoue, M., Sakuma, Z., Ogihara, Y., and Saracoglu, I., 1998, Induction of apoptotic cell death in HL-60 cells by acteoside, a phenylpropanoid glycoside, *Biol. Pharm. Bull.*, 21, 81–83.

Jaiswal, A.K., Venugopal, R., Mucha, J., Carothers, A.M., and Grunberger, D., 1997, Caffeic acid phenethyl ester stimulates human antioxidant response element-mediated expression of the NAD(P)H:quinone oxidoreductase (NQO1) gene, *Cancer Res.*, 57, 440–446.

Janicke, B., Onning, G., and Oredsson, S.M., 2005, Differential effects of ferulic acid and p-coumaric acid on S phase distribution and length of S phase in the human colonic cell line Caco-2, *J. Agric. Food Chem.*, 53, 6658–6665.

Jatana, M., Giri, S., Ansari, M.A., Elango, C., Singh, A.K., Singh, I., and Khan, M., 2006, Inhibition of NF-kappaB activation by 5-lipoxygenase inhibitors protects brain against injury in a rat model of focal cerebral ischemia, *J. Neuroinflammation*, 3, 1–13.

Jayaprakasam, B., Vanisree, M., Zhang, Y., Dewitt, D.L., and Nair, M.G., 2006, Impact of alkyl esters of caffeic and ferulic acids on tumor cell proliferation, cyclooxygenase enzyme, and lipid peroxidation, *J. Agric. Food Chem.*, 54, 5375–5381.

Jiang, J.G., Chen, R.J., Xiao, B., Yang, S., Wang, J.N., Wang, Y., Cowart, L.A., Xiao, X., Wang, D.W., and Xia, Y., 2007, Regulation of endothelial nitric-oxide synthase activity through phosphorylation in response to epoxyeicosatrienoic acids, *Prostaglandins Other Lipid Mediat.*, 82, 162–174.

Jin, G., Zhang, T., Wang, T., and Yang, L.P., 2002, Inhibition of alpha-interferon and cinnamic acid on proliferation of human lung cancer cell, *Ai Zheng*, 21, 860–862.

Jin, U.H., Chung, T.W., Kang, S.K., Suh, S.J., Kim, J.K., Chung, K.H., Gu, Y.H., Suzuki, I., and Kim, C.H., 2005, Caffeic acid phenyl ester in propolis is a strong inhibitor of matrix metalloproteinase-9 and invasion inhibitor: isolation and identification, *Clin. Chim. Acta*, 362, 57–64.

Jin, Y., Yan, E.Z., Fan, Y., Zong, Z.H., Qi, Z.M., and Li, Z., 2005, Sodium ferulate prevents amyloid-beta-induced neurotoxicity through suppression of p38 MAPK and upregulation of ERK-1/2 and Akt/protein kinase B in rat hippocampus, *Acta Pharmacol. Sin.*, 26, 43–51.

Joussen, A.M., Rohrschneider, K., Reichling, J., Kirchhof, B., and Kruse, F.E., 2000, Treatment of corneal neovascularization with dietary isoflavonoids and flavonoids, *Exp. Eye Res.*, 71, 483–487.

Kampa, M., Alexaki, V.I., Notas, G., Nifli, A.P., Nistikaki, A., Hatzoglou, A., Bakogeorgou, E., Kouimtzoglou, E., Blekas, G., Boskou, D., Gravanis, A., and Castanas, E., 2004, Antiproliferative and apoptotic effects of selective phenolic acids on T47D human breast cancer cells: potential mechanisms of action, *Breast Cancer Res.*, 6, R63–R74.

Kampa, M., Nifli, A.P., Notas, G., and Castanas, E., 2007, Polyphenols and cancer cell growth, *Rev. Physiol. Biochem. Pharmacol.*, 159, 79–113.

Kanazawa, K., Uehara, M., Yanagitani, H., and Hashimoto, T., 2006, Bioavailable flavonoids to suppress the formation of 8-OHdG in HepG2 cells, *Arch. Biochem. Biophys.*, 455, 197–203.

Kanda, Y., Richards, R.G., and Handwerger, S., 1998, Apolipoprotein A-I stimulates human placental lactogen release by activation of MAP kinase, *Mol. Cell. Endocrinol.*, 143, 125–131.

Kang, K.A., Lee, K.H., Zhang, R., Piao, M., Chae, S., Kim, K.N., Jeon, Y.J., Park, D.B., You, H.J., Kim, J.S., and Hyun, J.W., 2006, Caffeic acid protects hydrogen peroxide induced cell damage in WI-38 human lung fibroblast cells, *Biol. Pharm. Bull.*, 29, 1820–1824.

Karlsson, P.C., Huss, U., Jenner, A., Halliwell, B., Bohlin, L., and Rafter, J.J., 2005, Human fecal water inhibits COX-2 in colonic HT-29 cells: role of phenolic compounds, *J. Nutr.*, 135, 2343–2349.

Kasperczyk, H., La Ferla-Bruhl, K., Westhoff, M.A., Behrend, L., Zwacka, R.M., Debatin, K.M., and Fulda, S., 2005, Betulinic acid as new activator of NF-kappaB: molecular mechanisms and implications for cancer therapy, *Oncogene*, 24, 6945–6956.

Katsiki, M., Chondrogianni, N., Chinou, I., Rivett, A.J., and Gonos, E.S., 2007, The olive constituent oleuropein exhibits proteasome stimulatory properties in vitro and confers life span extension of human embryonic fibroblasts, *Rejuvenation Res.*, 10, 157–172.

Khan, M., Elango, C., Ansari, M.A., Singh, I., and Singh, A.K., 2007, Caffeic acid phenethyl ester reduces neurovascular inflammation and protects rat brain following transient focal cerebral ischemia, *J. Neurochem.*, 102, 365–377.

Kim, D.S., Pezzuto, J.M., and Pisha, E., 1998, Synthesis of betulinic acid derivatives with activity against human melanoma, *Bioorg. Med. Chem. Lett.*, 8, 1707–1712.

Kim, H.J., Lee, S.B., Park, S.K., Kim, H.M., Park, Y.I., and Dong, M.S., 2005, Effects of hydroxyl group numbers on the B-ring of 5,7-dihydroxyflavones on the differential inhibition of human CYP1A and CYP1B1 enzymes, *Arch. Pharm. Res.*, 28, 1114–1121.

Kim, J.A., Kim, D.K., Kang, O.H., Choi, Y.A., Park, H.J., Choi, S.C., Kim, T.H., Yun, K.J., Nah, Y.H., and Lee, Y.M., 2005, Inhibitory effect of luteolin on TNF-alpha-induced IL-8 production in human colon epithelial cells, *Int. Immunopharmacol.*, 5, 209–217.

Kim, J.H., Cho, Y.H., Park, S.M., Lee, K.E., Lee, J.J., Lee, B.C., Pyo, H.B., Song, K.S., Park, H.D., and Yun, Y.P., 2004, Antioxidants and inhibitor of matrix metalloproteinase-1 expression from leaves of *Zostera marina* L., *Arch. Pharm. Res.*, 27, 177–183.

Kim, J.H., Jin, Y.R., Park, B.S., Kim, T.J., Kim, S.Y., Lim, Y., Hong, J.T., Yoo, H.S., and Yun, Y.P., 2005, Luteolin prevents PDGF-BB-induced proliferation of vascular smooth muscle cells by inhibition of PDGF beta-receptor phosphorylation, *Biochem. Pharmacol.*, 69, 1715–1721.

Kim, J.S., Lee, H.J., Lee, M.H., Kim, J., Jin, C., and Ryu, J.H., 2006, Luteolin inhibits LPS-stimulated inducible nitric oxide synthase expression in BV-2 microglial cells, *Planta Med.*, 72, 65–68.

Kim, J.Y., Koo, H.M., and Kim, H.M., 2001, Development of C-20 modified betulinic acid derivatives as antitumor agents, *Bioorg. Med. Chem. Lett.*, 11, 2405–2408.

Kim, J.Y., Kwon, E.Y., Lee, Y.S., Kim, W.B., and Ro, J.Y., 2005, Eupatilin blocks mediator release via tyrosine kinase inhibition in activated guinea pig lung mast cells, *J. Toxicol. Environ. Health A*, 68(23-24), 2063–2080.

Kim, M.H., 2003, Flavonoids inhibit VEGF/bFGF-induced angiogenesis in vitro by inhibiting the matrix-degrading proteases, *J. Cell Biochem.*, 89, 529–538.

Kim, S.H., Shin, K.J., Kim, D., Kim, Y.H., Han, M.S., Lee, T.G., Kim, E., Ryu, S.H., and Suh, P.G., 2003, Luteolin inhibits the nuclear factor-kappa B transcriptional activity in Rat-1 fibroblasts, *Biochem. Pharmacol.*, 66, 955–963.

Kim, T.J., Zhang, Y.H., Kim, Y., Lee, C.K., Lee, M.K., Hong, J.T., and Yun, Y.P., 2002, Effects of apigenin on the serum- and platelet derived growth factor-BB-induced proliferation of rat aortic vascular smooth muscle cells, *Planta Med.*, 68, 605–609.

Kimata, M., Shichijo, M., Miura, T., Serizawa, I., Inagaki, N., and Nagai, H., 2000, Effects of luteolin, quercetin and baicalein on immunoglobulin E-mediated mediator release from human cultured mast cells, *Clin. Exp. Allergy*, 30, 501–508.

Kimura, Y., 2002, Carp oil or oleic acid, but not linoleic acid or linolenic acid, inhibits tumor growth and metastasis in Lewis lung carcinoma-bearing mice, *J. Nutr.*, 132, 2069–2075.

Kitts, D.D., Yuan, Y.V., Wijewickreme, A.N., and Thompson, L.U., 1999, Antioxidant activity of the flaxseed lignan secoisolariciresinol diglycoside and its mammalian lignan metabolites enterodiol and enterolactone, *Mol. Cell Biochem.*, 202, 91–100.

Klampfer, L., Huang, J., Sasazuki, T., Shirasawa, S., and Augenlicht, L., 2004, Oncogenic Ras promotes butyrate-induced apoptosis through inhibition of gelsolin expression, *J. Biol. Chem.*, 279, 36680–36688.

Ko, W.G., Kang, T.H., Lee, S.J., Kim, Y.C., and Lee, B.H., 2002, Effects of luteolin on the inhibition of proliferation and induction of apoptosis in human myeloid leukaemia cells, *Phytother. Res.,* 16, 295–298.

Kobayashi, T., Nakata, T., and Kuzumaki, T., 2002, Effect of flavonoids on cell cycle progression in prostate cancer cells, *Cancer Lett.,* 176, 17–23.

Kohyama, N., Nagata, T., Fujimoto, S., and Sekiya, K., 1997, Inhibition of arachidonate lipoxygenase activities by 2-(3,4-dihydroxyphenyl)ethanol, a phenolic compound from olives, *Biosci. Biotechnol. Biochem.,* 61, 347–350.

Koo, H.J., Lee, S., Shin, K.H., Kim, B.C., Lim, C.J., and Park, E.H., 2004a, Geniposide, an anti-angiogenic compound from the fruits of Gardenia jasminoides, *Planta Med.,* 70, 467–469.

Koo, H.J., Song, Y.S., Kim, H.J., Lee, Y.H., Hong, S.M., Kim, S.J., Kim, B.C., Jin, C., Lim, C.J., and Park, E.H., 2004b, Antiinflammatory effects of genipin, an active principle of gardenia, *Eur. J. Pharmacol.,* 495, 201–208.

Kossoy, G., Yarden, G., Ben-Hur, H., Kossoy, N., Stark, A., Madar, Z., and Zusman, I., 2001, Comparative effects of dimethylbenz(a)anthracene and a 15% olive-oil diet on cellular components and expression of apoptosis-related proteins in the spleen and mammary gland tumors of rats, *Oncol. Rep.,* 8, 435–439.

Kruk, I., Aboul-Enein, H.Y., Michalska, T., Lichszteld, K., and Kladna, A., 2005, Scavenging of reactive oxygen species by the plant phenols genistein and oleuropein, *Luminescence,* 20, 81–89.

Kuhn, D., Lam, W.H., Kazi, A., Daniel, K.G., Song, S., Chow, L.M., Chan, T.H., and Dou, Q.P., 2005, Synthetic peracetate tea polyphenols as potent proteasome inhibitors and apoptosis inducers in human cancer cells, *Front Biosci.,* 10, 1010–1023.

Kunvari, M., Paska, C., Laszlo, M., Orfi, L., Kovesdi, I., Eros, D., Bokonyi, G., Keri, G., and Gyurjan, I., 1999, Biological activity and structure of antitumor compounds from *Plantago media* L., *Acta Pharm. Hung.,* 69, 232–239.

Kuo, H.C., Kuo, W.H., Lee, Y.J., Lin, W.L., Chou, F.P., and Tseng, T.H., 2006, Inhibitory effect of caffeic acid phenethyl ester on the growth of C6 glioma cells *in vitro* and *in vivo, Cancer Lett.,* 234, 199–208.

Kuo, M.L. and Yang, N.C., 1995, Reversion of v-H-ras-transformed NIH 3T3 cells by apigenin through inhibiting mitogen activated protein kinase and its downstream oncogenes, *Biochem. Biophys. Res. Commun.,* 212(3), 767–775.

La Vecchia, C., 2004, Mediterranean diet and cancer, *Public Health Nutr.,* 7, 965–968.

La Vecchia, C., Negri, E., Franceschi, S., Decarli, A., Giacosa, A., and Lipworth, L., 1995, Olive oil, other dietary fats, and the risk of breast cancer (Italy), *Cancer Causes Control,* 6(6), 545–550.

Labieniec, M. and Gabryelak, T., 2007, Antioxidative and oxidative changes in the digestive gland cells of freshwater mussels *Unio tumidus* caused by selected phenolic compounds in the presence of H_2O_2 or Cu^{2+} ions, *Toxicol. In Vitro,* 21(1), 146–156.

Lai, M.Y., Leung, H.W., Yang, W.H., Chen, W.H., and Lee, H.Z., 2007, Up-regulation of matrix metalloproteinase family gene involvement in ursolic acid-induced human lung non-small carcinoma cell apoptosis, *Anticancer Res.,* 27, 145–153.

Lampe, J.W., Atkinson, C., and Hullar, M.A., 2006, Assessing exposure to lignans and their metabolites in humans, *J. O.A.C. Int.,* 89, 1174–1181.

Landis-Piwowar, K.R., Milacic, V., Chen, D., Yang, H., Zhao, Y., Chan, T.H., Yan, B., and Dou, Q.P., 2006, The proteasome as a potential target for novel anticancer drugs and chemosensitizers, *Drug Resist. Update,* 9, 263–273.

Lansky, E.P., Harrison, G., Froom, P., and Jiang, W.G., 2005, Pomegranate (*Punica granatum*) pure chemicals show possible synergistic inhibition of human PC-3 prostate cancer cell invasion across Matrigel, *Invest. New Drugs,* 23(2), 121–122.

Lasekan, J.B., Clayton, M.K., Gendron-Fitzpatrick, A., and Ney, D.M., 1990, Dietary olive and safflower oils in promotion of DMBA-induced mammary tumorigenesis in rats, *Nutr. Cancer,* 13(3), 153–163.

Lee, D.Y., Song, M.C., Yoo, K.H., Bang, M.H., Chung, I.S., Kim, S.H., Kim, D.K., Kwon, B.M., Jeong, T.S., Park, M.H., and Baek, N.I., 2007, Lignans from the fruits of *Cornus kousa* Burg. and their cytotoxic effects on human cancer cell lines, *Arch. Pharm. Res.,* 30, 402–407.

Lee, E.J., Min, H.Y., Joo Park, H., Chung, H.J., Kim, S., Nam Han, Y., and Lee, S.K., 2004, G2/M cell cycle arrest and induction of apoptosis by a stilbenoid, 3,4,5-trimethoxy-4′-bromo-cis-stilbene, in human lung cancer cells, *Life Sci.,* 75, 2829–2839.

Lee, H.J., Wang, C.J., Kuo, H.C., Chou, F.P., Jean, L.F., and Tseng, T.H., 2005, Induction apoptosis of luteolin in human hepatoma HepG2 cells involving mitochondria translocation of Bax/Bak and activation of JNK, *Toxicol. Appl. Pharmacol.,* 203, 124–131.

Lee, H.W., Ahn, D.H., Crawley, S.C., Li, J.D., Gum, J.R., Jr., Basbaum, C.B., Fan, N.Q., Szymkowski, D.E., Han, S.Y., Lee, B.H., Sleisenger, M.H., and Kim, Y.S., 2002, Phorbol 12-myristate 13-acetate up-regulates the transcription of MUC2 intestinal mucin via Ras, ERK, and NF-kappa B, *J. Biol. Chem.*, 27, 32624–32631.

Lee, L.T., Huang, Y.T., Hwang, J.J., Lee, P.P., Ke, F.C., Nair, M.P., Kanadaswam, C., and Lee, M.T., 2002, Blockade of the epidermal growth factor receptor tyrosine kinase activity by quercetin and luteolin leads to growth inhibition and apoptosis of pancreatic tumor cells, *Anticancer Res.*, 22, 1615–1627.

Lee, L.T., Huang, Y.T., Hwang, J.J., Lee, A.Y., Ke, F.C., Huang, C.J., Kandaswami, C., Lee, P.P., and Lee, M.T., 2004, Transinactivation of the epidermal growth factor receptor tyrosine kinase and focal adhesion kinase phosphorylation by dietary flavonoids: effect on invasive potential of human carcinoma cells, *Biochem. Pharmacol.*, 67, 2103–2114.

Lee, S.F. and Lin, J.K., 1997, Inhibitory effects of phytopolyphenols on TPA-induced transformation, PKC activation, and c-jun expression in mouse fibroblast cells, *Nutr. Cancer*, 28, 177–183.

Lee, W.J., Wu, L.F., Chen, W.K., Wang, C.J., and Tseng, T.H., 2006, Inhibitory effect of luteolin on hepatocyte growth factor/scatter factor-induced HepG2 cell invasion involving both MAPK/ERKs and PI3K-Akt pathways, *Chem. Biol. Interact.*, 160, 123–133.

Lee, W.R., Shen, S.C., Lin, H.Y., Hou, W.C., Yang, L.L., and Chen, Y.C., 2002, Wogonin and fisetin induce apoptosis in human promyeloleukemic cells, accompanied by a decrease of reactive oxygen species, and activation of caspase 3 and Ca(2+)-dependent endonuclease, *Biochem. Pharmacol.*, 63, 225–236.

Lee, Y.S., 2005, Role of NADPH oxidase-mediated generation of reactive oxygen species in the mechanism of apoptosis induced by phenolic acids in HepG2 human hepatoma cells, *Arch. Pharm. Res.*, 28, 1183–1189.

Lepley, D.M. and Pelling, J.C., 1997, Induction of p21/WAF1 and G1 cell-cycle arrest by the chemopreventive agent apigenin, *Mol. Carcinog.*, 19(2), 74–82.

Leung, H.W., Wu, C.H., Lin, C.H., and Lee, H.Z., 2005, Luteolin induced DNA damage leading to human lung squamous carcinoma CH27 cell apoptosis, *Eur. J. Pharmacol.*, 508, 77–83.

Li, P.G., Xu, J.W., Ikeda, K., Kobayakawa, A., Kayano, Y., Mitani, T., Ikami, T., and Yamori, Y., 2005, Caffeic acid inhibits vascular smooth muscle cell proliferation induced by angiotensin II in stroke-prone spontaneously hypertensive rats, *Hypertens. Res.*, 28, 369–377.

Li, Y. and Trush, M.A., 1994, Reactive oxygen-dependent DNA damage resulting from the oxidation of phenolic compounds by a copper-redox cycle mechanism, *Cancer Res.*, 54(7 Suppl.), 1895s–1898s.

Liang, Y.C., Huang, Y.T., Tsai, S.H., Lin-Shiau, S.Y., Chen, C.F., and Lin, J.K., 1999, Suppression of inducible cyclooxygenase and inducible nitric oxide synthase by apigenin and related flavonoids in mouse macrophages, *Carcinogenesis*, 20, 1945–1952.

Liang, Y.C., Tsai, S.H., Tsai, D.C., Lin-Shiau, S.Y., and Lin, J.K., 2001, Suppression of inducible cyclooxygenase and nitric oxide synthase through activation of peroxisome proliferator-activated receptor-gamma by flavonoids in mouse macrophages, *FEBS Lett.*, 496(1), 12–18.

Liao, H.F., Chen, Y.Y., Liu, J.J., Hsu, M.L., Shieh, H.J., Liao, H.J., Shieh, C.J., Shiao, M.S., and Chen, Y.J., 2003, Inhibitory effect of caffeic acid phenethyl ester on angiogenesis, tumor invasion, and metastasis, *J. Agric. Food Chem.*, 51, 7907–9712.

Lim do, Y., Jeong, Y., Tyner, A.L., and Park, J.H., 2007, Induction of cell cycle arrest and apoptosis in HT-29 human colon cancer cells by the dietary compound luteolin, *Am. J. Physiol. Gastrointest. Liver Physiol.*, 292, G66–G75.

Lima, C.F., Fernandes-Ferreira, M., and Pereira-Wilson, C., 2006, Phenolic compounds protect HepG2 cells from oxidative damage: relevance of glutathione levels, *Life Sci.*, 79, 2056–2068.

Lin, H.H., Chen, J.H., Huang, C.C., and Wang, C.J., 2007, Apoptotic effect of 3,4-dihydroxybenzoic acid on human gastric carcinoma cells involving JNK/p38 MAPK signaling activation, *Int. J. Cancer*, 120, 2306–2316.

Lin, J.K., Chen, Y.C., Huang, Y.T., and Lin-Shiau, S.Y., 1997, Suppression of protein kinase C and nuclear oncogene expression as possible molecular mechanisms of cancer chemoprevention by apigenin and curcumin, *J. Cell Biochem. Suppl.*, 28-29, 39–48.

Lin, L.C., Wang, Y.H., Hou, Y.C., Chang, S., Liou, K.T., Chou, Y.C., Wang, W.Y., and Shen, Y.C., 2006, The inhibitory effect of phenylpropanoid glycosides and iridoid glucosides on free radical production and beta2 integrin expression in human leucocytes, *J. Pharm. Pharmacol.*, 58, 129–135.

Lin, X., Switzer, B.R., and Demark-Wahnefried, W., 2001, Effect of mammalian lignans on the growth of prostate cancer cell lines, *Anticancer Res.*, 21, 3995–3999.

Lindenmeyer, F., Li, H., Menashi, S., Soria, C., and Lu, H., 2001, Apigenin acts on the tumor cell invasion process and regulates protease production, *Nutr. Cancer*, 39, 139–147.

Lipworth, L., Martinez, M.E., Angell, J., Hsieh, C.C., and Trichopoulos, D., 1997, Olive oil and human cancer: an assessment of the evidence, *Prev. Med.*, 26, 181–190.

Lirdprapamongkol, K., Sakurai, H., Kawasaki, N., Choo, M.K., Saitoh, Y., Aozuka, Y., Singhirunnusorn, P., Ruchirawat, S., Svasti, J., and Saiki, I., 2005, Vanillin suppresses in vitro invasion and in vivo metastasis of mouse breast cancer cells, *Eur. J. Pharm. Sci.*, 25, 57–65.

Liu, L., Hudgins, W.R., Shack, S., Yin, M.Q., and Samid, D., 1995, Cinnamic acid: a natural product with potential use in cancer intervention, *Int. J. Cancer*, 62, 345–350.

Liu, L.Z., Fang, J., Zhou, Q., Hu, X., Shi, X., and Jiang, B.H., 2005, Apigenin inhibits expression of vascular endothelial growth factor and angiogenesis in human lung cancer cells: implication of chemoprevention of lung cancer, *Mol. Pharmacol.*, 68, 635–643.

Liu, X.S. and Jiang, J., 2007, Induction of apoptosis and regulation of the MAPK pathway by ursolic acid in human leukemia k562 cells, *Planta Med.*, 73, 1192–1194.

Llor, X., Pons, E., Roca, A., Alvarez, M., Mane, J., Fernandez-Banares, F., and Gassull, M.A., 2003, The effects of fish oil, olive oil, oleic acid and linoleic acid on colorectal neoplastic processes, *Clin. Nutr.*, 22, 71–79.

Llorens, F., Garcia, L., Itarte, E., and Gomez, N., 2002, Apigenin and LY294002 prolong EGF-stimulated ERK1/2 activation in PC12 cells but are unable to induce full differentiation, *FEBS Lett.*, 510, 149–153.

Llorens, F., Miro, F.A., Casanas, A., Roher, N., Garcia, L., Plana, M., Gomez, N., and Itarte, E., 2004, Unbalanced activation of ERK1/2 and MEK1/2 in apigenin-induced HeLa cell death, *Exp. Cell Res.*, 299(1), 15–26.

Lotito, S.B. and Frei, B., 2006, Dietary flavonoids attenuate tumor necrosis factor alpha-induced adhesion molecule expression in human aortic endothelial cells. Structure-function relationships and activity after first pass metabolism, *J. Biol. Chem.*, 281, 37102–37110.

Maccaglia, A., Mallozzi, C., and Minetti, M., 2003, Differential effects of quercetin and resveratrol on Band 3 tyrosine phosphorylation signalling of red blood cells, *Biochem. Biophys. Res. Commun.*, 305, 541–547.

Magee, P.J., McGlynn, H., and Rowland, I.R., 2004, Differential effects of isoflavones and lignans on invasiveness of MDA-MB-231 breast cancer cells *in vitro*, *Cancer Lett.*, 208, 35–41.

Maiuri, M.C., De Stefano, D., Di Meglio, P., Irace, C., Savarese, M., Sacchi, R., Cinelli, M.P., and Carnuccio, R., 2005, Hydroxytyrosol, a phenolic compound from virgin olive oil, prevents macrophage activation, *Naunyn Schmiedebergs Arch. Pharmacol.*, 371, 457–465.

Manju, V. and Nalini, N., 2005, Chemopreventive potential of luteolin during colon carcinogenesis induced by 1,2-dimethylhydrazine, *Ital. J. Biochem.*, 54, 268–275.

Manju, V. and Nalini, N., 2007, Protective role of luteolin in 1,2-dimethylhydrazine induced experimental colon carcinogenesis, *Cell. Biochem. Funct.*, 25(2), 189–194.

Manna, C., Galletti, P., Maisto, G., Cucciolla, V., D'Angelo, S., and Zappia, V., 2000, Transport mechanism and metabolism of olive oil hydroxytyrosol in Caco-2 cells, *FEBS Lett.*, 470, 341–314.

Mansour, A., McCarthy, B., Schwander, S.K., Chang, V., Kotenko, S., Donepudi, S., Lee, J., and Raveche, E., 2004, Genistein induces G2 arrest in malignant B cells by decreasing IL-10 secretion, *Cell Cycle*, 3, 1597–1605.

Marks, F., Furstenberger, G., and Muller-Decker, K., 2007, Tumor promotion as a target of cancer prevention, *Recent Results Cancer Res.*, 174, 37–47.

Martin, T.A. and Jiang, W.G., 2001, Tight junctions and their role in cancer metastasis, *Histol. Histopathol.*, 16, 1183–1195.

Martinez, J., Gutierrez, A., Casas, J., Llado, V., Lopez-Bellan, A., Besalduch, J., Dopazo, A., and Escriba, P.V., 2005a, The repression of E2F-1 is critical for the activity of Minerval against cancer, *J. Pharmacol. Exp. Ther.*, 315, 466–474.

Martinez, J., Vogler, O., Casas, J., Barcelo, F., Alemany, R., Prades, J., Nagy, T., Baamonde, C., Kasprzyk, P.G., Teres, S., Saus, C., and Escriba, P.V., 2005b, Membrane structure modulation, protein kinase C alpha activation, and anticancer activity of minerval, *Mol. Pharmacol.*, 67, 531–540.

Matsukawa, Y., Marui, N., Sakai, T., Satomi, Y., Yoshida, M., Matsumoto, K., Nishino, H., and Aoike, A., 1993, Genistein arrests cell cycle progression at G2-M, *Cancer Res.*, 53, 1328–1331.

Matsuo, M., Sasaki, N., Saga, K., and Kaneko, T., 2005, Cytotoxicity of flavonoids toward cultured normal human cells, *Biol. Pharm. Bull.*, 28, 253–259.

McVean, M., Xiao, H., Isobe, K., and Pelling, J.C., 2000, Increase in wild-type p53 stability and transactivational activity by the chemopreventive agent apigenin in keratinocytes, *Carcinogenesis,* 21, 633–639.

Mendez-Samperio, P., Palma, J., and Vazquez, A., 2002, Signals involved in mycobacteria-induced CXCL-8 production by human monocytes, *J. Interferon Cytokine Res.,* 22, 189–197.

Menendez, J.A., Vellon, L., Colomer, R., and Lupu, R., 2005, Oleic acid, the main monounsaturated fatty acid of olive oil, suppresses Her-2/neu (erbB-2) expression and synergistically enhances the growth inhibitory effects of trastuzumab (Herceptin) in breast cancer cells with Her-2/neu oncogene amplification, *Ann. Oncol.,* 16, 359–371.

Menendez, J.A., Vazquez-Martin, A., Colomer, R., Brunet, J., Carrasco-Pancorbo, A., Garcia-Villalba, R., Fernandez-Gutierrez, A., and Segura-Carretero, A., 2007, Olive oil's bitter principle reverses acquired autoresistance to trastuzumab (Herceptin) in HER2-overexpressing breast cancer cells, *BMC Cancer,* 7, 80.

Menschikowski, M., Hagelgans, A., Hempel, U., and Siegert, G., 2004, Glycogen synthase kinase-3beta negatively regulates group IIA phospholipase A2 expression in human aortic smooth muscle and HepG2 hepatoma cells, *FEBS Lett.,* 577, 81–86.

Milder, I.E., Arts, I.C., van de Putte, B., Venema, D.P., and Hollman, P.C., 2005, Lignan contents of Dutch plant foods: a database including lariciresinol, pinoresinol, secoisolariciresinol and matairesinol, *Br. J. Nutr.,* 93, 393–402.

Milder, I.E., Kuijsten, A., Arts, I.C., Feskens, E.J., Kampman, E., Hollman, P.C., and Van 't Veer, P., 2007, Relation between plasma enterodiol and enterolactone and dietary intake of lignans in a Dutch endoscopy-based population, *J. Nutr.,* 137, 1266–1271.

Miro, F.A., Llorens, F., Roher, N., Plana, M., Gomez, N., and Itarte, E., 2002, Persistent nuclear accumulation of protein kinase CK2 during the G1-phase of the cell cycle does not depend on the ERK1/2 pathway but requires active protein synthesis, *Arch. Biochem. Biophys.,* 406, 165–172.

Molnar, J., Beladi, I., Domonkos, K., Foldeak, S., Boda, K., and Veckenstedt, A., 1981, Antitumor activity of flavonoids on NK/Ly ascites tumor cells, *Neoplasma,* 28, 11–18.

Moon, Y.J., Wang, X., and Morris, M.E., 2006, Dietary flavonoids: effects on xenobiotic and carcinogen metabolism, *Toxicol. In Vitro,* 20, 187–210.

Moral, R., Solanas, M., Garcia, G., Colomer, R., and Escrich, E., 2003, Modulation of EGFR and neu expression by n-6 and n-9 high-fat diets in experimental mammary adenocarcinomas, *Oncol. Rep.,* 10, 1417–1424.

Moreno, J.J., 2003, Effect of olive oil minor components on oxidative stress and arachidonic acid mobilization and metabolism by macrophages RAW 264.7, *Free Radic. Biol. Med.,* 35, 1073–1081.

Morrissey, C., O'Neill, A., Spengler, B., Christoffel, V., Fitzpatrick, J.M., and Watson, R.W., 2005, Apigenin drives the production of reactive oxygen species and initiates a mitochondrial mediated cell death pathway in prostate epithelial cells, *Prostate,* 63, 131–142.

Mottet, D., Ruys, S.P., Demazy, C., Raes, M., and Michiels, C., 2005, Role for casein kinase 2 in the regulation of HIF-1 activity, *Int. J. Cancer,* 117, 764–174.

Mounho, B.J. and Thrall, B.D., 1999, The extracellular signal-regulated kinase pathway contributes to mitogenic and antiapoptotic effects of peroxisome proliferators in vitro, *Toxicol. Appl. Pharmacol.,* 159, 125–133.

Nagao, T., Abe, F., and Okabe, H., 2001, Antiproliferative constituents in the plants 7. Leaves of *Clerodendron bungei* and leaves and bark of *C. trichotomum, Biol. Pharm. Bull.,* 24, 1338–1341.

Nagase, H. and Woessner, J.F., Jr., 1999, Matrix metalloproteinases, *J. Biol. Chem.,* 274, 21491–21494.

Nagase, H., Visse, R., and Murphy, G., 2006, Structure and function of matrix metalloproteinases and TIMPs, *Cardiovasc. Res.,* 69, 562–573.

Nangia-Makker, P., Tait, L., Shekhar, M.P., Palomino, E., Hogan, V., Piechocki, M.P., Funasaka, T., and Raz, A., 2007, Inhibition of breast tumor growth and angiogenesis by a medicinal herb: *Ocimum gratissimum, Int. J. Cancer,* 121, 884–894.

Nardini, M., Scaccini, C., Packer, L., and Virgili, F., 2000, In vitro inhibition of the activity of phosphorylase kinase, protein kinase C and protein kinase A by caffeic acid and a procyanidin-rich pine bark (*Pinus marittima*) extract, *Biochim. Biophys. Acta,* 1474, 219–225.

Nardini, M., Leonardi, F., Scaccini, C., and Virgili, F., 2001, Modulation of ceramide-induced NF-$_{kappa}$B binding activity and apoptotic response by caffeic acid in U937 cells: comparison with other antioxidants, *Free Radic. Biol. Med.,* 30, 722–733.

Natarajan, K., Singh, S., Burke, T.R., Jr., Grunberger, D., and Aggarwal, B.B., 1996, Caffeic acid phenethyl ester is a potent and specific inhibitor of activation of nuclear transcription factor NF-kappa B, *Proc. Natl. Acad. Sci. U.S.A.*, 93, 9090–9095.

Nelson, R., 2005, Oleic acid suppresses overexpression of ERBB2 oncogene, *Lancet Oncol.*, 6(2), 69.

Ng, T.B., Liu, F., and Wang, Z.T., 2000, Antioxidative activity of natural products from plants, *Life Sci.*, 66, 709–723.

Niisato, N., Ito, Y., and Marunaka, Y., 1999, Activation of Cl- channel and Na+/K+/2Cl- cotransporter in renal epithelial A6 cells by flavonoids: genistein, daidzein, and apigenin, *Biochem. Biophys. Res. Commun.*, 254, 368–371.

Noda, Y., Kaiya, T., Kohda, K., and Kawazoe, Y., 1997, Enhanced cytotoxicity of some triterpenes toward leukemia L1210 cells cultured in low pH media: possibility of a new mode of cell killing, *Chem. Pharm. Bull.* (Tokyo), 45, 1665–1670.

Noroozi, M., Angerson, W.J., and Lean, M.E., 1998, Effects of flavonoids and vitamin C on oxidative DNA damage to human lymphocytes, *Am. J. Clin. Nutr.*, 67, 1210–1218.

Nousis, L., Doulias, P.T., Aligiannis, N., Bazios, D., Agalias, A., Galaris, D., and Mitakou, S., 2005, DNA protecting and genotoxic effects of olive oil related components in cells exposed to hydrogen peroxide, *Free Radic. Res.*, 39, 787–795.

O'Leary, K.A., de Pascual-Tereasa, S., Needs, P.W., Bao, Y.P., O'Brien, N.M., and Williamson, G., 2004, Effect of flavonoids and vitamin E on cyclooxygenase-2 (COX-2) transcription, *Mutat. Res.*, 551, 245–254.

O'Prey, J., Brown, J., Fleming, J., and Harrison, P.R., 2003, Effects of dietary flavonoids on major signal transduction pathways in human epithelial cells, *Biochem. Pharmacol.*, 66, 2075–2088.

Oguro, T., Liu, J., Klaassen, C.D., and Yoshida, T., 1998, Inhibitory effect of oleanolic acid on 12-O-tetradecanoylphorbol-13-acetate-induced gene expression in mouse skin, *Toxicol. Sci.*, 45, 88–93.

Olszanecki, R., Gebska, A., Kozlovski, V.I., and Gryglewski, R.J., 2002, Flavonoids and nitric oxide synthase, *J. Physiol. Pharmacol.*, 53, 571–584.

Osada, M., Imaoka, S., and Funae, Y., 2004, Apigenin suppresses the expression of VEGF, an important factor for angiogenesis, in endothelial cells via degradation of HIF-1alpha protein, *FEBS Lett.*, 575, 59–63.

Ovesna, Z., Vachalkova, A., Horvathova, K., and Tothova, D., 2004, Pentacyclic triterpenoic acids: new chemoprotective compounds, *Minirev. Neoplasma*, 51(5), 327–333.

Owen, R.W., Mier, W., Giacosa, A., Hull, W.E., Spiegelhalder, B., and Bartsch, H., 2000, Identification of lignans as major components in the phenolic fraction of olive oil, *Clin. Chem.*, 46, 976–988.

Owen, R.W., Haubner, R., Mier, W., Giacosa, A., Hull, W.E., Spiegelhalder, B., and Bartsch, H., 2003, Isolation, structure elucidation and antioxidant potential of the major phenolic and flavonoid compounds in brined olive drupes, *Food Chem. Toxicol.*, 41(5), 703–717.

Pathak, A.K., Bhutani, M., Nair, A.S., Ahn, K.S., Chakraborty, A., Kadara, H., Guha, S., Sethi, G., and Aggarwal, B.B., 2007, Ursolic acid inhibits STAT3 activation pathway leading to suppression of proliferation and chemosensitization of human multiple myeloma cells, *Mol. Cancer Res.*, 5, 943–955.

Petridou, E., Zavras, A.I., Lefatzis, D., Dessypris, N., Laskaris, G., Dokianakis, G., Segas, J., Douglas, C.W., Diehl, S.R., and Trichopoulos, D., 2002, The role of diet and specific micronutrients in the etiology of oral carcinoma, *Cancer*, 94, 2981–2988.

Pettinari, A., Amici, M., Cuccioloni, M., Angeletti, M., Fioretti, E., and Eleuteri, A.M., 2006, Effect of polyphenolic compounds on the proteolytic activities of constitutive and immuno-proteasomes, *Antioxid. Redox Signal*, 8, 121–129.

Pisha, E., Chai, H., Lee, I.S., Chagwedera, T.E., Farnsworth, N.R., Cordell, G.A., Beecher, C.W., Fong, H.H., Kinghorn, A.D., Brown, D.M., et al., 1995, Discovery of betulinic acid as a selective inhibitor of human melanoma that functions by induction of apoptosis, *Nat. Med.*, 1, 1046–1051.

Plaumann, B., Fritsche, M., Rimpler, H., Brandner, G., and Hess, R.D., 1996, Flavonoids activate wild-type p53, *Oncogene*, 13, 1605–1614.

Poli, G., Leonarduzzi, G., Biasi, F., and Chiarpotto, E., 2004, Oxidative stress and cell signalling, *Curr. Med. Chem.*, 11, 1163–1682.

Prakash Chaturvedula, V. S., Gao, Z., Hecht, S.M., Jones, S.H., and Kingston, D.G., 2003, A new acylated oleanane triterpenoid from Couepia polyandra that inhibits the lyase activity of DNA polymerase beta, *J. Nat. Prod.*, 66, 1463–1465.

Qu, H., Madl, R.L., Takemoto, D.J., Baybutt, R.C., and Wang, W., 2005, Lignans are involved in the antitumor activity of wheat bran in colon cancer SW480 cells, *J. Nutr.*, 135, 598–602.

Raghuvar Gopal, D.V., Narkar, A.A., Badrinath, Y., Mishra, K.P., and Joshi, D.S., 2005, Betulinic acid induces apoptosis in human chronic myelogenous leukemia (CML) cell line K-562 without altering the levels of Bcr-Abl, *Toxicol. Lett.*, 155, 343–351.

Ragione, F.D., Cucciolla, V., Borriello, A., Pietra, V.D., Pontoni, G., Racioppi, L., Manna, C., Galletti, P., and Zappia, V., 2000, Hydroxytyrosol, a natural molecule occurring in olive oil, induces cytochrome c-dependent apoptosis, *Biochem. Biophys. Res. Commun.*, 278, 733–739.

Rao, C.V., Desai, D., Kaul, B., Amin, S., and Reddy, B.S., 1992, Effect of caffeic acid esters on carcinogen-induced mutagenicity and human colon adenocarcinoma cell growth, *Chem. Biol. Interact.*, 84, 277–290.

Rao, C.V., Desai, D., Simi, B., Kulkarni, N., Amin, S., and Reddy, B.S., 1993, Inhibitory effect of caffeic acid esters on azoxymethane-induced biochemical changes and aberrant crypt foci formation in rat colon, *Cancer Res.*, 53, 4182–4188.

Raso, G.M., Meli, R., Di Carlo, G., Pacilio, M., and Di Carlo, R., 2001, Inhibition of inducible nitric oxide synthase and cyclooxygenase-2 expression by flavonoids in macrophage J774A.1, *Life Sci.*, 68, 921–931.

Richardson, P.G., Schlossman, R., Hideshima, T., and Anderson, K.C., 2005, New treatments for multiple myeloma, *Oncology* (Williston Park), 19(14), 1781–1792; discussion 1792, 1795–1797.

Richter, M., Ebermann, R., and Marian, B., 1999, Quercetin-induced apoptosis in colorectal tumor cells: possible role of EGF receptor signaling, *Nutr. Cancer*, 34, 88–99.

Rigolio, R., Miloso, M., Nicolini, G., Villa, D., Scuteri, A., Simone, M., and Tredici, G., 2005, Resveratrol interference with the cell cycle protects human neuroblastoma SH-SY5Y cell from paclitaxel-induced apoptosis, *Neurochem. Int.*, 205–211.

Rodriguez, J., Yanez, J., Vicente, V., Alcaraz, M., Benavente-Garcia, O., Castillo, J., Lorente, J., and Lozano, J.A., 2002, Effects of several flavonoids on the growth of B16F10 and SK-MEL-1 melanoma cell lines: relationship between structure and activity, *Melanoma Res.*, 12, 99–107.

Ronchetti, D., Impagnatiello, F., Guzzetta, M., Gasparini, L., Borgatti, M., Gambari, R., and Ongini, E., 2006, Modulation of iNOS expression by a nitric oxide-releasing derivative of the natural antioxidant ferulic acid in activated RAW 264.7 macrophages, *Eur. J. Pharmacol.*, 532, 162–169.

Rosenberg, R.S., Grass, L., Jenkins, D.J., Kendall, C.W., and Diamandis, E.P., 1998, Modulation of androgen and progesterone receptors by phytochemicals in breast cancer cell lines, *Biochem. Biophys. Res. Commun.*, 248, 935–939.

Rossi, A., Longo, R., Russo, A., Borrelli, F., and Sautebin, L., 2002, The role of the phenethyl ester of caffeic acid (CAPE) in the inhibition of rat lung cyclooxygenase activity by propolis, *Fitoterapia*, 73(Suppl. 1), S30–S37.

Rouillier, P., Senesse, P., Cottet, V., Valleau, A., Faivre, J., and Boutron-Ruault, M.C., 2005, Dietary patterns and the adenomacarcinoma sequence of colorectal cancer, *Eur. J. Nutr.*, 44, 311–318.

Ruiz, P.A. and Haller, D., 2006, Functional diversity of flavonoids in the inhibition of the proinflammatory NF-kappaB, IRF, and Akt signaling pathways in murine intestinal epithelial cells, *J. Nutr.*, 136, 664–671.

Rzeski, W., Stepulak, A., Szymanski, M., Sifringer, M., Kaczor, J., Wejksza, K., Zdzisinska, B., and Kandefer-Szerszen, M., 2006, Betulinic acid decreases expression of bcl-2 and cyclin D1, inhibits proliferation, migration and induces apoptosis in cancer cells, *Naunyn Schmiedebergs Arch. Pharmacol.*, 374, 11–20.

Saenz, M.T., Garcia, M.D., Ahumada, M.C., and Ruiz, V., 1998, Cytostatic activity of some compounds from the unsaponifiable fraction obtained from virgin olive oil, *Farmaco*, 53(6), 448–449.

Samy, R.P., Gopalakrishnakone, P., and Ignacimuthu, S., 2006, Anti-tumor promoting potential of luteolin against 7,12-dimethylbenz(a)anthracene-induced mammary tumors in rats, *Chem. Biol. Interact.*, 164, 1–14.

Sang, Q.X., Jin, Y., Newcomer, R.G., Monroe, S.C., Fang, X., Hurst, D.R., Lee, S., Cao, Q., and Schwartz, M.A., 2006, Matrix metalloproteinase inhibitors as prospective agents for the prevention and treatment of cardiovascular and neoplastic diseases, *Curr. Top. Med. Chem.*, 6, 289–316.

Sato, F., Matsukawa, Y., Matsumoto, K., Nishino, H., and Sakai, T., 1994, Apigenin induces morphological differentiation and G2-M arrest in rat neuronal cells, *Biochem. Biophys. Res. Commun.*, 204, 578–584.

Schindler, R. and Mentlein, R., 2006, Flavonoids and vitamin E reduce the release of the angiogenic peptide vascular endothelial growth factor from human tumor cells, *J. Nutr.*, 136, 1477–482.

Schlupper, D., Giesa, S., and Gebhardt, R., 2006, Influence of biotransformation of luteolin, luteolin 7-O-glucoside, 3′,4′-dihydroxyflavone and apigenin by cultured rat hepatocytes on antioxidative capacity and inhibition of EGF receptor tyrosine kinase activity, *Planta Med.*, 72, 596–603.

Schmitt, C.A., Handler, N., Heiss, E.H., Erker, T., and Dirsch, V.M., 2007, No evidence for modulation of endothelial nitric oxide synthase by the olive oil polyphenol hydroxytyrosol in human endothelial cells, *Atherosclerosis*, 195, e58–e64.

Schultze-Mosgau, M.H., Dale, I.L., Gant, T.W., Chipman, J.K., Kerr, D.J., and Gescher, A., 1998, Regulation of c-fos transcription by chemopreventive isoflavonoids and lignans in MDA-MB-468 breast cancer cells, *Eur. J. Cancer*, 34, 1425–1431.

Schwartz, B., Birk, Y., Raz, A., and Madar, Z., 2004, Nutritional-pharmacological combinations — a novel approach to reducing colon cancer incidence, *Eur. J. Nutr.*, 43, 221–229.

Scott, B.C., Butler, J., Halliwell, B., and Aruoma, O.I., 1993, Evaluation of the antioxidant actions of ferulic acid and catechins, *Free Radic. Re. Commun.*, 19, 241–253.

Segaert, S., Courtois, S., Garmyn, M., Degreef, H., and Bouillon, R., 2000, The flavonoid apigenin suppresses vitamin D receptor expression and vitamin D responsiveness in normal human keratinocytes, *Biochem. Biophys. Res. Commun.*, 268(1), 237–241.

Selvendiran, K., Koga, H., Ueno, T., Yoshida, T., Maeyama, M., Torimura, T., Yano, H., Kojiro, M., and Sata, M., 2006, Luteolin promotes degradation in signal transducer and activator of transcription 3 in human hepatoma cells: an implication for the antitumor potential of flavonoids, *Cancer Res.*, 66(9), 4826–4834.

Sen, C.K., Khanna, S., Venojarvi, M., Trikha, P., Ellison, E.C., Hunt, T.K., and Roy, S., 2002, Copper-induced vascular endothelial growth factor expression and wound healing, *Am. J. Physiol. Heart Circ. Physiol.*, 282(5), H1821–H1827.

Shenouda, N.S., Zhou, C., Browning, J.D., Ansell, P.J., Sakla, M.S., Lubahn, D.B., and Macdonald, R.S., 2004, Phytoestrogens in common herbs regulate prostate cancer cell growth in vitro, *Nutr. Cancer*, 49(2), 200–208.

Shi, R., Huang, Q., Zhu, X., Ong, Y.B., Zhao, B., Lu, J., Ong, C.N., and Shen, H.M., 2007, Luteolin sensitizes the anticancer effect of cisplatin via c-Jun NH2-terminal kinase-mediated p53 phosphorylation and stabilization, *Mol. Cancer Ther.*, 6(4), 1338–1347.

Shi, R.X., Ong, C.N., and Shen, H.M., 2004, Luteolin sensitizes tumor necrosis factor-alpha-induced apoptosis in human tumor cells, *Oncogene*, 23(46), 7712–7721.

Shi, R.X., Ong, C.N., and Shen, H.M., 2005, Protein kinase C inhibition and x-linked inhibitor of apoptosis protein degradation contribute to the sensitization effect of luteolin on tumor necrosis factor-related apoptosis-inducing ligand-induced apoptosis in cancer cells, *Cancer Res.*, 65(17), 7815–7823.

Shigeoka, Y., Igishi, T., Matsumoto, S., Nakanishi, H., Kodani, M., Yasuda, K., Hitsuda, Y., and Shimizu, E., 2004, Sulindac sulfide and caffeic acid phenethyl ester suppress the motility of lung adenocarcinoma cells promoted by transforming growth factor-beta through Akt inhibition, *J. Cancer Res. Clin. Oncol.*, 130(3), 146–152.

Shin, K.M., Kim, I.T., Park, Y.M., Ha, J., Choi, J.W., Park, H.J., Lee, Y.S., and Lee, K.T., 2004, Anti-inflammatory effect of caffeic acid methyl ester and its mode of action through the inhibition of prostaglandin E2, nitric oxide and tumor necrosis factor-alpha production, *Biochem. Pharmacol.*, 68(12), 2327–2336.

Shishodia, S., Sethi, G., Konopleva, M., Andreeff, M., and Aggarwal, B.B., 2006, A synthetic triterpenoid, CDDO-Me, inhibits IkappaBalpha kinase and enhances apoptosis induced by TNF and chemotherapeutic agents through down-regulation of expression of nuclear factor kappaB-regulated gene products in human leukemic cells, *Clin. Cancer Res.*, 12(6), 1828–1838.

Shoulars, K., Brown, T., Alejandro, M.A., Crowley, J., and Markaverich, B.M., 2002, Identification of nuclear type II [(3)H]estradiol binding sites as histone H4, *Biochem. Biophys. Res. Commun.*, 296(5), 1083–1090.

Shoulars, K., Rodrigues, M.A., Crowley, J.R., Turk, J., Thompson, T., and Markaverich, B.M., 2005, Nuclear type II [3H]estradiol binding sites: a histone H3-H4 complex, *J. Steroid Biochem. Mol. Biol.*, 96(1), 19–30.

Shoulars, K., Rodriguez, M.A., Crowley, J., Turk, J., Thompson, T., and Markaverich, B.M., 2006, Reconstitution of the type II [3H]estradiol binding site with recombinant histone H4, *J. Steroid Biochem. Mol. Biol.*, 99(1), 1–8.

Shukla, S. and Gupta, S., 2004a, Molecular mechanisms for apigenin-induced cell-cycle arrest and apoptosis of hormone refractory human prostate carcinoma DU145 cells, *Mol. Carcinog.*, 39(2), 114–126.

Shukla, S. and Gupta, S., 2004b, Suppression of constitutive and tumor necrosis factor alpha-induced nuclear factor (NF)-kappaB activation and induction of apoptosis by apigenin in human prostate carcinoma PC-3 cells: correlation with down-regulation of NF-kappaB-responsive genes, *Clin. Cancer Res.*, 10(9), 3169–3178.

Shukla, S. and Gupta, S., 2006, Molecular targets for apigenin-induced cell cycle arrest and apoptosis in prostate cancer cell xenograft, *Mol. Cancer Ther.*, 5(4), 843–852.

Shukla, S. and Gupta, S., 2007, Apigenin-induced cell cycle arrest is mediated by modulation of MAPK, PI3K-Akt, and loss of cyclin D1 associated retinoblastoma dephosphorylation in human prostate cancer cells, *Cell Cycle*, 6(9), 1102–1114.

Shukla, S., Mishra, A., Fu, P., MacLennan, G.T., Resnick, M.I., and Gupta, S., 2005, Up-regulation of insulin-like growth factor binding protein-3 by apigenin leads to growth inhibition and apoptosis of 22Rv1 xenograft in athymic nude mice, *FASEB J.*, 19(14), 2042–2044.

Sieri, S., Krogh, V., Pala, V., Muti, P., Micheli, A., Evangelista, A., Tagliabue, G., and Berrino, F., 2004, Dietary patterns and risk of breast cancer in the ORDET cohort, *Cancer Epidemiol. Biomarkers Prev.*, 13(4), 567–572.

Sim, G.S., Lee, B.C., Cho, H.S., Lee, J.W., Kim, J.H., Lee, D.H., Kim, J.H., Pyo, H.B., Moon, D.C., Oh, K.W., Yun, Y.P., and Hong, J.T., 2007, Structure activity relationship of antioxidative property of flavonoids and inhibitory effect on matrix metalloproteinase activity in UVA-irradiated human dermal fibroblast, *Arch. Pharm. Res.*, 30(3), 290–298.

Smith, T.J., Yang, G.Y., Seril, D.N., Liao, J., and Kim, S., 1998, Inhibition of 4-(methylnitrosamino)-1-(3-pyridyl)-1-butanone-induced lung tumorigenesis by dietary olive oil and squalene, *Carcinogenesis*, 19(4), 703–706.

Snyder, R.D. and Gillies, P.J., 2002, Evaluation of the clastogenic, DNA intercalative, and topoisomerase II-interactive properties of bioflavonoids in Chinese hamster V79 cells, *Environ. Mol. Mutagen*, 40(4), 266–276.

Sohn, K.H., Lee, H.Y., Chung, H.Y., Young, H.S., Yi, S.Y., and Kim, K.W., 1995, Anti-angiogenic activity of triterpene acids, *Cancer Lett.*, 94(2), 213–218.

Soleas, G.J., Goldberg, D.M., Grass, L., Levesque, M., and Diamandis, E.P., 2001, Do wine polyphenols modulate p53 gene expression in human cancer cell lines? *Clin. Biochem.*, 34(5), 415–420.

Soler, M., Chatenoud, L., La Vecchia, C., Franceschi, S., and Negri, E., 1998, Diet, alcohol, coffee and pancreatic cancer: final results from an Italian study, *Eur. J. Cancer Prev.*, 7(6), 455–460.

Song, Y.S., Park, E.H., Hur, G.M., Ryu, Y.S., Lee, Y.S., Lee, J.Y., Kim, Y.M., and Jin, C., 2002, Caffeic acid phenethyl ester inhibits nitric oxide synthase gene expression and enzyme activity, *Cancer Lett.*, 175(1), 53–61.

Spencer-Cisek, P.A., 2002, The role of growth factors in malignancy: a focus on the epidermal growth factor receptor, *Semin. Oncol. Nurs.*, 18(Suppl. 2), 13–19.

Stagos, D., Kazantzoglou, G., Magiatis, P., Mitaku, S., Anagnostopoulos, K., and Kouretas, D., 2005, Effects of plant phenolics and grape extracts from Greek varieties of Vitis vinifera on Mitomycin C and topoisomerase I-induced nicking of DNA, *Int. J. Mol. Med.*, 15(6), 1013–1022.

Stupans, I., Murray, M., Kirlich, A., Tuck, K.L., and Hayball, P.J., 2001, Inactivation of cytochrome P450 by the food-derived complex phenol oleuropein, *Food Chem. Toxicol.*, 39(11), 1119–1124.

Stupans, L., Tan, H.W., Kirlich, A., Tuck, K., Hayball, P., and Murray, M., 2002, Inhibition of CYP3A-mediated oxidation in human hepatic microsomes by the dietary derived complex phenol, gallic acid, *J. Pharm. Pharmacol.*, 54(2), 269–275.

Sultana, R., Ravagna, A., Mohmmad-Abdul, H., Calabrese, V., and Butterfield, D.A., 2005, Ferulic acid ethyl ester protects neurons against amyloid beta-peptide(1-42)-induced oxidative stress and neurotoxicity: relationship to antioxidant activity, *J. Neurochem.*, 92(4), 749–758.

Suzuki, I., Iigo, M., Ishikawa, C., Kuhara, T., Asamoto, M., Kunimoto, T., Moore, M.A., Yazawa, K., Araki, E., and Tsuda, H., 1997, Inhibitory effects of oleic and docosahexaenoic acids on lung metastasis by colon-carcinoma-26 cells are associated with reduced matrix metalloproteinase-2 and -9 activities, *Int. J. Cancer*, 73(4), 607–612.

Syrovets, T., Buchele, B., Gedig, E., Slupsky, J.R., and Simmet, T., 2000, Acetyl-boswellic acids are novel catalytic inhibitors of human topoisomerases I and IIalpha, *Mol. Pharmacol.*, 58(1), 71–81.

Szaefer, H., Kaczmarek, J., Rybczynska, M., and Baer-Dubowska, W., 2007, The effect of plant phenols on the expression and activity of phorbol ester-induced PKC in mouse epidermis, *Toxicology*, 230(1), 1–10.

Takagaki, N., Sowa, Y., Oki, T., Nakanishi, R., Yogosawa, S., and Sakai, T., 2005, Apigenin induces cell cycle arrest and p21/WAF1 expression in a p53-independent pathway, *Int. J. Oncol.*, 26(1), 185–189.

Tang, D.G., Chen, Y.Q., and Honn, K.V., 1996, Arachidonate lipoxygenases as essential regulators of cell survival and apoptosis, *Proc. Natl. Acad. Sci. U.S.A.*, 93(11), 5241–5246.

Tatsuta, A., Iishi, H., Baba, M., Yano, H., Murata, K., Mukai, M., and Akedo, H., 2000, Suppression by api-genin of peritoneal metastasis of intestinal adenocarcinomas induced by azoxymethane in Wistar rats, *Clin. Exp. Metastasis,* 18(8), 657–662.

Thurnher, D., Turhani, D., Pelzmann, M., Wannemacher, B., Knerer, B., Formanek, M., Wacheck, V., and Selzer, E., 2003, Betulinic acid: a new cytotoxic compound against malignant head and neck cancer cells, *Head Neck,* 25(9), 732–740.

Tong, X., Van Dross, R.T., Abu-Yousif, A., Morrison, A.R., and Pelling, J.C., 2007, Apigenin prevents UVB-induced cyclooxygenase 2 expression: coupled mRNA stabilization and translational inhibition, *Mol. Cell. Biol.,* 27(1), 283–296.

Torkin, R., Lavoie, J.F., Kaplan, D.R., and Yeger, H., 2005, Induction of caspase-dependent, p53-mediated apoptosis by apigenin in human neuroblastoma, *Mol. Cancer Ther.,* 4, 1–11.

Trichopoulou, A., Katsouyanni, K., Stuver, S., Tzala, L., Gnardellis, C., Rimm, E., and Trichopoulos, D., 1995, Consumption of olive oil and specific food groups in relation to breast cancer risk in Greece, *J. Natl. Cancer Inst.,* 87(2), 110–116.

Trochon, V., Blot, E., Cymbalista, F., Engelmann, C., Tang, R.P., Thomaidis, A., Vasse, M., Soria, J., Lu, H., and Soria, C., 2000, Apigenin inhibits endothelial-cell proliferation in G(2)/M phase whereas it stimu-lates smooth-muscle cells by inhibiting P21 and P27 expression, *Int. J. Cancer,* 85(5), 691–696.

Tseng, T.H., Kao, T.W., Chu, C.Y., Chou, F.P., Lin, W.L., and Wang, C.J., 2000, Induction of apoptosis by hibiscus protocatechuic acid in human leukemia cells via reduction of retinoblastoma (RB) phosphory-lation and Bcl-2 expression, *Biochem. Pharmacol.,* 60, 307–315.

Tzonou, A., Lipworth, L., Kalandidi, A., Trichopoulou, A., Gamatsi, I., Hsieh, C.C., Notara, V., and Tricho-poulos, D., 1996, Dietary factors and the risk of endometrial cancer: a case-control study in Greece, *Br. J. Cancer,* 73, 1284–1290.

Ujiki, M.B., Ding, X.Z., Salabat, M.R., Bentrem, D.J., Golkar, L., Milam, B., Talamonti, M.S., Bell, R.H., Jr., Iwamura, T., and Adrian, T.E., 2006, Apigenin inhibits pancreatic cancer cell proliferation through G2/M cell cycle arrest, *Mol. Cancer,* 5, 76.

Van Dross, R.T., Hong, X., Essengue, S., Fischer, S.M., and Pelling, J.C., 2007, Modulation of UVB-induced and basal cyclooxygenase 2 (COX-2) expression by apigenin in mouse keratinocytes: role of USF tran-scription factors, *Mol. Carcinog.,* 46(4), 303–314.

Van Dross, R.T., Hong, X., and Pelling, J.C., 2005, Inhibition of TPA-induced cyclooxygenase-2 (COX-2) expression by apigenin through downregulation of Akt signal transduction in human keratinocytes, *Mol. Carcinog.,* 44(2), 83–91.

van Nimwegen, M.J. and van de Water, B., 2007, Focal adhesion kinase: a potential target in cancer therapy, *Biochem. Pharmacol.,* 73(5), 597–609.

van Rijn, J. and van den Berg, J., 1997, Flavonoids as enhancers of x-ray-induced cell damage in hepatoma cells, *Clin. Cancer Res.,* 3(10), 1775–1779.

Vargo, M.A., Voss, O.H., Poustka, F., Cardounel, A.J., Grotewold, E., and Doseff, A.I., 2006, Apigenin-induced-apoptosis is mediated by the activation of PKCdelta and caspases in leukemia cells, *Biochem. Pharmacol.,* 72(6), 681–692.

Visioli, F., Bellosta, S., and Galli, C., 1998, Oleuropein, the bitter principle of olives, enhances nitric oxide production by mouse macrophages, *Life Sci.,* 62(6), 541–546.

von Moltke, L.L., Weemhoff, J.L., Bedir, E., Khan, I.A., Harmatz, J.S., Goldman, P., and Greenblatt, D.J., 2004, Inhibition of human cytochromes P450 by components of Ginkgo biloba, *J. Pharm. Pharmacol.,* 56(8), 1039–1044.

Wahle, K.W., Caruso, D., Ochoa, J.J., and Quiles, J.L., 2004, Olive oil and modulation of cell signaling in disease prevention, *Lipids,* 39(12), 1223–1231.

Wallerath, T., Li, H., Godtel-Ambrust, U., Schwarz, P.M., and Forstermann, U., 2005, A blend of polypheno-lic compounds explains the stimulatory effect of red wine on human endothelial NO synthase, *Nitric Oxide,* 12(2), 97–104.

Wang, B.H. and Polya, G.M., 1996, Selective inhibition of cyclic AMP-dependent protein kinase by amphi-philic triterpenoids and related compounds, *Phytochemistry,* 41(1), 55–63.

Wang, C. and Kurzer, M.S., 1997, Phytoestrogen concentration determines effects on DNA synthesis in human breast cancer cells, *Nutr. Cancer,* 28(3), 236–247.

Wang, L.Q., 2002, Mammalian phytoestrogens: enterodiol and enterolactone, *J. Chromatogr. B Analyt. Tech-nol. Biomed. Life Sci.,* 777(1–2), 289–309.

Wang, W., Heideman, L., Chung, C.S., Pelling, J.C., Koehler, K.J., and Birt, D.F., 2000, Cell-cycle arrest at G2/M and growth inhibition by apigenin in human colon carcinoma cell lines, *Mol. Carcinog.*, 28(2), 102–110.

Wang, W., VanAlstyne, P.C., Irons, K.A., Chen, S., Stewart, J.W., and Birt, D.F., 2004, Individual and interactive effects of apigenin analogs on G2/M cell-cycle arrest in human colon carcinoma cell lines, *Nutr. Cancer*, 48(1), 106–114.

Wartenberg, M., Budde, P., De Marees, M., Grunheck, F., Tsang, S.Y., Huang, Y., Chen, Z.Y., Hescheler, J., and Sauer, H., 2003, Inhibition of tumor-induced angiogenesis and matrix-metalloproteinase expression in confrontation cultures of embryoid bodies and tumor spheroids by plant ingredients used in traditional Chinese medicine, *Lab. Invest.*, 83(1), 87–98.

Way, T.D., Kao, M.C., and Lin, J.K., 2004, Apigenin induces apoptosis through proteasomal degradation of HER2/neu in HER2/neu-overexpressing breast cancer cells via the phosphatidylinositol 3-kinase/Akt-dependent pathway, *J. Biol. Chem.*, 279(6), 4479–4489.

Way, T.D., Kao, M.C., and Lin, J.K., 2005, Degradation of HER2/neu by apigenin induces apoptosis through cytochrome c release and caspase-3 activation in HER2/neu-overexpressing breast cancer cells, *FEBS Lett.*, 579(1), 145–152.

Wei, H., Tye, L., Bresnick, E., and Birt, D.F., 1990, Inhibitory effect of apigenin, a plant flavonoid, on epidermal ornithine decarboxylase and skin tumor promotion in mice, *Cancer Res.*, 50(3), 499–502.

Weldon, C.B., McKee, A., Collins-Burow, B.M., Melnik, L.I., Scandurro, A.B., McLachlan, J.A., Burow, M.E., and Beckman, B.S., 2005, PKC-mediated survival signaling in breast carcinoma cells: a role for MEK1-AP1 signaling, *Int. J. Oncol.*, 26(3), 763–768.

Weyant, M.J., Carothers, A.M., Bertagnolli, M.E., and Bertagnolli, M.M., 2000, Colon cancer chemopreventive drugs modulate integrin-mediated signaling pathways, *Clin. Cancer Res.*, 6(3), 949–956.

Wick, W., Grimmel, C., Wagenknecht, B., Dichgans, J., and Weller, M., 1999, Betulinic acid-induced apoptosis in glioma cells: a sequential requirement for new protein synthesis, formation of reactive oxygen species, and caspase processing, *J. Pharmacol. Exp. Ther.*, 289(3), 1306–1312.

Williams, E.L. and Djamgoz, M.B., 2005, Nitric oxide and metastatic cell behaviour, *Bioessays*, 27(12), 1228–1238.

Wu, K., Yuan, L.H., and Xia, W., 2005, Inhibitory effects of apigenin on the growth of gastric carcinoma SGC-7901 cells, *World J. Gastroenterol.*, 11(29), 4461–4464.

Xagorari, A., Roussos, C., and Papapetropoulos, A., 2002, Inhibition of LPS-stimulated pathways in macrophages by the flavonoid luteolin, *Br. J. Pharmacol.*, 136, 1058–1064.

Xu, F., Song, D., and Zhen, Y., 2004, Inhibition of tumor metastasis by sodium caffeate and its effect on angiogenesis, *Oncology*, 67(1), 88–92.

Yamashita, N. and Kawanishi, S., 2000, Distinct mechanisms of DNA damage in apoptosis induced by quercetin and luteolin, *Free Radic. Res.*, 33(5), 623–633.

Yanez, J., Vicente, V., Alcaraz, M., Castillo, J., Benavente-Garcia, O., Canteras, M., and Teruel, J.A., 2004, Cytotoxicity and antiproliferative activities of several phenolic compounds against three melanocytes cell lines: relationship between structure and activity, *Nutr. Cancer*, 49(2), 191–199.

Yano, S., Tachibana, H., and Yamada, K., 2005, Flavones suppress the expression of the high-affinity IgE receptor FcepsilonRI in human basophilic KU812 cells, *J. Agric. Food Chem.*, 53(5), 1812–1817.

Yasukawa, K., Takido, M., Matsumoto, T., Takeuchi, M., and Nakagawa, S., 1991, Sterol and triterpene derivatives from plants inhibit the effects of a tumor promoter, and sitosterol and betulinic acid inhibit tumor formation in mouse skin two-stage carcinogenesis, *Oncology*, 48, 72–76.

Ye, Y.N., Liu, E.S., Shin, V.Y., Wu, W.K., and Cho, C.H., 2004, Contributory role of 5-lipoxygenase and its association with angiogenesis in the promotion of inflammation-associated colonic tumorigenesis by cigarette smoking, *Toxicology*, 203(1-3), 179–188.

Yee, S.B., Lee, J.H., Chung, H.Y., Im, K.S., Bae, S.J., Choi, J.S., and Kim, N.D., 2003, Inhibitory effects of luteolin isolated from Ixeris sonchifolia Hance on the proliferation of HepG2 human hepatocellular carcinoma cells, *Arch. Pharm. Res.*, 26(2), 151–156.

Yin, F., Giuliano, A.E., and Van Herle, A.J., 1999a, Growth inhibitory effects of flavonoids in human thyroid cancer cell lines, *Thyroid*, 9(4), 369–376.

Yin, F., Giuliano, A.E., and Van Herle, A.J., 1999b, Signal pathways involved in apigenin inhibition of growth and induction of apoptosis of human anaplastic thyroid cancer cells (ARO), *Anticancer Res.*, 19(5B), 4297–4303.

Yin, F., Giuliano, A.E., Law, R.E., and Van Herle, A.J., 2001, Apigenin inhibits growth and induces G2/M arrest by modulating cyclin-CDK regulators and ERK MAP kinase activation in breast carcinoma cells, *Anticancer Res.*, 21(1A), 413–420.

Yip, E.C., Chan, A.S., Pang, H., Tam, Y.K., and Wong, Y.H., 2006, Protocatechuic acid induces cell death in HepG2 hepatocellular carcinoma cells through a c-Jun N-terminal kinase-dependent mechanism, *Cell. Biol. Toxicol.*, 22(4), 293–302.

Zhang, F., Jia, Z., Deng, Z., Wei, Y., Zheng, R., and Yu, L., 2002, In vitro modulation of telomerase activity, telomere length and cell cycle in MKN45 cells by verbascoside, *Planta Med.*, 68(2), 115–118.

Zhang, G.P., Lu, Y.Y., Lv, J.C., and Ou, H.J., 2006, [Effect of ursolic acid on caspase-3 and PARP expression of human MCF-7 cells], *Zhongguo Zhong Yao Za Zhi*, 31, 141–144.

Zhang, W., Turner, D.J., Segura, B.J., Cowles, R., and Mulholland, M.W., 2000, ATP induces c-fos expression in C6 glioma cells by activation of P(2Y) receptors, *J. Surg. Res.*, 94(1), 49–55.

Zhang, Z., Wei, T., Hou, J., Li, G., Yu, S., and Xin, W., 2003, Iron-induced oxidative damage and apoptosis in cerebellar granule cells: attenuation by tetramethylpyrazine and ferulic acid, *Eur. J. Pharmacol.*, 467, 41–47.

Zhao, C., Dodin, G., Yuan, C., Chen, H., Zheng, R., Jia, Z., and Fan, B.T., 2005, "In vitro" protection of DNA from Fenton reaction by plant polyphenol verbascoside, *Biochim. Biophys. Acta*, 1723, 114–123.

Zheng, P.W., Chiang, L.C., and Lin, C.C., 2005, Apigenin induced apoptosis through p53-dependent pathway in human cervical carcinoma cells, *Life Sci.*, 76(12), 1367–1379.

Zheng, Q.S., Sun, X.L., Xu, B., Li, G., and Song, M., 2005, Mechanisms of apigenin-7-glucoside as a hepatoprotective agent, *Biomed. Environ. Sci.*, 18, 65–70.

Zheng, Z.S., Xue, G.Z., Grunberger, D., and Prystowsky, J.H., 1995, Caffeic acid phenethyl ester inhibits proliferation of human keratinocytes and interferes with the EGF regulation of ornithine decarboxylase, *Oncol. Res.*, 7(9), 445–452.

Zhou, B.N., Bahler, B.D., Hofmann, G.A., Mattern, M.R., Johnson, R.K., and Kingston, D.G., 1998, Phenylethanoid glycosides from Digitalis purpurea and Penstemon linarioides with PKCalpha-inhibitory activity, *J. Nat. Prod.*, 61(11), 1410–1412.

Zhou, S., Koh, H.L., Gao, Y., Gong, Z.Y., and Lee, E.J., 2004, Herbal bioactivation: the good, the bad and the ugly, *Life Sci.*, 74(8), 935–968.

Zhu, F., Liu, X.G., and Liang, N.C., 2003, [Effect of emodin and apigenin on invasion of human ovarian carcinoma HO-8910PM cells *in vitro*], *Ai Zheng*, 22(4), 358–362.

Zhu, Y.P., Su, Z.W., and Li, C.H., 1989, Growth-inhibition effects of oleic acid, linoleic acid, and their methyl esters on transplanted tumors in mice, *J. Natl. Cancer Inst.*, 81(17), 1302–1306.

Ziyan, L., Yongmei, Z., Nan, Z., Ning, T., and Baolin, L., 2007, Evaluation of the anti-inflammatory activity of luteolin in experimental animal models, *Planta Med.*, 73(3), 221–226.

Zou, Y. and Chiou, G.C., 2006, Apigenin inhibits laser-induced choroidal neovascularization and regulates endothelial cell function, *J. Ocul. Pharmacol. Ther.*, 22(6), 425–430.

Zusman, I., 1998, Comparative anticancer effects of vaccination and dietary factors on experimentally-induced cancers, *In Vivo*, 12, 675–689.

8 Antithrombotic and Antiatherogenic Lipid Minor Constituents from Olive Oil

Smaragdi Antonopoulou, Haralabos C. Karantonis, and Tzortzis Nomikos

CONTENTS

8.1 INTRODUCTION

From ancient times until now human nutritional habits have been adopted from developmental experience and various other factors, mainly geographical location, social-economical status, and religious traditions. Systematic observation and record of the dietary habits around the world have demonstrated the existence of distinct dietary models. The study of these models has been focused on the establishment of an etiological relation between the dietary habits of different populations and the incidence of pathological conditions.

The first international study investigating the possible correlation between diet and cardiovascular disease (CVD) was held in 1960 by Professor Ancel Keys and it is well known as the Study of the Seven Countries (Aravanis et al., 1970). The correlation between the Mediterranean diet (MD) and the distribution of cardiovascular morbidity and mortality was established and showed that populations which consumed the above diet rarely presented CVDs and that this favorable effect is probably due to the consumption of olive oil.

On the other hand, other similar trials, such as the Study of Australian Immigrants (Hu, 2003), demonstrated that environmental and hereditary factors are not implicated in atherogenesis. Experimental data from a variety of clinical intervention studies have shown that a change in cholesterol intake slightly alters plasma total cholesterol; they have also shown that fat restriction does not result in a proportional reduction of risk factors for coronary heart disease.

The MD is considered a model of a health-beneficial diet exerting a protective role in various pathological conditions such as CVDs, cancer, rheumatoid arthritis, kidney diseases, Alzheimer disease and other neurodegenerative diseases, Parkinson disease, disturbances of the gastrointestinal tract, and diabetes. Although differences in dietary traditions exist between the various Mediterranean populations, there are common nutritional characteristics such as olive oil as the main fat source; high consumption of fruits, vegetables, and legumes; moderate consumption of fish, wine, and dairy products; and low intake of animal proteins.

Epidemiological and experimental studies attribute the beneficial effect of MD to the consumption of olive oil and especially to the presence of monounsaturated fatty acids (MUFAs), mainly oleic acid. During the last decades, data have provided increasing evidence that the existence of bioactive components — usually present in minor quantities — in the MD may be responsible for its protective effect against chronic diseases. Under the term "bioactive minor components" essential unsaturated fatty acids, dietary antioxidants, vitamins, phenolic compounds, and other lipid microconstituents are included. To establish their contribution to the beneficial role of the MD, their implication in each pathological condition should be further studied.

The relation between CVDs and the MD is the most studied one. In addition, prevention of atherosclerosis is a major objective of modern medical investigation. Despite the complexity of this disease, it is clear that atherosclerosis is a chronic inflammatory condition that can lead to an acute clinical event through plaque rupture and thrombosis. Several theories have been formulated in order to explain the pathogenesis of atherosclerosis. The most important theories are those of inflammation, oxidation, and response-to-retention. Thrombosis, inflammation, and oxidation are critical points in the above hypotheses. The above theories can be unified to form one single theory by a molecular mechanism orchestrated by PAF (Demopoulos et al., 2003). PAF is the common name for 1-O-alkyl-2-acetyl-sn-glycero-3-phosphocholine and its structure was identified in 1979 (Demopoulos et al., 1979). PAF is a mediator of crucial importance in the inflammatory response and is synthesized by several different cell types upon activation, e.g., platelets, monocytes, macrophages, foam cells, and endothelial cells (Demopoulos et al., 2003).

The "PAF-implicated atherosclerosis theory" proposes a new biochemical mechanism for the initiation of atheromatosis and it interprets the epidemiological observations demonstrating the protective role of the MD against atherogenesis, atherosclerosis, and CVDs. The proposed mechanism is the following.

Oxidation of low density lipoprotein (LDL) takes place in human blood and depends on several factors such as diet (total intake of antioxidants) and lifestyle factors (such as smoking, sedentary lifestyle, etc.). Even though PAF production is under strict control, unregulated production of PAF is observed during LDL oxidation. The PAF produced during LDL oxidization has been isolated and identified (Liapikos et al., 1994). When LDL oxidation or pathological conditions induce the unregulated increase of PAF levels, then PAF — among other mediators — can initiate a rapid local inflammatory response in the vessel. This action leads to endothelium dysfunction, which shows increased permeability for blood cells and oxidized LDL (OxLDL) along with foam cell formation and proliferation of smooth muscle cells. All the above steps are well-known biological activities of PAF that lead to early atherosclerotic lesions (Demopoulos et al., 2003).

This mechanism is also supported by *in vivo* experiments in which atherogenesis was not detected in the experimental animals fed a cholesterol-rich diet along with specific inhibitors of PAF. It also should be noted that oxidative modification of LDL leads to progressive loss of associated PAF acetylhydrolase (PAF-AH) activity, the only enzyme that can hydrolyze and inactivate PAF, minimizing by this way the physical defense system of the human organism. The above findings show that specific PAF inhibitors may protect from atherogenesis. It should also be mentioned that the antioxidants, which are found in high quantities in foods of the MD, partly prevent LDL oxidation and therefore PAF production.

The presence of PAF inhibitors in foods of the MD has been well established. Olive oil was the first among them where lipid molecules exerting strong anti-PAF activity were detected.

"PAF implicated atherosclerosis theory" could also explain the so-called "French paradox" or the lower mortality rates of the French due to CVDs despite the high consumption of saturated fat and cholesterol. This observation was attributed to the daily moderate consumption of red wine. The presence of PAF inhibitors in different varieties of wines that has already been reported may explain this paradox (Demopoulos et al., 2003). It is of interest that PAF inhibitors are not always found in higher amounts in red wines compared to white ones (Fragopoulou et al., 2001).

PAF inhibitors were also found in several other foods of the MD, such as honey, yogurt, plants, garlic, onion, and fish (Demopoulos et al., 2003). The existence of PAF inhibitors in fish also explains the low mortality rates observed in Japan as well as the hematological disorders resulting from fish overconsumption. In addition, vitamin E, an antioxidant and antiatherogenic compound of plant foods, also inhibits PAF actions (Kakishita et al., 1990).

In addition, dietary intervention studies have shown that the administration of traditional MD meals, rich in PAF-antagonists, to either normal volunteers or type 2 diabetic patients, resulted in the attenuation of platelet reactivity induced by PAF (Antonopoulou et al., 2006).

The existence of PAF inhibitors in MD foods may offer an alternative explanation of the MD protective effect in the aforementioned pathological conditions since PAF is implicated in all of them.

8.2 ANTIATHEROGENIC PROPERTIES OF OLIVE OIL MINOR CONSTITUENTS

Atherosclerosis constitutes an inflammatory disease. One of the earliest signs of atherosclerosis development is the activation of endothelium, accompanied by adhesion and trans-endothelial migration of monocytes. Within the endothelium, monocytes acquire a macrophage-like phenotype and scavenge OxLDL and triglyceride-rich lipoproteins (TRLs), thus becoming foam cells. This contributes to the formation of early atherosclerotic lesions (Ross, 1999; Demopoulos et al., 2003).

Major causes of endothelium dysfunction are inflammatory molecules that exist on OxLDL or are derived from activated monocytes and platelets. Such inflammatory molecules are PAF, interleukin-1β (IL-1β), and tumor necrosis factor α (TNFα). Endothelium activation is accompanied by an increase in the expression of specific cytokines and adhesion molecules such as P- and E-selectin, intracellular adhesion molecule-1 (ICAM-1), vascular cell adhesion molecule-1 (VCAM-1), IL-6 released from macrophages, and C reactive protein (CRP) released from the liver (Davies et al., 1993; Ross, 1999; Demopoulos et al., 2003; Jialal et al., 2004).

Olive oil is recognized as a food with beneficial effects on CVDs. At present, the beneficial effects of olive oil are mainly attributed to its minor components that exert significant biological effects, despite the fact that they are of limited amount (Covas et al., 2006a). The importance of minor olive oil components on atherosclerosis has been implied by studies with monounsaturated dietary oils that have reported conflicting effects; these studies indicate that other compounds beyond MUFAs may exert antiatherogenic activities. Indeed, minor olive oil components have been shown to exert antiatherogenic properties. These properties are due to their antioxidant effects that protect LDL from its oxidation or to their direct anti-inflammatory effects on endothelium or even to their hypolipidemic or hypotensive activity (Perona et al., 2006).

Olive oil minor components constitute about 1–2% of the total content of virgin olive oil (Boskou, 2006). After saponification of olive oil the remaining unsaponifiable fraction contains minor components including hydrocarbons, like squalene and β-carotene; tocopherols, such as α-tocopherol; fatty alcohols; triterpenic alcohols, such as erythrodiol and uvaol; triterpenic acids, such as oleanolic and maslinic acid; other terpenic compounds; sterols, such as β-sitosterol, campesterol, and 4-methylsterols; and pigments, like chlorophylls and pheophytins. Other olive oil minor compounds are the well-studied phenolic compounds such as oleuropein aglycons, tyrosol, and hydroxytyrosol secoiridoids; other phenols (see also Chapter 3), waxes, sterol-esters, mono- and diacylglycerols, phosphatides, unusual glycero-glycolipids, and other unidentified components (Kiritakis, 1990; Boskou, 2000; Harwood and Aparicio, 2000; Karantonis et al., 2002; Boskou et al., 2006).

8.2.1 ANTIATHEROGENIC PROPERTIES OF OLIVE OIL MINOR CONSTITUENTS OF THE UNSAPONIFIABLE FRACTION

Several experimental data demonstrate that the unsaponifiable fraction of olive oil exerts antioxidant and anti-inflammatory activities (Perona et al., 2006).

In endothelial cells incubated with postprandial TRLs, isolated from the plasma of healthy subjects who had consumed a meal with virgin olive oil enriched with its unsaponifiable fraction (Perona et al., 2004), prostaglandin E_2 (PGE_2) and thromboxane B_2 (TxB_2) production was reduced.

In rabbits, a diet high in olive oil unsaponifiable fraction leads to a higher antioxidant content in LDLs and lowers its susceptibility to oxidation (Ochoa et al., 2002).

Squalene or triterpenes exert *in vitro* antioxidant activity (Covas et al., 2006a). Moreover, in rodents supplementation of their diet with squalene strongly inhibits the activity of beta-hydroxy-beta-methylglutaryl-CoA reductase (HMG-CoA reductase), a key enzyme in cholesterol biosynthesis, thus indicating a hypolipidemic action of these molecules (Bellosta et al., 2000).

In rat aorta, oleanolic acid and erythrodiol, two olive oil triterpenoids, have been used to evoke an endothelium-dependent vasorelaxation through nitric oxide (NO) production by the endothelium (Rodriguez-Rodriguez et al., 2004). Moreover, oleanolic acid possesses anti-inflammatory properties since it inhibits the activity of lipoxygenase (LOX) and cyclooxygenase-2 (COX-2) (Ringbom et al., 1998; Simon et al., 1992), thus reducing the production of PGE_2 and leukotriene B_4 (LTB_4) and also inhibits superoxide anion generation by human neutrophils (Leu et al., 2004). In addition, erythrodiol reduces the 12-*O*-tetradecanoylphorbol-13-acetate (TPA)-caused edema, thus exerting anti-inflammatory activities (De la Puerta et al., 2000).

Human and animal studies demonstrate that plant sterol supplementation decreases serum cholesterol concentration (Jones et al., 1997). Mechanisms for this effect include inhibition of cholesterol absorption (Quilez et al., 2003) and decreased production of apoB-containing lipoproteins from liver and intestine (Ho and Pal, 2005). In familial hypercholesterolemic children, administration of a phytosterol mixture containing β-sitosterol, campesterol, and stigmasterol led to LDL-cholesterol reduction (de Jongh et al., 2003). However, it is questionable whether the low sterol content of olive oil is able to modulate serum cholesterol levels.

In RAW 264.7 macrophages stimulated by phorbol esters, β-sitosterol reduces reactive oxygen species (ROS) production by regulating the glutathione (GSH) redox cycle, enhancing GSH peroxidase and superoxide dismutase (SOD) activities. ROS modulate arachidonic acid (AA) release and COX-2 induction through phospholipase A_2 (PLA_2) and nuclear factor kappa beta (NFκB) activation, respectively. Indeed, this reduction of ROS by β-sitosterol leads to the reduction of AA release as well as PGE_2 and LTB_4 production (Moreno, 2003). In mice, β-sitosterol also exerts anti-inflammatory effects by reducing auricular edema induced by TPA (De la Puerta et al., 2000).

Vitamin E (α-tocopherol) is one of the most studied minor constituents of olive oil. Dietary intervention studies with α-tocopherol in humans produced controversial results regarding its ability to reduce the risk of cardiovascular events. The conflicting results may be attributed to differences in vitamin E doses used (Pryor, 2000). However, a dose of 1200 IU, which is a therapeutically safe dosage, seems to be necessary in order to modulate the inflammatory processes related to atherosclerosis (Kappus and Diplock, 1992).

Vitamin E constitutes the major lipid-soluble antioxidant and its antioxidant activities are mediated by its ability to scavenge free radicals, to react with NO, and to deactivate single oxygen (Esterbauer et al., 1991; Kamal-Eldin and Appelqvist, 1996; Giugliano, 2000). Vitamin E levels (especially α-tocopherol) that are ingested by the daily consumption of virgin olive oil are low. Nevertheless, its chronic ingestion contributes to antioxidant activity in the human body, thus protecting LDL from lipid peroxidation (Princen et al., 1995), a key point in the initiation of atherosclerosis. Beyond its antioxidant effects, it has a plethora of other biological activities (Azzi et al., 2003). α-Tocopherol inhibits the production and expression of adhesion molecules induced by LDLs or cytokines (Offermann and Medford, 1994; Zapolska-Downar et al., 2000) and inhibits the monocytic adhesion onto endothelial cells (Faruqi et al., 1994; Martin et al., 1997). This effect is due to the inhibition of cell adhesion molecule expression such as ICAM-1, VCAM-1 (Yoshikawa et al., 1998), and E-selectin (Faruqi et al., 1994). Moreover, in the monocytic cell line THP-1 α-tocopherol regulates the production of IL-1β by downregulating its gene expression (Akeson et al., 1991).

Vitamin E also modulates the metabolism of eicosanoids in endothelial cells. In vitamin E-deficient mice prostacyclin I_2 (PGI_2) synthesis is reduced (Okuma et al., 1980; Chan and Leith, 1981), while in endothelial cells, vitamin E restores the reduced synthesis of PGI_2 (Kunisaki et al., 1992a; Kunisaki et al., 1992b). Moreover, α-tocopherol inhibits LOX (Jialal et al., 2001) and COX-2 (Wu et al., 2001). In mouse macrophages stimulated by bacterial lipopolysaccharide (LPS), α-tocopherol reduces COX activity, thus prohibiting PGE_2, TxB_2 increment (Meydani et al., 1986; Meydani et al., 1990). This effect of α-tocopherol on COX is due to the scavenging of hydroperoxides and NO that lead to lower OONO⁻ production. OONO⁻ modulates COX activation via Ca^{2+}-dependent PLA_2 activity and AA release (Kim, 2005). In addition, pretreatment of cultured human coronary artery endothelial cells with vitamin E decreases IκB degradation and OxLDL-induced apoptosis (Li et al., 2000).

8.2.2 ANTIATHEROGENIC PROPERTIES OF OTHER OLIVE OIL MINOR CONSTITUENTS

8.2.2.1 Olive Oil Phenolics

In vivo studies in humans and in apolipoprotein E-deficient mice have shown that olive oil phenolic extract delays atherogenesis (Aviram, 1996). The protective effect of olive oil phenolics against atherogenesis can be attributed to several mechanisms.

Olive oil phenolics increase the total phenolic content of LDL after olive oil consumption, thus increasing the resistance of LDL to oxidation even in areas where other antioxidants are not present, such as in the arterial intima (Gimeno et al., 2002). In addition, several studies have shown that phenolics from extra virgin olive oil significantly inhibit the oxidation of LDL *in vitro, ex vivo* (Wiseman, 1996; Visioli and Galli, 1998; Caruso et al., 1999; Fito et al., 2000), and *in vivo* during postprandial oxidative stress (Covas et al., 2006b) and in hypertensive stable coronary heart disease (CHD) patients (Fito et al., 2005; see also Chapter 6).

Other interventional studies as well as the EUROLIVE study focused on the antioxidant role of olive oil phenolics in humans, and showed that oxidative stress markers as well as the total cholesterol–high density lipoprotein (HDL) cholesterol ratio were decreased linearly with increasing phenolic content of olive oil (Weinbrenner et al., 2004a; Weinbrenner et al., 2004b; Covas et al., 2006c).

Consumption of a diet rich in olive oil phenolics favorably modulates eicosanoid production, thus exerting an anti-inflammatory effect. In healthy and mildly dyslipidemic subjects, this diet lowers the postprandial levels of LTB_4 and TxB_2 (Weinbrenner et al., 2004b; Visioli et al., 2005a) as well as TxB_2 levels in post-menopausal women (Oubina et al., 2001).

Minor olive oil components — probably phenolics — as part of a diet also have been reported to reduce blood pressure in hypertensive women (Ruiz-Gutierrez et al., 1996) and in mild to moderate hypertensive patients (Ferrara et al., 2000). In addition, oleuropein has also been demonstrated to have hypotensive properties in humans (Panizzi et al., 1960). In support of the above studies, the administration of a high-phenolic olive oil diet induced a decrease in systolic blood pressure, in contrast to a low-phenolic olive oil diet in hypertensive stable CHD patients (Fito et al., 2005). Moreover, olive oil phenolics improve endothelial-dependent vasodilatation during the postprandial state (Covas et al., 2006c). This effect is accompanied by a decrease in NO metabolites, thus indicating a beneficial effect of olive oil phenolics on blood pressure through a protective effect on the vascular endothelial function.

Studies with specific phenolic compounds also demonstrate their beneficial effects on the atherosclerosis mechanisms. Hydroxytyrosol (HT) and oleuropein derivatives in concentrations of 10^{-6} to 10^{-4} M inhibit *in vitro* LDL oxidation in a dose-dependent manner (Visioli and Galli, 1994;

Visioli et al., 1995). Oleuropein and protocatechuic acid also inhibit the cell-mediated oxidation of LDL by increasing the mRNA transcription of glutathione-related enzymes (Masella et al., 2004).

In murine macrophages stimulated by LPS, oleuropein increases the production of NO. This increase is achieved through a direct effect of oleuropein on both activity and expression of the inducible form of NO synthase (iNOS) (Visioli et al., 1998b). In this way oleuropein protects LDL from its oxidative modification at the site of inflammation (Bloodsworth et al., 2000).

In rat leukocytes, oleuropein glycoside, caffeic acid, and tyrosol inhibit LTB_4 generation at the 5-LOX level and reduce the generation of ROS (De La Puerta et al., 1999). In neutrophils, oleuropein and HT potently scavenge ROS (Visioli et al., 1998a; Briante et al., 2001) and reactive nitrogen species (RNS) (NO$^\bullet$ and OONO$^-$) in a concentration-dependent manner (Tuck and Hayball, 2002). In human leukocytes, HT inhibits LOX activity and concomitantly leukotriene production (Petroni et al., 1997).

HT increases plasma antioxidant capacity (Visioli et al., 2001) and inhibits passive smoking-induced oxidative stress in rats (Visioli et al., 2000a). Antioxidant activities of HT, in terms of isoprostane excretion, also have been reported in human volunteers (Visioli et al., 2000b). More-over in humans the postprandial increment of plasma HT after olive oil intake is concomitant to a postprandial decrease in plasma OxLDLs (Sutherland et al., 2002).

HT, oleuropein, and tyrosol have been reported to inhibit the expression of VCAM-1, ICAM-1, and E-selectin and the adhesion of monocytes in LPS- or cytokine-stimulated human umbilical vein endothelial cells (HUVECs) (Carluccio et al., 2003). This effect is mediated by the repression of NFκB and AP-1, two transcription factors that amplify VCAM-1 promoter activation, as well as reduction in VCAM-1 mRNA expression (Ahmad et al., 1998).

Oleocanthal, a novel phenolic compound from olive oil, also inhibits COX-1 and COX-2 similarly with the potent anti-inflammatory molecule ibuprofen (Beauchamp et al., 2005).

The above results demonstrate that phenolics exert antioxidant activities, improve endothelial function, transcriptionally inhibit endothelial adhesion molecule expression, increase the disposal of NO, and quench intracellular free radicals, thus protecting from atherosclerosis development.

At this point, it should be mentioned that the biological metabolites of olive oil phenolics, synthesized (Khymenets et al., 2006) after their ingestion, might show a different antioxidant activity than their precursor molecules. Usually these metabolites are in the form of methylated, glucuronide, or glutathionyl conjugated derivatives (Tuck et al., 2002; Corona et al., 2006). The bioactivity of metabolites that are synthesized after the ingestion of minor compounds, other than phenolics, is interesting and promising, yet unexplored.

8.2.2.2 Polar Lipid Minor Constituents with Anti-PAF Activity

PAF is the strongest inflammatory lipid mediator. Its presence is essential for the activation of leukocytes and their binding in endothelial cells (Demopoulos et al., 2003). PAF antagonists have been shown to exert a protective action against atherosclerotic development (Feliste et al., 1989; Demopoulos et al., 2003).

Olive oils, independently from their extraction procedure, are rich in PAF antagonists. Olive oil polar lipids, rich in PAF antagonists, can be extracted by a modified method of Galanos and Kapoulas (Galanos and Kapoulas, 1962) as previously described (Karantonis et al., 2002). This method uses petroleum ether (bp 40–70°C) and ethanol 87% pre-equilibrated with each other. Specifically, 100 ml of olive oil is placed in a separatory funnel and diluted in 400 ml of petroleum ether. This mixture is then successively washed three times by 100 ml ethanol 87% each time. The combined ethanol extracts are washed twice with 300 ml petroleum ether solvent and after equilibration the two phases are separated. The combined ethanol phases contain olive oil polar lipids, rich in PAF antagonist, while neutral lipids remain in the petroleum ether phases (Figure 8.1).

The PAF antagonistic activity of the olive oil polar lipids can be determined by the washed platelet aggregation assay (Demopoulos et al., 1979). This assay demonstrates the ability of the

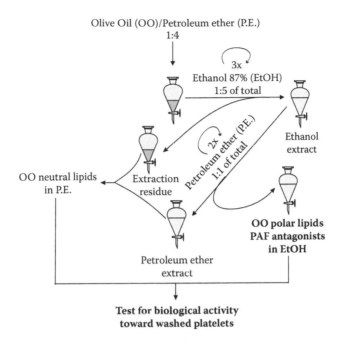

Olive Oil (OO)/Petroleum ether (P.E.)
1:4

3x
Ethanol 87% (EtOH)
1:5 of total

Ethanol
extract

OO neutral lipids
in P.E.

Extraction
residue

2x
Petroleum ether (P.E.)
1:1 of total

OO polar lipids
PAF antagonists
in EtOH

Petroleum ether
extract

Test for biological activity
toward washed platelets

FIGURE 8.1 Schematic representation of the extracting procedure for the isolation of olive oil polar lipids.

samples to inhibit PAF-induced washed rabbit platelet aggregation. Briefly, PAF and the examined samples are dissolved in a solution of 2.5 mg bovine serum albumin (BSA) per milliliter of saline. In order to study the inhibitory activities of the lipid fractions, platelets are preincubated with the samples for 1 min prior to the addition of PAF (2.5×10^{-11} M, final concentration in the cuvette). The platelet aggregation induced by PAF is measured as PAF-induced aggregation before (considered as 0% inhibition) and after the addition of various concentrations of the examined sample. Consequently, the plot of percent inhibition vs. different concentrations of the sample is constructed and from this plot the concentration of the sample that inhibited 50% PAF-induced aggregation (IC_{50}) is calculated.

Olive oil PAF antagonists can be purified from the polar lipid fraction by HPLC on a normal phase aminopropyl-modified silica column with a gradient elution system using a flow rate of 1 ml/min and a UV spectrophotometric detection at 208 nm at room temperature (Antonopoulou and Karantonis, 2002). The solvent gradient includes acetonitrile/methanol (70/30 v/v; solvent A), methanol (100%; solvent B), and water (100%; solvent C). An isocratic elution of 100% solvent A is applied for the first 35 min followed by a 5-min linear gradient to 100% of solvent B, a 5-min isocratic elution of 100% of solvent B, a 5-min linear gradient to 100% of solvent C, and a 5-min isocratic elution of 100% solvent C (Figure 8.2).

Structural elucidation of these minor olive oil components can be performed by electrospray mass spectrometry (ESMS). Each bioactive purified compound is dissolved in 1:1 v/v aqueous methanol at a concentration of 10 ng/μl. The ionization experiments must be performed in both positive and negative mode.

Simple chemical determinations are also useful for the structure elucidation of the polar lipids of olive oil. In this sense phosphorus, sugar, ester (Kates, 1972), and phenolic determination (Gutfinger, 1981) may be applied to the HPLC purified fractions.

The amount of PAF antagonists in olive oils is higher than that of seed oils with the exception of sesame oil (Karantonis et al., 2002). Depending on the extraction procedure, the olive oil polar lipid extracts (OOPLs) obtained from 6- to 18-μl initial olive oil volume are able to induce 50% inhibition of PAF-elicited washed rabbit platelet aggregation. Further purification of the OOPL fraction

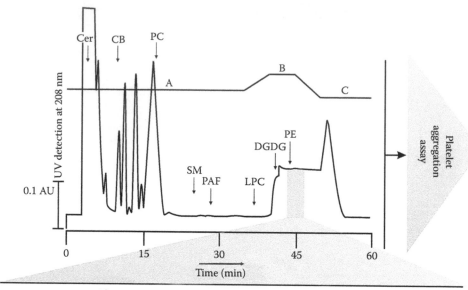

FIGURE 8.2 HPLC fractionation of olive oil polar lipids on a normal phase NH$_2$ column at 208 nm with a gradient elution system. A: acetonitrile/methanol (70/30 v/v); B: methanol (100%); C: water (100%); Cer: Ceramides; CB: Cerebrosides; PC: Phospatidylocholine; SM: Sphingomyelin; PAF: Platelet Activating Factor; LPC: Lysophosphatidylcholine; DGDG: Digalactosyldiglycerides; PE: Phosphatidylethanolimine.

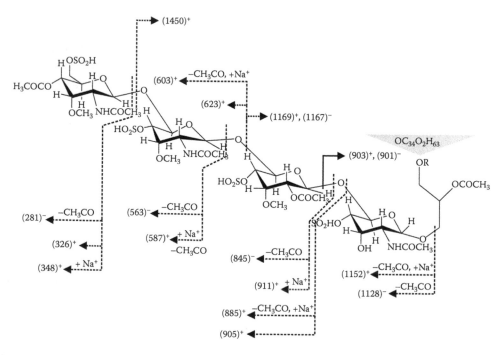

FIGURE 8.3 Proposed structure of the most potent PAF antagonist, isolated from the olive oil polar lipid fraction along with its MS fragmentation.

on HPLC revealed that the most active PAF antagonist has the structure of an alkylacetylglycero-acetylated glycolipid (Karantonis et al., 2002) (Figure 8.3).

Olive pomace polar lipid extract (PPL) also inhibits PAF activity *in vitro* and the most potent antagonist has been identified as a glycerylether-sn-2-acetyl glycolipid with common structural characteristics with the respective potent antagonist of OOPL (Karantonis et al., 2007). Radioligand binding studies demonstrated that OOPL and PPL fractions also inhibit specific PAF binding on rabbit platelets. The specific PAF receptor antagonist, BN 52021, inhibited PAF binding on rabbit platelets at a concentration of 2.3 ($\pm$0.8) $\times$ 10^{-7} M. In the same way, the most diluted concentrations of OOPL and PPL that resulted in 50% inhibition of PAF binding were 1.5 ($\pm$0.2) $\times$ 10^{-7} M and 0.42 ($\pm$0.11) $\times$ 10^{-7} M, respectively, based on sugar determination (Tsantila et al., 2007).

When rabbits are fed with an atherogenic diet supplemented with olive oil or OOPL, rich in PAF antagonists, they develop less severe early atherosclerotic lesions in terms of thickness compared to rabbits of the control group. Rabbits fed with an atherogenic diet supplemented with olive oil neutral lipid extract, poor in PAF antagonist, develop early atherosclerotic lesions comparable to those of the control group. In rabbits fed olive oil or OOPL fraction, the antiatherogenic effect is accompanied by retention of the elasticity of their vessel wall. During the study plasma PAF-AH activity increased in all experimental groups including the control group, while platelet sensitivity to PAF, in terms of agreggation, was decreased in rabbits fed olive oil or OOPL fraction and increased in

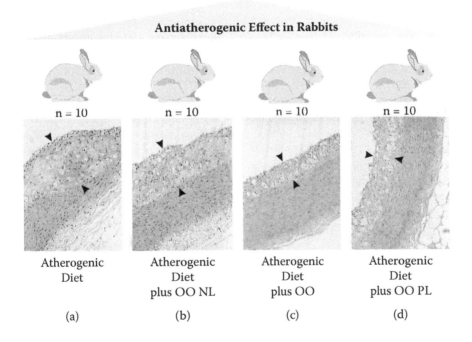

FIGURE 8.4 Representative optic micrographs ($\times$100) of rabbit aortic wall sections stained with hematoxylin and eosin. The four different groups of rabbits consumed an (a) atherogenic diet, (b) atherogenic diet enriched with olive oil neutral lipids, (c) atherogenic diet enriched with olive oil, (d) atherogenic diet enriched with olive oil polar lipids. Atherosclerotic lesions appear as foam cells (▲). Rabbits fed an atherogenic diet supplemented with olive oil or olive oil polar lipids, rich in PAF inhibitors, develop lower early atherosclerotic lesions compared to those fed only an atherogenic diet or an atherogenic diet supplemented with olive oil neutral lipids.

the control group (Karantonis et al., 2006) (Figure 8.4). Similar results were obtained when rabbits' atherogenic diet was enriched with PPL fraction (Tsantila et al., 2007)

8.3 ANTITHROMBOTIC PROPERTIES OF OLIVE OIL MINOR CONSTITUENTS

8.3.1 INTRODUCTION

The hemostatic system is responsible for the integrity of vasculature and normal blood flow within the circulation. It is regulated by the delicate balance between blood clotting mechanisms, which include the activation of platelets and coagulation pathways, and the fibrinolytic system.

The intact endothelium prevents initiation of thrombotic mechanisms since it functions as a physical barrier between circulating blood and thrombotic subendothelial molecules while it releases mediators (PGI_2 and NO), which are strong inhibitors of platelet activation. As soon as the blood vessel is injured both endothelial- and subendothelial- derived mechanisms induce activation of circulating cells, among them platelets, and their recruitment to the damaged site, where they aggregate, forming a loose plug (primary hemostasis). This plug is strengthened by the incorporation of the fibrin polymer in it. The formation of fibrin polymer is the final step of the blood coagulation cascade, which is initiated by contact of blood with a procoagulant surface and involves sequential proteolytic activation of several coagulation enzymes (secondary hemostasis). The unregulated activation of the blood clotting mechanisms is prevented by simultaneous release of several coagulation inhibitors by the endothelium and degradation of the coagulation factors by the liver. Clot lysis is achieved by fibrinolysis. Endothelial cells secrete tissue plasminogen activator and urokinase, which hydrolyze fibrin-bound plasminogen to plasmin that in turn degrades the fibrin clot. Any disruption of balance between blood clotting and anticlotting mechanisms in favor of the first (hyperaggregability of platelets, unregulated activation of the coagulation pathway, and/or impaired fibrinolysis) may lead to the formation of intravascular blood clots and thrombosis (Andreoli et al., 2003).

A chronic activation of thrombotic mechanisms is observed in individuals at high risk of CVDs; population-based studies have demonstrated that a prothrombotic state is a predictor of CVD (Lowe et al., 2002). The most common prothrombotic markers measured in these studies are the aggregating activity of platelets, TxB_2 (the stable metabolite of the potent activator of platelets TxA_2, which is secreted by the endothelium and platelets) levels in plasma and urine, the coagulating factor VII (FVII), which significantly contributes to the development of coronary disease, and tissue factor (TF), which is expressed in the vascular wall increasing coagulating activity. On the other hand, the most important markers of fibrinolytic activity are the tissue plasminogen activator (tPA), which favors the production of plasmin and clot lysis, and plasminogen activator inhibitor-1 (PAI-1), which regulates tPA activity (Iacoviello et al., 1998; Breddin et al., 1999; Choi et al., 2006). Elevated markers of thrombosis, such as fibrinogen (Ernst and Resch, 1993), factor VII coagulant activity (Junker et al., 1997), PAI-1 (Hamsten et al., 1987), and platelet aggregability (Elwood et al., 1991), are positively associated with CHD. *In vitro* studies have also shown that atherosclerotic plaque contains platelet fragments and fibrin, which may contribute to the propagation of atheromatous plaque (Pearson et al., 1997).

Despite intense research in the field of dietary modification of CVD risk factors, the effect of nutritional patterns and food components on hemostatic variables is much less studied. However, the strong relationship between prothrombotic state and CVD makes the thrombotic mechanisms an attractive target for food nutrients.

Concerning olive oil–rich diets of the Mediterranean region, it was soon realized that apart from their ability to improve the lipoprotein profile, they also have a wide array of beneficial effects on low-grade inflammation, endothelial function, and hemostasis (Simopoulos, 2001; Visioli et al., 2005b; Davis et al., 2007). Our knowledge on the effect of olive oil on hemostatic variables is largely based on observational and dietary intervention studies, while *in vitro* mechanistic studies are rather limited. The results so far imply a role for both oleic acid and olive oil microconstituents on the modification of thrombotic markers, although their mode of action has been rather speculative until now (Perez-Jimenez et al., 2006).

8.3.2 OLIVE OIL– AND MUFA-RICH DIETS AND HEMOSTASIS

Several dietary intervention studies with olive oil– or MUFA-rich diets have investigated the effect of increased consumption of either olive oil or MUFAs on hemostatic variables. The results produced from these studies are rather conflicting in the sense that both favorable and unfavorable effects on the prothrombotic markers were observed. Several studies have shown that increased consumption of MUFAs has no significant effect on platelet aggregation (Freese et al., 1994; Vicario et al., 1998), while other investigators have found that platelet sensitivity to ADP and collagen and the urinary levels of TxB2 were increased after MUFA-rich diets when compared with saturated fat–rich diets (Mutanen et al., 1992; Turpeinen et al., 1998). In contrast to these results, other studies have shown that a high oleic acid diet attenuated the aggregating potential of platelets to AA, collagen, and ADP (Kelly et al., 2001; Smith et al., 2003). Moreover, a high MUFA diet was able to reduce the plasma levels of Von Willebrand factor (vWF), which favors adherence of platelets to the disrupted endothelium (Rasmussen et al., 1994; Perez-Jimenez et al., 1999).

Olive oil–rich diets are able to decrease plasma levels of FVII, XIIa, and α2-antiplasmin along with the activity of TF in mononuclear cells in comparison with saturated fat–rich diets (Larsen et al., 1999; Junker et al., 2001). Concerning the fibrinolytic system, Lopez-Segura et al. demonstrated that a Mediterranean type of diet, rich in olive oil, was able to reduce PAI-1 levels in comparison with a carbohydrate-rich, low-fat diet (Lopez-Segura et al., 1996), while Tholstrup et al. found no effect of MUFA-rich diets on t-PA activity or PAI-1 antigen levels (Tholstrup et al., 1999).

Similar conflicting results were also observed when the effect of olive oil and MUFAs on postprandial activation of hemostatic parameters was studied. Postprandial lipemia is able to induce activation of the coagulation pathways mainly through activation of platelets and elevation of plasma levels of activated FVII and PAI-1. There are studies showing no difference in the postprandial response of plasma FVII after consumption of various meals differing in their fatty acid content, while other investigators have demonstrated an increased postprandial activation of FVII after high oleate meals (Duttaroy, 2005). On the other hand, a long-term isoenergetic substitution of MUFA for saturated fatty acids (SFA) is able to reduce the postprandial activation of FVII after an oral fat load, while the postprandial levels of TF, fibrinogen, and PAI-1 are associated with the ratio of oleic to palmitic acid in dietary fats (Pacheco et al., 2006).

8.3.3 BEYOND OLEIC ACID: THE EFFECT OF OLIVE OIL MICROCONSTITUENTS ON HEMOSTASIS

The modulation of hemostatic mechanisms by olive oil could not be wholly attributed to its oleic acid content since the latter is also found in high quantities in animal foods and other seed oils; therefore its content in other Western diets is not as low as was initially believed (Dougherty et al., 1987). Moreover, the conflicting results obtained by the above intervention studies can be partly explained by the fact that the degree of olive oil's refinement and the content of olive micronutrients were not taken into account in many of these studies. However, solid evidence for the ability of olive oil micronutrients to modulate hemostasis comes from studies that directly compare the effects of extra virgin olive oils (rich in micronutrients) and refined olive oils (poor in micronutrients) on hemostatic parameters. Visioli et al. compared the vasoprotective potential of virgin olive oil (rich in phenolic compounds) and refined olive oil in mildly dyslipidemic patients and they clearly showed the superiority of virgin olive oil in decreasing serum TxB$_2$ production (Visioli et al., 2005a). The same authors extended this study to the postprandial state and found that extra virgin olive oil is able to decrease postprandial levels of TxB$_2$ and LTB$_4$ in comparison to olive oil and corn oil (Bogani et al., 2007). Moreover, in contrast to MUFA-rich diets (Tholstrup et al., 1999), an extra virgin olive oil diet was able to decrease fasting plasma levels of t-PA antigen, PAI-1 antigen, and prothrombin fragment 1+2 in hypertensive patients (Trifiletti et al., 2005). The supplementation of rats with an extra virgin olive oil–enriched diet resulted in a beneficial modulation of their thrombotic profile since a significant delay in the aortic thrombotic occlusion, a lower incidence of venous thrombosis, and a prolonged bleeding time were observed in comparison with their usual diet (Brzosko et al., 2002). A comparative study between a saturated fat diet and olive oil diet showed decreased platelet hyperactivity and subendothelial thrombogenicity in the olive oil group (De La Cruz et al., 2000). Even more persuasive results on the antithrombotic potential of microconstituents of virgin olive oil have been produced from a study investigating the effect of postprandial blood fractions, obtained after the consumption of different types of olive oil, on cellular functions. Perona et al. isolated postprandial TRLs from volunteers who had consumed extra virgin olive oil, virgin olive oil, or high oleic sunflower oil. The TRLs obtained after consumption of extra virgin olive demonstrated a reduced ability to induce secretion of TxB_2 and PGE_2 by endothelial cells (Perona et al., 2004). The above comparative studies clearly imply that other bioactive micronutrients, apart from oleic acid, are able to modulate hemostatic variables. However, their exact role is still unknown because of the limited mechanistic studies conducted so far.

8.3.3.1 Effect of Olive Oil Phenolics on Hemostasis

Apart from their well-known antioxidant properties (Visioli and Galli, 2002), olive oil phenolics seem to possess antithrombotic properties, mainly through their ability to attenuate platelet aggregation. HT is able to inhibit ADP- and collagen-induced platelet aggregation in platelet-rich plasma of healthy volunteers with IC_{50} values 23 and 67 μM, respectively. Oleuropein was much less active than HT (Petroni et al., 1995). Tyrosol and its monoacetylated derivatives are able to inhibit PAF-induced washed rabbit platelet aggregation. Tyrosol showed an IC_{50} value of 2160 μM, while its monoacetylated derivatives were almost two orders of magnitude more potent inhibitors of PAF-induced aggregation than tyrosol, demonstrating IC_{50} values of 40 and 27 μM (Fragopoulou et al., 2007). It should be mentioned that acetylated tyrosol has been found in minor quantities in black olives and olive oils. Tyrosol in the free form but mainly as a secoiridoid derivative is one of the major constituents of the olive oil polar fraction (see Chapter 3). Oleuropein was also able to inhibit PAF-induced platelet aggregation in platelet rich plasma (PRP) of healthy donors showing an IC_{50} of 410 μM (Andrikopoulos et al., 2002). Caffeic acid is also able to inhibit arachidonic acid–induced platelet aggregation (Koshihara et al., 1984). Moreover, isochromans, which are naturally present HT derivatives produced by its reaction with aldehydes and ketones, are potent inhibitors of platelet aggregation (Togna et al., 2003) (also see Chapter 9).

The antiplatelet activity of olive oil's phenolics seems to be partly attributed to their ability to modulate eicosanoid metabolism in the endothelium and platelets resulting in a decreased production of potent aggregating agents such as thromboxanes. HT reduces TxB_2 production by collagen- or thrombin-stimulated PRP and the accumulation of TxB_2 and 12-hydroxy-eicosatetraenoic acid (12-HETE) during blood clotting (Petroni et al., 1995). The *in vitro* results were recently verified by a dietary intervention study where HT-rich phenolic extracts were administrated to diabetic patients for 4 days. An immediate 46% decrease in serum levels of TxB_2 was observed (Leger et al., 2005). However, a large part of the antiplatelet activity of olive oil phenolics seems to be derived from their antioxidant properties and their ability to inhibit LDL oxidation. It is well known that the oxidatively modified LDL is able to induce platelet aggregation and shape change, while the LDL oxidation generates prothrombotic mediators with platelet stimulatory properties such as PAF, oxidized phospholipids, F(2)-isoprostanes, and lysophosphatidic acid (Siess, 2006). Moreover, these molecules can impair the function of tissue factor pathway inhibitor (TFPI) and the fibrinolytic capacity of endothelial cells by downregulating tPA and upregulating PAI-1, while at the same time reducing the anticoagulant function of endothelium by downregulating thrombomodulin (Kim et al., 2004; Ohkura et al., 2004). Therefore, the ability of olive oil phenolics to inhibit LDL oxidation prevents the formation of those potent prothrombotic molecules and minimizes activation of thrombotic mechanisms. However, no studies relating the antioxidant potential of phenolics with their antithrombotic action have been made yet.

8.3.3.2 Effect of Other Olive Oil Micronutrients on Hemostasis

Although the daily amount of antioxidant vitamins α-tocopherol (vitamin E) and β-carotene (vitamin A) supplied by the consumption of olive oil is rather low, it may contribute to the antioxidant status of humans. Acting in a similar fashion as phenolics, antioxidant vitamins of olive oil inhibit oxidation of LDL and activation of thrombotic mechanisms induced by OxLDL and its derivatives (Lapointe et al., 2006). Moreover, vitamin E modulates NO and eicosanoid synthesis in the endothelium, retaining plasma levels of NO and PGI_2 in adequate quantities to exert their physiological antithrombotic actions. In addition, α-tocopherol inhibits COX-2 and attenuates the LPS-induced increase of aggregating eicosanoid TxA_2 from mice macrophages (Perona et al., 2006). α-Tocopherol also exerts a more direct action on platelets inhibiting human and rabbit platelet aggregation both *in vivo* and *in vitro* and delays intra-arterial thrombus formation. Inhibition of platelet aggregation by α-tocopherol is independent of its antioxidant properties but it is protein kinase C (PKC)-dependent (Freedman and Keaney, 2001).

Both dietary intervention studies and cell studies demonstrated the anti-coagulant effects of phytosterols, especially β-sitosterol, the main phytosterol of olive oil. Phytosterols are able to reduce platelet counts and fibrinogen levels and enhance the fibrinolytic activity and capacity of the endothelium (Moghadasian, 2000).

Finally, a novel class of bioactive nutrients of olive oil that may contribute to its antithrombotic potential are lipids derived from its polar lipid fraction that possess PAF antagonistic activity toward washed rabbit platelet aggregation. Olive oil and sesame oil contain higher amounts of these lipids among all vegetables oils. The most potent of them was identified as a glycero-glycolipid as mentioned above (Karantonis et al., 2002).

8.4 CONCLUSIONS

The studies conducted so far clearly indicate a role of olive oil microconstituents on hemostatic mechanisms. However, several questions should be addressed in order to clarify the real role of microconstituents on thrombotic mechanisms. For example, it is not clear yet whether doses ingested by daily consumption of olive oil are adequate to exert a significant action *in vivo*, considering the low amounts of these molecules in olive oil and their limited bioavailability. A possible synergistic effect of the microconstituents may compensate for the low levels of these molecules. Moreover, most cell studies conducted so far have utilized bioactive molecules found in olive oil but not their metabolites in blood, which may have a completely different mode of action. In addition, we don't know yet the relative contribution of oleic acid, in comparison to microconstituents, on modulation of hemostatic mechanisms. Therefore, more cell studies with both pure olive oil components and extracts in combination with dietary intervention studies, carefully controlled for the amounts of microconstituents, may shed more light on the thus far putative antithrombotic actions of olive oil.

REFERENCES

Ahmad, M., Theofanidis, P., and Medford, R.M., 1998, Role of activating protein-1 in the regulation of the vascular cell adhesion molecule-1 gene expression by tumor necrosis factor-alpha, *J. Biol. Chem.*, 273, 4616–4621.

Akeson, A.L., Woods, C.W., Mosher, L.B., Thomas, C.E., and Jackson, R.L., 1991, Inhibition of IL-1 beta expression in THP-1 cells by probucol and tocopherol, *Atherosclerosis*, 86, 261–270.

Andreoli, T.E., Carpenter, C.C.J., Griggs, R.C., and Loscalzo, J., 2003, *Cecil Essentials of Medicine,* Saunders Book Company, Collingwood, Ontario, Canada.

Andrikopoulos, N.K., Antonopoulou, S., and Kaliora, A.C., 2002, Oleuropein inhibits LDL oxidation induced by cooking oil frying by-products and platelet aggregation induced by platelet-activating factor, *Lebensm. Wiss. Technol.*, 35, 479–484.

Antonopoulou, S. and Karantonis, H.C., 2002, Separation of polar lipids from soybean oil and cotton seed oil by one-step HPLC system. Biological activity of isolated lipids, *J. Liq. Chrom. Rel. Technol.*, 25, 771–779.

Antonopoulou, S., Fragopoulou, E., Karantonis, H.C., Mitsou, E., Sitara, M., Rementzis, J., Mourelatos, A., Ginis, A., and Phenekos, C., 2006, Effect of traditional Greek Mediterranean meals on platelet aggregation in normal subjects and in patients with type 2 diabetes mellitus, *J. Med. Food*, 9, 356–362.

Aravanis, C., Corcondilas, A., Dontas, A.S., Lekos, D., and Keys, A., 1970, Coronary heart disease in seven countries. IX. The Greek islands of Crete and Corfu, *Circulation*, 41(Suppl. 4), 188–100.

Aviram, M., 1996, Interaction of oxidized low density lipoprotein with macrophages in atherosclerosis, and the antiatherogenicity of antioxidants, *Eur. J. Clin. Chem. Clin. Biochem.*, 34, 599–608.

Azzi, A., Gysin, R., Kempna, P., Ricciarelli, R., Villacorta, L., Visarius, T., and Zingg, J.M., 2003, The role of alpha-tocopherol in preventing disease: from epidemiology to molecular events, *Mol. Aspects Med.*, 24, 325–336.

Beauchamp, G.K., Keast, R.S., Morel, D., Lin, J., Pika, J., Han, Q., Lee, C.H., Smith, A.B., and Breslin, P.A., 2005, Phytochemistry: ibuprofen-like activity in extra-virgin olive oil, *Nature*, 437, 45–46.

Bellosta, S., Ferri, N., Bernini, F., Paoletti, R., and Corsini, A., 2000, Non-lipid-related effects of statins, *Ann. Med.*, 32, 164–176.

Bloodsworth, A., O'Donnell, V.B., and Freeman, B.A., 2000, Nitric oxide regulation of free radical- and enzyme-mediated lipid and lipoprotein oxidation, *Arterioscler. Thromb. Vasc. Biol.*, 20, 1707–1715.

Bogani, P., Galli, C., Villa, M., and Visioli, F., 2007, Postprandial anti-inflammatory and antioxidant effects of extra virgin olive oil, *Atherosclerosis*, 190, 181–186.

Boskou, D., 2000, Olive oil, in *Mediterranean Diets. World Review. Nutrition Diet*, Vol. 87, Simopoulos, A. and Visioli, F., Eds., S. Karger, Basel, 56–77.

Boskou, D., 2006, *Olive Oil, Chemistry and Technology*, Boskou, D., Ed., AOCS Press, Champaign, IL.

Breddin, H.K., Lippold, R., Bittner, M., Kirchmaier, C.M., Krzywanek, H.J., and Michaelis, J., 1999, Spontaneous platelet aggregation as a predictive risk factor for vascular occlusions in healthy volunteers? Results of the HAPARG Study. Haemostatic parameters as risk factors in healthy volunteers, *Atherosclerosis*, 144, 211–219.

Briante, R., La, C.F., Tonziello, M.P., Febbraio, F., and Nucci, R., 2001, Antioxidant activity of the main bioactive derivatives from oleuropein hydrolysis by hyperthermophilic beta-glycosidase, *J. Agric. Food Chem.*, 49, 3198–3203.

Brzosko, S., De Curtis, A., Murzilli, S., de Gaetano, G., Donati, M.B., and Iacoviello, L., 2002, Effect of extra virgin olive oil on experimental thrombosis and primary hemostasis in rats, *Nutr. Metab. Cardiovasc. Dis.*, 12, 337–342.

Carluccio, M.A., Siculella, L., Ancora, M.A., Massaro, M., Scoditti, E., Storelli, C., Visioli, F., Distante, A., and De Caterina, R., 2003, Olive oil and red wine antioxidant polyphenols inhibit endothelial activation: antiatherogenic properties of Mediterranean diet phytochemicals, *Arterioscler. Thromb. Vasc. Biol.*, 23, 622–629.

Caruso, D., Berra, B., Giavarini, F., Cortesi, N., Fedeli, E., and Galli, G., 1999, Effect of virgin olive oil phenolic compounds on in vitro oxidation of human low density lipoproteins, *Nutr. Metab. Cardiovasc. Dis.*, 9, 102–107.

Chan, A.C. and Leith, M.K., 1981, Decreased prostacyclin synthesis in vitamin E-deficient rabbit aorta, *Am. J. Clin. Nutr.*, 34, 2341–2347.

Choi, B.G., Vilahur, G., Ibanez, B., Zafar, M.U., Rodriguez, J., and Badimon, J.J., 2006, Measures of thrombosis and fibrinolysis, *Clin. Lab. Med.*, 26, 655–678.

Corona, G., Tzounis, X., Assunta, D.M., Deiana, M., Debnam, E.S., Visioli, F., and Spencer, J.P., 2006, The fate of olive oil polyphenols in the gastrointestinal tract: implications of gastric and colonic microflora-dependent biotransformation, *Free Radic. Res.*, 40, 647–658.

Covas, M.I., Ruiz, G., De La Torre, R., Kafatos, A., Lamuela, R., Osada, J., Owen, R.W., and Visioli, F., 2006a, Minor components of olive oil: evidence to date of health benefits in humans, *Nutr. Rev.*, 64, 20–30.

Covas, M.I., de la Torre, K., Farre-Albaladejo, M., Kaikkonen, J., Fito, M., Lopez-Sabater, C., Pujadas-Bastardes, M.A., Joglar, J., Weinbrenner, T., Lamuela-Raventos, R.M., and de la Torre, R., 2006b, Postprandial LDL phenolic content and LDL oxidation are modulated by olive oil phenolic compounds in humans, *Free Radic. Biol. Med.*, 40, 608–616.

Covas, M.I., Nyyssonen, K., Poulsen, H.E., Kaikkonen, J., Zunft, H.J., Kiesewetter, H., Gaddi, A., de la Torre, R., Mursu, J., Baumler, H., Nascetti, S., Salonen, J.T., Fito, M., Virtanen, J., Marrugat, J., and EUROL-IVE Study Group, 2006c, The effect of polyphenols in olive oil on heart disease risk factors: a randomized trial, *Ann. Intern. Med.*, 145, 333–341.

Davies, M.J., Gordon, J.L., Gearing, A.J., Pigott, R., Woolf, N., Katz, D., and Kyriakopoulos, A., 1993, The expression of the adhesion molecules ICAM-1, VCAM-1, PECAM, and E-selectin in human atherosclerosis, *J. Pathol.*, 171, 223–229.

Davis, N., Katz, S., and Wylie-Rosett, J., 2007, The effect of diet on endothelial function, *Cardiol. Rev.*, 15, 62–66.

de Jongh, S., Vissers, M.N., Rol, P., Bakker, H.D., Kastelein, J.J., and Stroes, E.S., 2003, Plant sterols lower LDL cholesterol without improving endothelial function in prepubertal children with familial hypercholesterolaemia, *J. Inherit. Metab. Dis.*, 26, 343–351.

De la Cruz, J.P., Villalobos, M.A., Carmona, J.A., Martin-Romero, M., Smith-Agreda, J.M., and de la Cuesta, F.S., 2000, Antithrombotic potential of olive oil administration in rabbits with elevated cholesterol, *Thromb. Res.*, 100, 305–315.

De la Puerta, R., Gutierrez, V.R., and Hoult, J.R.S., 1999, Inhibition of leukocyte 5-lipoxygenase by phenolics from virgin olive oil, *Biochem. Pharmacol.*, 57, 445–449.

De la Puerta, R., Martinez-Dominguez, E., and Ruiz-Gutierrez, V., 2000, Effect of minor components of virgin olive oil on topical antiinflammatory assays, *Z. Naturforsch. C*, 55, 814–819.

Demopoulos, C.A., Pinckard, R.N., and Hanahan, D.J., 1979, Platelet-activating factor. Evidence for 1-O-alkyl-2-acetyl-sn-glyceryl-3-phosphorylcholine as the active component (a new class of lipid chemical mediators), *J. Biol. Chem.*, 254, 9355–9358.

Demopoulos, C.A., Karantonis, H.C., and Antonopoulou, S., 2003, Platelet activating factor — a molecular link between atherosclerosis theories, *Eur. J. Lipid Sci. Technol.*, 105, 705–716.

Dougherty, R.M., Galli, C., Ferro-Luzzi, A., and Iacono, J.M., 1987, Lipid and phospholipid fatty acid composition of plasma, red blood cells, and platelets and how they are affected by dietary lipids: a study of normal subjects from Italy, Finland, and the USA, *Am. J. Clin. Nutr.*, 45, 443–455.

Duttaroy, A.K., 2005, Postprandial activation of hemostatic factors: role of dietary fatty acids, *Prostaglandins Leukot. Essent. Fatty Acids*, 72, 381–391.

Elwood, P.C., Renaud, S., Sharp, D.S., Beswick, A.D., O'Brien, J.R., and Yarnell, J.W., 1991, Ischemic heart disease and platelet aggregation. The Caerphilly Collaborative Heart Disease Study, *Circulation*, 83, 38–44.

Ernst, E. and Resch, K.L., 1993, Fibrinogen as a cardiovascular risk factor: a meta-analysis and review of the literature, *Ann. Intern. Med.*, 118, 956–963.

Esterbauer, H., Eber-Rotheneder, M., Striegl, G., and Waeg, G., 1991, Role of vitamin E in preventing the oxidation of low-density lipoprotein, *Am. J. Clin. Nutr.*, 53, 314S–321S.

Faruqi, R., de la Motte, C., and DiCorleto, P.E., 1994, Alpha-tocopherol inhibits agonist-induced monocytic cell adhesion to cultured human endothelial cells, *J. Clin. Invest.*, 94, 592–600.

Feliste, R., Perret, B., Braquet, P., and Chap, H., 1989, Protective effect of BN 52021, a specific antagonist of platelet-activating factor (PAF-acether) against diet-induced cholesteryl ester deposition in rabbit aorta, *Atherosclerosis*, 78, 151–158.

Ferrara, L.A., Raimondi, A.S., d'Episcopo, L., Guida, L., Dello, R.A., and Marotta, T., 2000, Olive oil and reduced need for antihypertensive medications, *Arch. Intern. Med.*, 160, 837–842.

Fito, M., Covas, M.I., Lamuela-Raventos, R.M., Vila, J., Torrents, L., de la Torre, C., and Marrugat, J., 2000, Protective effect of olive oil and its phenolic compounds against low density lipoprotein oxidation, *Lipids*, 35, 633–638.

Fito, M., Cladellas, M., de la Torre, R., Marti, J., Alcantara, M., Pujadas-Bastardes, M., Marrugat, J., Bruguera, J., Lopez-Sabater, M.C., Vila, J., and Covas, M.I., 2005, Antioxidant effect of virgin olive oil in patients with stable coronary heart disease: a randomized, crossover, controlled, clinical trial, *Atherosclerosis*, 181, 149–158.

Fragopoulou, E., Nomikos, T., Tsantila, N., Mitropoulou, A., Zabetakis, I., and Demopoulos, C.A., 2001, Biological activity of total lipids from red and white wine/must, *J. Agric. Food Chem.*, 49, 5186–5193.

Fragopoulou, E., Nomikos, T., Karantonis, H.C., Apostolakis, C., Pliakis, E., Samiotaki, M., Panayotou, G., and Antonopoulou, S., 2007, Biological activity of acetylated phenolic compounds, *J. Agric. Food Chem.*, 55, 80–89.

Freedman, J.E. and Keaney, J.F., Jr., 2001, Vitamin E inhibition of platelet aggregation is independent of antioxidant activity, *J. Nutr.*, 131, 374S–377S.

Freese, R., Mutanen, M., Valsta, L.M., and Salminen, I., 1994, Comparison of the effects of two diets rich in monounsaturated fatty acids differing in their linoleic/alpha-linolenic acid ratio on platelet aggregation, *Thromb. Haemost.*, 71, 73–77.

Galanos, D.S. and Kapoulas, V.M., 1962, Isolation of polar lipids from triglyceride mixtures, *J. Lipid Res.*, 3, 134–136.

Gimeno, E., Fito, M., Lamuela-Raventos, R.M., Castellote, A.I., Covas, M., Farre, M., de La Torre-Boronat, M.C., and Lopez-Sabater, M.C., 2002, Effect of ingestion of virgin olive oil on human low-density lipoprotein composition, *Eur. J. Clin. Nutr.*, 56, 114–120.

Giugliano, D., 2000, Dietary antioxidants for cardiovascular prevention, *Nutr. Metab. Cardiovasc. Dis.*, 10, 38–44.

Gutfinger, T., 1981, Phenols in olive oils, *J. Amer. Oil Chem. Soc.*, 58, 966–998.

Hamsten, A., de Faire, U., Walldius, G., Dahlen, G., Szamosi, A., Landou, C., Blomback, M., and Wiman, B., 1987, Plasminogen activator inhibitor in plasma: risk factor for recurrent myocardial infarction, *Lancet*, 2, 3–9.

Harwood, J. and Aparicio, R., 2000, *Handbook of Olive Oil, Analysis and Properties,* Aspen Publishers, Gaithersburg, MD.

Ho, S.S. and Pal, S., 2005, Margarine phytosterols decrease the secretion of atherogenic lipoproteins from HepG2 liver and Caco2 intestinal cells, *Atherosclerosis*, 182, 29–36.

Hu, F.B., 2003, The Mediterranean Diet and mortality — olive oil and beyond, *N. Engl. J. Med.*, 348, 2595–2596.

Iacoviello, L., Zito, F., Di Castelnuovo, A., De Maat, M., Kluft, C., and Donati, M.B., 1998, Contribution of factor VII, fibrinogen and fibrinolytic components to the risk of ischaemic cardiovascular disease: their genetic determinants, *Fibrinol. Proteol.*, 12, 259–276.

Jialal, I., Devaraj, S., and Kaul, N., 2001, The effect of alpha-tocopherol on monocyte proatherogenic activity, *J. Nutr.*, 131, 389S–394S.

Jialal, I., Devaraj, S., and Venugopal, S.K., 2004, C-reactive protein: risk marker or mediator in atherothrombosis? *Hypertension*, 44, 6–11.

Jones, P.J., MacDougall, D.E., Ntanios, F., and Vanstone, C.A., 1997, Dietary phytosterols as cholesterol-lowering agents in humans, *Can. J. Physiol. Pharmacol.*, 75, 217–227.

Junker, R., Heinrich, J., Schulte, H., van de Loo, J., and Assmann, G., 1997, Coagulation factor VII and the risk of coronary heart disease in healthy men, *Arterioscler. Thromb. Vasc. Biol.*, 17, 1539–1544.

Junker, R., Pieke, B., Schulte, H., Nofer, R., Neufeld, M., Assmann, G., and Wahrburg, U., 2001, Changes in hemostasis during treatment of hypertriglyceridemia with a diet rich in monounsaturated and n-3 polyunsaturated fatty acids in comparison with a low-fat diet, *Thromb. Res.*, 101, 355–366.

Kakishita, E., Suehiro, A., Oura, Y., and Nagai, K., 1990, Inhibitory effect of vitamin E (alpha-tocopherol) on spontaneous platelet aggregation in whole blood, *Thromb. Res.*, 60, 489–499.

Kamal-Eldin, A. and Appelqvist, L.A., 1996, The chemistry and antioxidant properties of tocopherols and tocotrienols, *Lipids*, 31, 671–701.

Kappus, H. and Diplock, A.T., 1992, Tolerance and safety of vitamin E: a toxicological position report, *Free Radic. Biol. Med.*, 13, 55–74.

Karantonis, H.C., Antonopoulou, S., and Demopoulos, C.A., 2002, Antithrombotic lipid minor constituents from vegetable oils. Comparison between olive oils and others, *J. Agric. Food Chem.*, 50, 1150–1160.

Karantonis, H.C., Antonopoulou, S., Perrea, D.N., Sokolis, D.P., Theocharis, S.E., Kavantzas, N., Iliopoulos, D.G., and Demopoulos, C.A., 2006, *In vivo* antiatherogenic properties of olive oil and its constituent lipid classes in hyperlipidemic rabbits, *Nutr. Metab. Cardiovasc. Dis.*, 16, 174–185.

Karantonis, H.C., Tsantila, N., Stamatakis, G., Samiotaki, M., Panayotou, G., Antonopoulou, S., and Demopoulos, C.A., in press, Bioactive polar lipids in olive oil, pomace and waste byproducts, *J. Food Biochem.*

Kates, M., 1972, Analysis, isolation and identification of lipids, in *Techniques of Lipidology*, Kates, M., Ed., Elsevier, New York.

Kelly, C.M., Smith, R.D., and Williams, C.M., 2001, Dietary monounsaturated fatty acids and haemostasis, *Proc. Nutr. Soc.*, 60, 161–170.

Khymenets, O., Joglar, J., Clapés, P., Parella, T., Covas, M.I., and De La Torre, R., 2006, Biocatalyzed synthesis and structural characterization of monoglucuronides of hydroxytyrosol, tyrosol, homovanillic alcohol, and 3-(4'-hydroxyphenyl) propanol, *Adv. Synth. Catal.*, 348, 2155–2162.

Kim, J.A., Tran, N.D., Berliner, J.A., and Fisher, M.J., 2004, Minimally oxidized low-density lipoprotein regulates hemostasis factors of brain capillary endothelial cells, *J. Neurol. Sci.*, 217, 135–141.

Kim, J.Y., Lee, K.H., Lee, B.K., and Ro, J.Y., 2005, Peroxynitrite modulates release of inflammatory mediators from guinea pig lung mast cells activated by antigen-antibody reaction, *Int. Arch. Allergy Immunol.*, 137, 104–114.

Kiritsakis, A., 1990, Chemistry of olive oil, in *Olive Oil*, Kiritsakis, A.K., Ed., AOCS Press, Champaign, IL, 25–55.

Koshihara, Y., Neichi, T., Murota, S., Lao, A., Fujimoto, Y., and Tatsuno, T., 1984, Caffeic acid is a selective inhibitor for leukotriene biosynthesis, *Biochim. Biophys. Acta*, 792, 92–97.

Kunisaki, M., Umeda, F., Inoguchi, T., and Nawata, H., 1992a, Vitamin E binds to specific binding sites and enhances prostacyclin production by cultured aortic endothelial cells, *Thromb. Haemost.*, 68, 744–751.

Kunisaki, M., Umeda, F., Inoguchi, T., and Nawata, H., 1992b, Vitamin E restores reduced prostacyclin synthesis in aortic endothelial cells cultured with a high concentration of glucose, *Metabolism*, 41, 613–621.

Lapointe, A., Couillard, C., and Lemieux, S., 2006, Effects of dietary factors on oxidation of low-density lipoprotein particles, *J. Nutr. Biochem.*, 17, 645–658.

Larsen, L.F., Jespersen, J., and Marckmann, P., 1999, Are olive oil diets antithrombotic? Diets enriched with olive, rapeseed, or sunflower oil affect postprandial factor VII differently, *Am. J. Clin. Nutr.*, 70, 976–982.

Leger, C.L., Carbonneau, M.A., Michel, F., Mas, E., Monnier, L., Cristol, J.P., and Descomps, B., 2005, A thromboxane effect of a hydroxytyrosol-rich olive oil wastewater extract in patients with uncomplicated type I diabetes, *Eur. J. Clin. Nutr.*, 59, 727–730.

Leu, Y.L., Kuo, S.M., Hwang, T.L., and Chiu, S.T., 2004, The inhibition of superoxide anion generation by neutrophils from Viscum articulactum, *Chem. Pharm. Bull.* (Tokyo), 52, 858–860.

Li, D., Saldeen, T., and Mehta, J.L., 2000, Effects of alpha-tocopherol on ox-LDL-mediated degradation of IkappaB and apoptosis in cultured human coronary artery endothelial cells, *J. Cardiovasc. Pharmacol.*, 36, 297–301.

Liapikos, T.A., Antonopoulou, S., Karabina, S.A.P., Tsoukatos, D.C., Demopoulos, C.A., and Tselepis, A.D., 1994, Platelet-activating factor formation during oxidative modification of low-density lipoprotein when PAF-acetylhydrolase has been inactivated, *Biochim. Biophys. Acta*, 1212, 353–360.

Lopez-Segura, F., Velasco, F., Lopez-Miranda, J., Castro, P., Lopez-Pedrera, R., Blanco, A., Jimenez-Pereperez, J., Torres, A., Trujillo, J., Ordovas, J.M., and Perez-Jimenez, F., 1996, Monounsaturated fatty acid-enriched diet decreases plasma plasminogen activator inhibitor type 1, *Arterioscler. Thromb. Vasc. Biol.*, 16, 82–88.

Lowe, G.D., Rumley, A., Whincup, P.H., and Danesh, J., 2002, Hemostatic and rheological variables and risk of cardiovascular disease, *Semin. Vasc. Med.*, 2, 429–439.

Martin, A., Foxall, T. , Blumberg, J.B., and Meydani, M., 1997, Vitamin E inhibits low-density lipoprotein-induced adhesion of monocytes to human aortic endothelial cells in vitro, *Arterioscler. Thromb. Vasc. Biol.*, 17, 429–436.

Masella, R., Vari, R., D'Archivio, M., Di, B.R., Matarrese, P., Malorni, W., Scazzocchio, B., and Giovannini, C., 2004, Extra virgin olive oil biophenols inhibit cell-mediated oxidation of LDL by increasing the mRNA transcription of glutathione-related enzymes, *J. Nutr.,* 134, 785–791.

Meydani, S.N., Meydani, M., Verdon, C.P., Shapiro, A.A., Blumberg, J.B., and Hayes, K.C., 1986, Vitamin E supplementation suppresses prostaglandin E1(2) synthesis and enhances the immune response of aged mice, *Mech. Ageing Dev.*, 34, 191–201.

Meydani, S.N., Lipman, R., Blumberg, J.B., and Taylor, A., 1990, Dietary energy restriction decreases ex vivo spleen prostaglandin E2 synthesis in Emory mice, *J. Nutr.*, 120, 112–115.

Moghadasian, M.H., 2000, Pharmacological properties of plant sterols in vivo and in vitro observations, *Life Sci.*, 67, 605–615.

Moreno, J.J., 2003, Effect of olive oil minor components on oxidative stress and arachidonic acid mobilization and metabolism by macrophages RAW 264.7, *Free Radic. Biol. Med.*, 35, 1073–1081.

Mutanen, M., Freese, R., Valsta, L.M., Ahola, I., and Ahlstrom, A., 1992, Rapeseed oil and sunflower oil diets enhance platelet in vitro aggregation and thromboxane production in healthy men when compared with milk fat or habitual diets, *Thromb. Haemost.*, 67, 352–356.

Ochoa, J.J., Quiles, J.L., Ramirez-Tortosa, M.C., Mataix, J., and Huertas, J.R., 2002, Dietary oils high in oleic acid but with different unsaponifiable fraction contents have different effects in fatty acid composition and peroxidation in rabbit LDL, *Nutrition,* 18, 60–65.

Offermann, M.K. and Medford, R.M., 1994, Antioxidants and atherosclerosis: a molecular perspective, *Heart Dis. Stroke*, 3, 52–57.

Ohkura, N., Hiraishi, S., Itabe, H., Hamuro, T., Kamikubo, Y., Takano, T., Matsuda, J., and Horie, S., 2004, Oxidized phospholipids in oxidized low-density lipoprotein reduce the activity of tissue factor pathway inhibitor through association with its carboxy-terminal region, *Antioxid. Redox. Signal.*, 6, 705–712.

Okuma, M., Takayama, H., and Uchino, H., 1980, Generation of prostacyclin-like substance and lipid peroxidation in vitamin E-deficient rats, *Prostaglandins*, 19, 527–536.

Oubina, P., Sanchez-Muniz, F.J., Rodenas, S., and Cuesta, C., 2001, Eicosanoid production, thrombogenic ratio, and serum and LDL peroxides in normo- and hypercholesterolaemic post-menopausal women consuming two oleic acid-rich diets with different content of minor components, *Br. J. Nutr.*, 85, 41–47.

Pacheco, Y.M., Bermudez, B., Lopez, S., Abia, R., Villar, J., and Muriana, F.J., 2006, Ratio of oleic to palmitic acid is a dietary determinant of thrombogenic and fibrinolytic factors during the postprandial state in men, *Am. J. Clin. Nutr.*, 84, 342–349.

Panizzi, L.M., Scarpati, J.M., and Oriente, E.G., 1960, Costituzione dell'oleuropeina, glucoside amaro ed ad azione ipotensiva dell'olivo, *Gazz. Chim. Ital.*, 1449–1485.

Pearson, T.A., LaCava, J., and Weil, H.F., 1997, Epidemiology of thrombotic-hemostatic factors and their associations with cardiovascular disease, *Am. J. Clin. Nutr.*, 65, 1674S–1682S.

Perez-Jimenez, F., Castro, P., Lopez-Miranda, J., Paz-Rojas, E., Blanco, A., Lopez-Segura, F., Velasco, F., Marin, C., Fuentes, F., and Ordovas, J.M., 1999, Circulating levels of endothelial function are modulated by dietary monounsaturated fat, *Atherosclerosis*, 145, 351–358.

Perez-Jimenez, F., Lista, J.D., Perez-Martinez, P., Lopez-Segura, F., Fuentes, F., Cortes, B., Lozano, A., and Lopez-Miranda, J., 2006, Olive oil and haemostasis: a review on its healthy effects, *Public Health Nutr.*, 9, 1083–1088.

Perona, J.S., Nez, G., Sanchez, D., Badimon, L., and Ruiz-Gutierrez, V., 2004, The unsaponifiable fraction of virgin olive oil in chylomicrons from men improves the balance between vasoprotective and prothrombotic factors released by endothelial cells, *J. Nutr.*, 134, 3284–3289.

Perona, J.S., Cabello-Moruno, R., and Ruiz-Gutierrez,V., 2006, The role of virgin olive oil components in the modulation of endothelial function, *J. Nutr. Biochem.*, 17, 429–445.

Petroni, A., Blasevich, M., Salami, M., Papini, N., Montedoro, G.F., and Galli, C., 1995, Inhibition of platelet aggregation and eicosanoid production by phenolic components of olive oil, *Thromb. Res.*, 78, 151–160.

Petroni, A., Blasevich, M., Papini, N., Salami, M., Sala, A., and Galli, C., 1997, Inhibition of leukocyte leukotriene B4 production by an olive oil-derived phenol identified by mass-spectrometry, *Thromb. Res.*, 87, 315–322.

Princen, H.M., van Duyvenvoorde, W., Buytenhek, R., van der Laarse, A., van Poppel, G., Gevers Leuven, J.A., and van Hinsbergh, V., 1995, Supplementation with low doses of vitamin E protects LDL from lipid peroxidation in men and women, *Arterioscler. Thromb. Vasc. Biol.*, 15, 325–333.

Pryor, W.A., 2000, Vitamin E and heart disease: basic science to clinical intervention trials, *Free Radic. Biol. Med.*, 28, 141–164.

Quilez, J., Garcia-Lorda, P., and Salas-Salvado, J., 2003, Potential uses and benefits of phytosterols in diet: present situation and future directions, Clin. Nutr., 22, 343–351.

Rasmussen, O., Thomsen, C., Ingerslev, J., and Hermansen, K., 1994, Decrease in von Willebrand factor levels after a high-monounsaturated-fat diet in non-insulin-dependent diabetic subjects, *Metabolism*, 43, 1406–1409.

Ringbom, T., Segura, L., Noreen, Y., Perera, P., and Bohlin, L., 1998, Ursolic acid from Plantago major, a selective inhibitor of cyclooxygenase-2 catalyzed prostaglandin biosynthesis, *J. Nat. Prod.*, 61, 1212–1215.

Rodriguez-Rodriguez, R., Herrera, M.D., Perona, J.S., and Ruiz-Gutierrez, V., 2004, Potential vasorelaxant effects of oleanolic acid and erythrodiol, two triterpenoids contained in "orujo" olive oil, on rat aorta, *Br. J. Nutr.*, 92, 635–642.

Ross, R., 1999, Atherosclerosis is an inflammatory disease, *Am. Heart J.*, 138, S419–S420.

Ruano, J., Lopez-Miranda, J., Fuentes, F., Moreno, J.A., Bellido, C., Perez-Martinez, P., Lozano, A., Gomez, P., Jimenez, Y., and Perez, J.F., 2005, Phenolic content of virgin olive oil improves ischemic reactive hyperemia in hypercholesterolemic patients, *J. Am. Coll. Cardiol.*, 46, 1864–1868.

Ruiz-Gutierrez, V., Muriana, F.J., Guerrero, A., Cert, A.M., and Villar, J., 1996, Plasma lipids, erythrocyte membrane lipids and blood pressure of hypertensive women after ingestion of dietary oleic acid from two different sources, *J. Hypertens.*, 14, 1483–1490.

Siess, W., 2006, Platelet interaction with bioactive lipids formed by mild oxidation of low density lipoprotein, *Pathophysiol. Haemost. Thromb.*, 35, 292–304.

Simon, A., Najid, A., Chulia, A.J., Delage, C., and Rigaud, M., 1992, Inhibition of lipoxygenase activity and HL60 leukemic cell proliferation by ursolic acid isolated from heather flowers (Calluna vulgaris), *Biochim. Biophys. Acta*, 1125, 68–72.

Simopoulos, A.P., 2001, The Mediterranean diets: What is so special about the diet of Greece? The scientific evidence, *J. Nutr.*, 131, 3065S–3073S.

Smith, R.D., Kelly, C.N., Fielding, B.A., Hauton, D., Silva, K.D., Nydahl, M.C., Miller, G.J., and Williams, C.M., 2003, Long-term monounsaturated fatty acid diets reduce platelet aggregation in healthy young subjects, *Br. J. Nutr.*, 90, 597–606.

Sutherland, W.H., De Jong, S.A., Walker, R.J., Williams, M.J., Murray, S.C., Duncan, A., and Harper, M., 2002, Effect of meals rich in heated olive and safflower oils on oxidation of postprandial serum in healthy men, *Atherosclerosis*, 160, 195–203.

Tholstrup, T., Marckmann, P., Hermansen, J., Holmer, G., and Sandstrom, B., 1999, Effect of modified dairy fat on fasting and postprandial haemostatic variables in healthy young men, *Br. J. Nutr.*, 82, 105–113.

Togna, G.I., Togna, A.R., Franconi, M., Marra, C., and Guiso, M., 2003, Olive oil isochromans inhibit human platelet reactivity, *J. Nutr.*, 133, 2532–2536.

Trifiletti, A., Scamardi, R., Gaudio, A., Lasco, A., and Frisina, N., 2005, Hemostatic effects of diets containing olive or soy oil in hypertensive patients, *J. Thromb. Haemost.*, 3, 179–180.

Tsantila, N., Karantonis, H.C., Perrea, D.N., Theocharis, S.E., Iliopoulos, D.G., Antonopoulou, S., and Demopoulos, C.A., 2007, Antithrombotic and antiatherosclerotic properties of olive oil and olive pomace polar extracts in rabbits, *Mediators Inflamm.*, Article ID 36204.

Tuck, K.L. and Hayball, P.J., 2002, Major phenolic compounds in olive oil: metabolism and health effects, *J. Nutr. Biochem.*, 13, 636–644.

Tuck, K.L., Hayball, P.J., and Stupans, I., 2002, Structural characterization of the metabolites of hydroxytyrosol, the principal phenolic component in olive oil, in rats, *J. Agric. Food Chem.*, 50, 2404–2409.

Turpeinen, A.M., Pajari, A.M., Freese, R., Sauer, R., and Mutanen, M., 1998, Replacement of dietary saturated by unsaturated fatty acids: effects of platelet protein kinase C activity, urinary content of 2,3-dinor-TXB2 and in vitro platelet aggregation in healthy man, *Thromb. Haemost.*, 80, 649–655.

Vicario, I.M., Malkova, D., Lund, E.K., and Johnson, I.T., 1998, Olive oil supplementation in healthy adults: effects in cell membrane fatty acid composition and platelet function, *Ann. Nutr. Metab.*, 42, 160–169.

Visioli, F. and Galli, C., 1994, Oleuropein protects low density lipoprotein from oxidation, *Life Sci.*, 55, 1965–1971.

Visioli, F. and Galli, C., 1998, The effect of minor constituents of olive oil on cardiovascular disease: new findings, *Nutr. Rev.*, 56, 142–147.

Visioli, F. and Galli, C., 2002, Biological properties of olive oil phytochemicals, *Cri. Rev. Food Sci. Nutr.*, 42, 209–221.

Visioli, F., Bellomo, G., Montedoro, G.F., and Galli, C., 1995, Low density lipoprotein oxidation is inhibited in vitro by olive oil constituents, *Atherosclerosis*, 117, 25–32.

Visioli, F., Bellomo, G., and Galli, C., 1998a, Free radical-scavenging properties of olive oil polyphenols, *Biochem. Biophys. Res. Commun.*, 247, 60–64.

Visioli, F., Bellosta, S., and Galli, C., 1998b, Oleuropein, the bitter principle of olives, enhances nitric oxide production by mouse macrophages, *Life Sci.*, 62, 541–546.

Visioli, F., Galli, C., Plasmati, E., Viappiani, S., Hernandez, A., Colombo, C., and Sala, A., 2000a, Olive phenol hydroxytyrosol prevents passive smoking-induced oxidative stress, *Circulation*, 102, 2169–2171.

Visioli, F., Caruso, D., Galli, C., Viappiani, S., Galli, G., and Sala, A., 2000b, Olive oils rich in natural catecholic phenols decrease isoprostane excretion in humans, *Biochem. Biophys. Res. Commun.*, 278, 797–799.

Visioli, F., Caruso, D., Plasmati, E., Patelli, R., Mulinacci, N., Romani, A., Galli, G., and Galli, C., 2001, Hydroxytyrosol, as a component of olive mill waste water, is dose-dependently absorbed and increases the antioxidant capacity of rat plasma, *Free Radic. Res.*, 34, 301–305.

Visioli, F., Caruso, D., Grande, S., Bosisio, R., Villa, M., Galli, G., Sirtori, C., and Galli, C., 2005a, Virgin Olive Oil Study (VOLOS): vasoprotective potential of extra virgin olive oil in mildly dyslipidemic patients, *Eur. J. Nutr.*, 44, 121–127.

Visioli, F., Bogani, P., Grande, S., and Galli, C., 2005b, Mediterranean food and health: building human evidence, *J. Physiol. Pharmacol.*, 56(Suppl. 1), 37–49.

Weber, C., Erl, W., Pietsch, A., and Weber, P.C., 1995, Aspirin inhibits nuclear factor-kappa B mobilization and monocyte adhesion in stimulated human endothelial cells, *Circulation*, 91, 1914–1917.

Weinbrenner, T., Fito, M., De La Torre, R., Saez, G.T., Rijken, P., Tormos, C., Coolen, S., Albaladejo, M.F., Abanades, S., Schroder, H., Marrugat, J., and Covas, M.I., 2004a, Olive oils high in phenolic compounds modulate oxidative/antioxidative status in men, *J. Nutr.*, 134, 2314–2321.

Weinbrenner, T., Fito, M., Farre, A.M., Saez, G.T., Rijken, P., Tormos, C., Coolen, S., De La Torre, R., and Covas, M.I., 2004b, Bioavailability of phenolic compounds from olive oil and oxidative/antioxidant status at postprandial state in healthy humans, *Drugs Exp. Clin. Res.,* 30, 207–212.

Wiseman, S.A., Mathot, J.N.N.J., De Fouw, N.J., and Tijburg, L.B.M., 1996, Dietary non-tocopherol antioxidants present in extra virgin olive oil increase the resistance of low density lipoproteins to oxidation in rabbits, *Atherosclerosis*, 120, 15–23.

Yoshikawa, T., Yoshida, N., Manabe, H., Terasawa, Y., Takemura, T., and Kondo, M., 1998, Alpha-tocopherol protects against expression of adhesion molecules on neutrophils and endothelial cells, *Biofactors,* 7, 15–19.

Zapolska-Downar, D., Zapolski-Downar, A., Markiewski, M., Ciechanowicz, A., Kaczmarczyk, M., and Naruszewicz, M., 2000, Selective inhibition by alpha-tocopherol of vascular cell adhesion molecule-1 expression in human vascular endothelial cells, *Biochem. Biophys. Res. Commun.*, 274, 609–615.

9 Olive Oil Hydroxy-Isochromans

Giuseppina I. Togna, Giuliana Trefiletti, and Marcella Guiso

CONTENTS

9.1 INTRODUCTION

Natural antioxidants present in the diet increase the resistance toward damages due to oxidation and may have a substantial impact on human health. Dietary antioxidants include ascorbate, tocopherols, carotenoids, and bioactive plant phenols (Boskou, 2006). Widely distributed in the plant kingdom and abundant in our diet, today plant phenols are among the most talked about classes of phytochemicals (Boskou, 2006); the beneficial health effect of the Mediterranean diet has been partly ascribed to the presence of these compounds. In fact, the high content of vegetables, fruits, cereals, wine, and olive oil, typical of the Mediterranean diet, has been associated with a lower risk of coronary heart disease, neurodegenerative diseases, and cancer (Keys, 1995; Owen et al., 2000a; Visioli et al., 2000; Harwood and Yaqoob, 2002; Huxley and Neil, 2003; Visioli et al., 2004; Arts and Hollman, 2005).

Several studies have shown that extra virgin olive oil contains an abundance of phenolic antioxidants including simple phenols (hydroxytyrosol, tyrosol), aldehydic secoiridoids, flavonoids, and lignans (acetoxypinoresinol, pinoresinol) (Owen et al., 2000b). The polar phenolic compounds present in olive oil are a very important class of minor constituents and they are related to the stability of the oil but also to its biological properties (Visioli et al., 2004; Boskou et al., 2005; Bendini et al., 2007).

Olive oil, the main fat component of the Mediterranean diet, consists primarily of triacylglycerols rich in the monounsaturated fatty acid, oleic acid. The nonglyceride constituents of extra virgin olive oil, which comprise approximately 0.5–1.0%, include at least 30 phenolic compounds (Tuck and Hayball, 2002). These phenolic compounds are responsible for its typical taste and contribute to the resistance of the oil to oxidative rancidity (Boskou, 1996). The phenolic content of olive oil depends on a number of factors, including cultivar, degree of maturation, possible infestation by the olive fly *Dacus olea*, climate, and mainly production and storage of the oil (Brenes et al., 1999; Boskou, 2000; Manach et al., 2004).

Phenols are compounds with an aromatic ring structure with one or more hydroxyl groups. Phenols with two or more hydroxyl groups show antioxidant capacity *in vitro*, whereas phenols with one hydroxyl group have little or none (Rice-Evans et al., 1996; Leenen et al., 2002). Extra virgin oil contains phenolic substances with either one or more hydroxyl groups. The types of phenols in extra virgin oil are different from those of the olive fruit. The olives mainly contain the polar glycosides oleuropein and ligstroside, which are the parent compounds of the less polar oleuropein and ligstroside aglycones. These aglycones and their derivatives are the most abundant phenols in olive oil (see Chapter 3).

9.2 HYDROXY-ISOCHROMANS

Recently, a new group of orthodiphenols, 6,7-dihydroxy-isochromans, has been found in extra virgin olive oil by Bianco and co-workers (Bianco et al., 2001).

Isochromans are 3,4-dihydro-1H-benzo[c]pyran derivatives generally present in nature as a part of complex fused ring systems (Peng et al., 1999). The isochroman template is present in structures of drugs (medicines, agrochemicals, etc.) and drug candidates, as well as among natural products. A natural compound, 6,7-dihydroxy-1,1-dimethylisochroman, found in the leaves of *Tectaria sub-trifilla* (Hsu and Chen, 1993; Ralph et al., 1998) and stephaoxocanine, obtained from *Stephania cepharantha*, is a selected example of isochromans of vegetable origin. Furthermore, there are some other examples of natural isochromans obtained from insects and microorganisms such as DMHI, a plant growth regulator isolated from *Penicillium steckii* of terrestrial and marine origin, an anticoccidial isochroman originally found in a hybrid strain of *P. citreo-vitride*, later in *Penicillium* sp. FO-2295 and in *P. expansum* (Masuma et al., 1994), the pseudodeflectusin, a selective human cancer cytotoxin from *Aspergillus pseudodeflectus* (Ogawa et al., 2004), and bioxanthracene (Isaka et al., 2001), a promising antimalarial agent.

Isochroman derivatives also exhibit plant-growth regulatory and herbicidal activities (Bianchi et al., 2004), and they are estrogen receptors (Liu et al., 2005) and dopamine receptor ligands (TenBrink et al., 1996). The synthetic isochroman galaxolide and the tricyclic etodolac bearing the related pyrano {3,4 b} indole ring are isochromans with commercial importance in the cosmetic and drug industries (Larghi and Kaufman, 2006). 1-Phenyl-6,7-dihydroxy-isochroman (1) and 1-(3-methoxy-4-hydroxy-phenyl)-6,7-dihydroxy-isochroman (2) (Figure 9.1) are two 6,7-dihydroxy-isochromans identified in extra virgin olive oil (Bianco et al., 2001).

Guiso and co-workers (2001a) and Guiso et al. (2001b) demonstrated that hydroxytyrosol, a simple polyphenol found in olives (Romani et al., 1999; Bianco and Uccella, 2000) and in olive oil (Montedoro et al., 1992), can react with aldehydes and ketones under very mild conditions to produce 6,7-dihydroxy-isochromans by a modified oxa-Pictet-Spengler reaction. Because of the concurrent presence of many carbonyl compounds in olive oil (Kubo and Kinst-Hori, 1999; Cartoni et al., 2000), the same authors were able to demonstrate the occurrence of this reaction in olive oil by preparing isochromans in this medium (Guiso et al., 2001b).

Isochromans (1) and (2) have been identified in extra virgin olive oil by high performance liquid chromatography–mass/mass spectroscopy (HPLC-MS/MS) (Bianco et al., 2001). Olive oil samples were extracted three times by a solution of methanol/water (4:1). The alcoholic extracts were evaporated under reduced pressure and at a temperature below 35°C to eliminate the methanol. The obtained water solution was acidified (pH = 2.2) and passed through a C_{18} cartridge. The phenolic substances were then eluted by methanol; the obtained solution was evaporated under N_2 and the residue, dissolved in methanol, was analyzed by HPLC-MS/MS.

The levels of these compounds in samples of extra virgin olive oil are very low and extremely variable, ranging from 8–1400 ng/kg for 1-phenyl-6,7-dihydroxy-isochroman and 20–390 ng/kg for 1-(3-methoxy-4-hydroxy-phenyl)-6,7-dihydroxy-isochroman (Bianco et al., 2001).

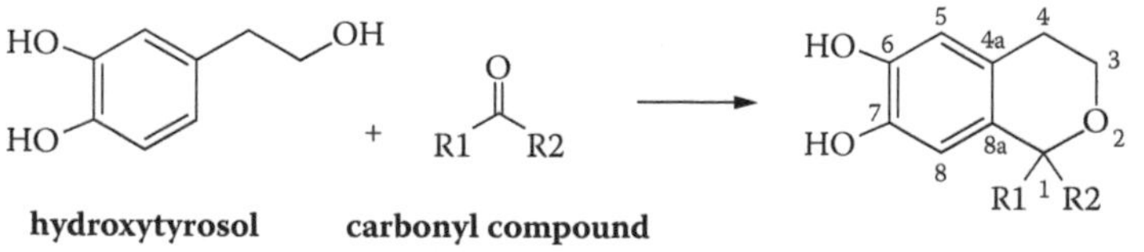

1-Phenyl-6, 7-dihydroxy-isochroman R_1 = H, R_2 = phenyl

1-(3-methoxy-4-hydroxy-phenyl)-6, 7-dihydroxy-isochroman R_1 = H, R_2 = (4-hydroxy-3-methoxy-phenyl)

FIGURE 9.1   Formation of dihydroxy-isochromans.

The presence in olive oil samples of 1-phenyl-6,7-dihydroxy-isochroman and 1-(3′-methoxy-4′-hydroxy-phenyl)-6,7-dihydroxy-isochroman was demonstrated by a comparison between HPLC–MS/MS spectra of the above fraction (Bianco et al., 2001) and those of related standards synthesized from hydroxytyrosol and benzaldehyde and vanillin, respectively, by a modification of the oxa-Pictet-Spengler reaction catalyzed by a small quantity of oleic acid (Guiso et al., 2001a; Guiso et al., 2003).

The scheme of the reaction and the structure of these 6,7-dihydroxy-isochromans are presented in Figure 9.1.

The synthesis of isochromans and derivatives by oxa-Pictet-Spengler cyclization has been widely reviewed by Larghi and Kaufman (2006). It has also been demonstrated (Guiso et al., paper submitted) that these compounds are not present in fresh olive fruits nor in just prepared olive paste. The absence of (1) and (2) in olives and olive paste demonstrates that these compounds are not initially present but they are formed during extraction procedures and storage.

Only 1-(3-methoxy-4-hydroxy-phenyl)-6,7-dihydroxy-isochroman (2) is present in extra-virgin olive oil immediately after extraction. In particular, the presence in olive oil of compound (2) immediately after its extraction coincides with a greater amount of vanillin instead of benzaldehyde in this matrix. Obviously hydroxytyrosol, aldehydes, and free fatty acids are mainly produced by enzymatic and chemical reactions during extraction procedures. During oil preparation, in particular in the "kneader" (malaxation) step, hydrolytic processes due to the uncontrolled action of hydrolytic enzymes (glycosidases and esterases) increase the quantity of free hydroxytyrosol as well as carbonylic compounds, favoring the co-occurrence of all compounds necessary for the formation of isochroman derivatives (Bianco et al., 2001). Compound (1) was found in olive oil stored for 1 month.

Guiso and co-workers (Guiso et al., paper submitted) demonstrated that the amounts of compounds (1) and (2) increase in the initial phase of storage, then the concentrations of both compounds decrease, more rapidly in the case of compound (2).

A different behavior was found between artisan monocultivar and commercial polycultivar oil. In this case the decrease was faster. The difference could depend on several factors such as different polyphenol amounts in the original cultivars, different extraction procedures, etc. It is interesting to note that the highest amount of (1) and (2) was reached after about 1 year in commmercial oil and after about 24 months or more in the examined artisan oil.

9.3 PHARMACOLOGICAL PROPERTIES

Numerous studies have shown that the phenolic fraction of olive oil is endowed with "pharmacological" properties. Among these compounds, hydroxytyrosol and oleuropein aglycone exhibit a series of *in vitro* biological activities, such as protection of low-density lipoprotein (LDL) against peroxyl radical- or copper-induced oxidation (Visioli and Galli, 1995; Caruso et al., 1999; Andrikopoulos et al., 2002; Benkhalti et al., 2003; Ferroni et al., 2004), inhibition of platelet aggregation (Petroni et al., 1995), and potentiation of the nitric oxide-mediated macrophagic immune response (Visioli et al., 1998). Some phenolics have been shown to inhibit eicosanoid production *in vitro*, suggesting that they might exert anti-inflammatory effects (Miles et al., 2005). Thus, olive oil phenols have been beneficially linked to processes that contribute to the pathogenesis of heart diseases and atherosclerosis as well as to inflammatory pathologies (Martinez-Dominguez et al., 2001). Moreover, experimental evidence has shown that minor components of olive oil are able to inhibit endothelial activation and to modulate the expression of proatherogenic adhesion molecules (Carluccio et al., 2003; Dell'Agli et al., 2006; Perona et al., 2006).

Extra virgin olive oil dihydroxy-isochromans are a class of compounds little studied and thus it is not surprising that there is not much available information about their functions and biological properties. The antioxidant power of the olive oil dihydroxy-isochromans and their ability to inhibit human platelet aggregation were first investigated by Togna et al. (2003), who demonstrated that these compounds are effective free radical scavengers and inhibit human platelet aggregation and thromboxane release evoked by agonists that induce reactive oxygen species-mediated platelet activation (Togna et al., 2003).

The free radical-scavenging capacities of 1-(3′-methoxy-4′-hydroxy-phenyl)-6,7-dihydroxy-iso-chroman and 1-phenyl-6,7-dihydroxy-isochroman were determined by the 1,1-diphenyl-2-picryl-hydrazyl (DPPH) test. 1-(3′-Methoxy-4′-hydroxy-phenyl)-6,7-dihydroxy-isochroman elicited an antioxidant activity lower than hydroxytyrosol, comparable to that of quercetin but greater than 1-phenyl-6,7-dihydroxy-isochroman and resveratrol (in this study hydroxytyrosol, quercetin, and resveratrol were used as reference compounds).

The relation between structure and scavenging properties was assessed by Lorenz et al. (2005) by comparing the naturally occurring 1-(3′-methoxy-4′-hydroxy-phenyl)-6,7-dihydroxy-isochroman (ISO-3: three OH groups) with three newly synthesized derivatives that differ in their degree of hydroxylation by substitution with methoxy groups (from ISO-0 to ISO-4 with 4 OH groups). These authors demonstrated that the tetrahydroxy-substituted derivative ISO-4 [1-(3,4-dihydroxy-phenyl)-6,7-dihydroxyisochroman] possesses the highest scavenging activity for the artificial radical DPPH and that a successive blocking of the OH groups by methoxylation results in a complete loss of antioxidant activity.

Moreover, ISO-4 and ISO-2 (Lorenz et al., 2005) elicited high efficiency to reduce intracellular oxidative stress (rat glioma cell cultures), showing excellent scavenging activity for pathophysiolog-ically relevant free radicals and reactive oxygen or nitrogen (O^-_2, $ONOO^-$, and H_2O_2). Surprisingly, the natural compound ISO-3 caused only half the protection in comparison to the new derivatives. The difference in the effects may not only result from their chemical properties but may also depend on the different intracellular bioavailability, due to their methoxylation degree and lipophilicity (Togna et al., 2003; Lorenz et al., 2005). The authors conclude that for the good radical- and ROS/RNS-scavenging features and their simple synthesis the hydroxy-isochromans appear to be inter-esting candidates for pharmaceutical interventions that protect against oxidative/nitrosative stress (Lorenz et al., 2005).

The antiplatelet activity of 1-(3′-methoxy-4′-hydroxy-phenyl)-6,7-dihydroxy-isochroman and 1-phenyl-6,7-dihydroxy-isochroman was demonstrated by Togna et al. (2003) in human platelet-rich plasma, *in vitro*. The dihydroxy-isocromans were able to inhibit platelet aggregation induced by sodium arachidonate (SA) and collagen, while no effect was recorded on platelet response to ADP. The fact that production of oxygen radicals appears to be more important during the initial phases of platelet activation when induced by SA and collagen than by the other agonists, such as ADP (Iuliano et al., 1992; Pratico et al., 1992; Caccese et al., 2000), suggests that the capability of these isochromans to interfere with platelet function is related to their radical-scavenging activity.

It is interesting to note that these dihydroxy-isochromans appear to be more active than the parent compound, hydroxytyrosol (Petroni et al., 1995), and that their antiaggregating effect is comparable to or even higher than that reported for quercetin (Tzeng et al., 1991; Pignatelli et al., 2000) and resveratrol (Bertelli et al., 1996; Fremont, 2000), which were extensively investigated to determine the relationship between dietary phenolic compounds and decreased risk of cardiovas-cular diseases.

The described effect of these dihydroxy-isochromans on arachidonic acid mobilization from platelet membrane (Togna et al., 2003) could also be ascribed to their scavenging activity. Actually, 1-(3′-methoxy-4′-hydroxy-phenyl)-6,7-dihydroxy-isochroman and 1-phenyl-6,7-dihydroxy-isochro-man inhibited arachidonic acid mobilization from platelet membrane phospholipids induced by thrombin and, to a greater extent, by collagen. This result indicates that these dihydroxy-isochro-mans are able to inhibit the directly induced (thrombin) and/or ROS-mediated (collagen) phospholi-pase A_2 activation (Hashizume et al., 1991; Kramer et al., 1993; Pignatelli et al., 1998).

A protective effect by 1-phenyl-6,7-dihydroxy-isochroman on vascular endothelial function has also been demonstrated (Orlando et al., 2003). The experiments performed to investigate the vascular effect of this isochroman showed that the compound is able to induce endothelium-dependent relaxation in isolated rabbit aorta by preserving nitric oxide (NO) from destruction by superoxide anion (the biological activity of NO can be effectively increased by scavengers of oxygen-free radicals [Bouloumié et al., 1997]).

Running investigations would suggest that the compound may also enhance endothelial NO synthesis by increasing intracellular Ca^{2+} concentrations (unpublished data).

9.4 CONCLUDING REMARKS

The biological activities of olive oil dihydroxy-isochromans, as shown by experimental data available up to now, appear to be very similar to those of other phenolic compounds studied more extensively. Although this new class of compounds has been poorly investigated, dihydroxy-isochromans appear promising compounds for antioxidant strategies.

The levels of 1-phenyl-6,7-dihydroxy-isochroman and 1-(3'-methoxy-4'-hydroxy-phenyl)-6,7-dihydroxy-isochroman in extra virgin olive oil are very low and extremely variable due to the different amounts of hydroxytyrosol and carbonyl compounds, which is related to the harvesting times of different cultivars and olives. Nevertheless, the possibility that other isochromans, in addition to those discovered up to now, are present in extra virgin olive oil cannot be excluded. In fact, as mentioned above, carbonylic compounds are numerous in this matrix and nearly all of them can react with hydroxytyrosol to produce isochromans.

Therefore, it would be of interest to carry out additional studies to verify the presence of other isochromans in extra virgin olive oil, and to investigate the influence of different factors (i.e., cultivar, initial amount of polyphenols and carbonylic compounds, oil extraction procedures, storage conditions, etc.) on their levels. Their biological activity as well as their possible synergistic or interactive effects should also be more thoroughly investigated.

It is clear that significant pharmacodynamically active concentrations of hydroxy-isochromans and other biologically active compounds cannot be achieved in men with normal diets. The possibility that olive oil may contribute to the prevention of several human diseases appears more likely to be due to the simultaneous presence of various biologically active compounds and to possible synergistic effects of olive oil phenolic constituents, as already demonstrated for other phenolic compounds (Pignatelli et al., 2000), rather than to one single component.

REFERENCES

Andrikopoulos, N.K., Kaliora, A.C., Assimopoulou, A., and Papageorgiou, V.P., 2002, Inhibitory activity of minor polyphenolic and nonpolyphenolic constituents of olive oil against *in vitro* low-density lipoprotein oxidation, *J. Med. Food*, 5(1), 1–7.

Arts, I.C. and Hollman, P.C., 2005, Polyphenols and disease risk in epidemiologic studies, *Am. J. Clin. Nutr.*, 81(Suppl. 1), 317S–325S.

Bendini, A., Cerretani, L., Carrasco-Pancorbo, A., Gómez-Caravaca, A.M., Segura-Carretero, A., Fernández-Gutiérrez, A., and Lercker, G., 2007, Phenolic molecules in virgin olive oils: a survey of their sensory properties, health effects, antioxidant activity and analytical methods. An overview of the last decade, *Molecules*, 12, 1679–1719.

Benkhalti, F., Legssyer, A., Gomez, P., Paz, E., Lopez-Miranda, J., Perez-Jimenez, F., and el Boustani, E.S., 2003, Effects of virgin olive oil phenolic compounds on LDL oxidation and vasorelaxation activity, *Therapie*, 58(2), 133–137.

Bertelli, A.A., Giovannini, L., Bernini, W., Migliori, M., Fregoni, M., Bavaresco, L., and Bertelli, A., 1996, Antiplatelet activity of cis-resveratrol, *Drug Exp. Clin. Res.*, 22, 61–63.

Bianchi, D.A., Blanco, N.E., Carrillo, N., Kaufman, T.S., 2004, Synthesis of 4-hydroxy-7,8-dimetoxyisochroman-3-one and its plant growth-regulating properties on tobacco (*Nicotiana tabacum* cv. Petit Havana), *J. Agric. Food Chem.*, 52(7), 1923–1927.

Bianco, A. and Uccella, N., 2000, Biophenolic components of olives, *Food Res. Int.*, 33, 475–485.

Bianco, A., Coccioli, F., Guiso, M., and Marra, C., 2001, The occurrence in olive oil of a new class of phenolic compounds: hydroxy-isochromans, *Food Chem.*, 77, 405–411.

Boskou, D., 1996, *Olive Oil: Chemistry and Technology*, AOCS Press, Champaign, IL.

Boskou, D., 2000, Olive oil, in *Mediterranean Diets*, Simopoulus, A.P. and Visioli, F., Eds., S. Karger, Basel, 56–77.

Boskou, D., Blekas, G., and Tsimidou, M., 2005, Phenolic compounds in olive oil and olives, *Curr. Top. Nutraceut. Res.*, 3, 125–136.

Boskou, D., 2006, Sources of natural phenolic antioxidants, *Trends Food Sci. Technol.*, 17, 505–512.

Bouloumié, A., Bauersachs, J., Linz, W., Scholkens, B.A., Wiemer, G., Fleming, I., and Busse, R., 1997, Endothelial dysfunction coincides with an enhanced nitric oxide synthase expression and superoxide anion production, *Hypertension*, 30(4), 934–941.

Brenes, M., Garcia, A., Garcia, P., Rios, J.J., and Garrido, A., 1999, Phenolic compounds in Spanish olive oils, *J. Agric. Food Chem.*, 47(9), 3535–3540.

Caccese, D., Praticò, D., Ghiselli, A., Natoli, S., Pignatelli, P., Sanguigni, V., Iuliano, L., and Violi, F., 2000, Superoxide anion and hydroxyl radical release by collagen-induced platelet aggregation. Role of arachidonic acid metabolism, *Thromb. Haemost.*, 83, 485–490.

Carluccio, M.A., Siculella, L., Ancora, M.A., Massaro, M., Scoditti, E., Storelli, C., Visioli, F., Distante, A., and De Caterina, R., 2003, Olive oil and red wine antioxidant polyphenols inhibit endothelial activation: antiatherogenic properties of Mediterranean diet phytochemicals, *Arterioscler. Thromb. Vasc. Biol.*, 23(4), 622–629.

Cartoni, G.P., Coccioli, F., Jasionowska, R., and Ramirez, D., 2000, HPLC analysis of the benzoic and cinnamic acids in edible vegetable oils, *It. J. Food Sci.*, 12, 163–167.

Caruso, D., Berra, B., Giavarini, F., Cortesi, N., Fedeli, E., and Galli, G., 1999, Effect of virgin olive oil phenolic compounds on *in vitro* oxidation of human low density lipoproteins, *Nutr. Metab. Cardiovasc. Dis.*, 9(3), 102–107.

Dell'Agli, M., Fagnani, R., and Mitro, N., 2006, Minor components of olive oil modulate proatherogenic adhesion molecules involved in endothelial activation, *J. Agric. Food Chem.*, 54(9), 3259–3264.

Ferroni, F., Maccaglia, A., Pietraforte, D., Turco, L., and Minetti, M., 2004, Phenolic antioxidants and the protection of low density lipoprotein from peroxynitrite-mediated oxidations at physiologic CO_2, *J. Agric. Food Chem.*, 52(10), 2866–2874.

Fremont, L., 2000, Biological effects of resveratrol, *Life Sci.*, 66(8), 663–673.

Guiso, M., Marra, C., and Cavarischia, C., 2001a, Isochromans from 2-(3′,4′-dihydroxy) phenylethanol, *Tetrahedron Lett.*, 42, 6531–6534.

Guiso, M., Marra, C., Togna, G.I., Coccioli, F., 2001b, L'Olea Europaea: un'occasione d'incontro tra ricerca scientifica e alimenti, 27th National Convention of the Division of Organic Chemistry, P146, Trieste, Italy, 3–7, September 2001.

Guiso, M., Bianco, A., Marra, C., and Cavarischia, C., 2003, One-pot synthesis of 6-hydroxyisochromans: the example of demethyl-oxa-coclaurine, *Eur. J. Org. Chem.*, 17, 3407–3411.

Guiso, M. et al., paper submitted, Natural Products Research.

Guiso, M., Marra, C., and Rodriguez Aras, R., in press, An investigation on dihydroxy-isochromans in extra-virgin olive oil, *Nat. Prod. Res.*

Harwood, J.L. and Yaqoob, P., 2002, Nutritional and health aspects of olive oil, *Eur. J. Lipid Sci. Technol.*, 104, 685–697.

Hashizume, T., Yamaguchi, H., Kawamoto, A., Tamura, A., Sato, T., and Fujii, T., 1991, Lipid peroxide makes rabbit platelet hyperaggregable to agonists through phospholipase A_2 activation, *Arch. Biochem. Biophys.*, 289, 47–52.

Hsu, F.Y. and Chen, J.Y., 1993, Phenolics from *Tectaria subtriphylla*, *Phytochemistry*, 34, 1625–1627.

Huxley, R.R. and Neil, H.A.W., 2003, The relation between dietary flavonoid intake and coronary heart disease mortality: a meta-analysis of prospective cohort studies, *Eur. J. Clin. Nutr.*, 57, 904–908.

Isaka, M., Kongsaeree, P., and Thebtaranonth, Y., 2001, Bioxanthracenes from the insect pathogenic fungus *Cordyceps pseudomilitaris* BCC 1620. II. Structure elucidation, *J. Antibiot.*, 54(1), 36–43.

Iuliano, L., Pedersen, J.Z., Praticò, D., Rotilio, G., and Violi, F., 1992, Role of hydroxyl radicals in the activation of human platelets, *Eur. J. Biochem.*, 221, 695–704.

Keys, A., 1995, Mediterranean diet and public health: personal reflections, *Am. J. Clin. Nutr.*, 61(Suppl. 6), 1321S–1323S.

Kramer, R.M., Roberts, E.F., Manetta, J.V., Hylsop, P.A., and Jakubowski, J.A., 1993, Thrombin-induced phosphorylation and activation of Ca^{++}-sensitive cytosolic phospholipase A_2 in human platelets, *J. Biol. Chem.*, 268, 26796–26804.

Kubo, I. and Kinst-Hori, I., 1999, Tyrosinase inhibitory activity of the olive oil flavor compounds, *J. Agric. Food Chem.*, 47(11), 4574–4578.

Larghi, E.L. and Kaufman, T.S., 2006, The Oxa-Pictet-Spengler cyclization: synthesis of isochromans and related pyran-type heterocycles, *Synthesis*, 2, 187–220.

Leenen, R., Roodenburg, A.J., Vissers, M.N., Schuurbiers, J.A., van Putte, K.P., Wiseman, S.A., and van de Put, F.H., 2002, Supplementation of plasma with olive oil phenols and extracts: influence on LDL oxidation, *J. Agric. Food Chem.*, 50(5), 1290–1297.

Liu, J., Birzin, E.T., Chan, W., Yang, Y.T., Pai, L.Y., Dasilva, C., Hayes, E.C., Mosley, R.T., Dininno, F., Rohrer, S.P., Schaeffer, J.M., and Hammond, M.L., 2005, Estrogen receptor ligands. Part 11. Synthesis and activity of isochromans and isothiochromans, *Bioorg. Med. Chem. Lett.*, 15(3), 715–718.

Lorenz, P., Zeh, M., Martens-Lobenhoffer, J., Schmidt, H., Wolf, G., and Horn, T.F., 2005, Natural and newly synthesized hydroxy-1-aryl-isochromans: a class of potential antioxidants and radical scavengers, *Free Radic. Res.*, 39(5), 535–545.

Manach, C., Scalbert, P., Morand, C., Rémésy, C., and Jiménez, L., 2004, Polyphenols: food sources and bioavailability, *Am. J. Clin. Nutr.*, 79(5), 727–747.

Martinez-Dominguez, E., de la Puerta, R., and Ruiz-Gutierrez, V., 2001, Protective effects upon experimental inflammation models of a polyphenol-supplemented virgin olive oil diet, *Inflamm. Res.*, 50(2), 102–106.

Masuma, R., Tabata, N., Tomoda, H., Haneda, K., Iwai, Y., and Omura, S., 1994, Arohynapenes A and B, new anticoccidial agents produced by *Penicillium* sp. Taxonomy, fermentation, and structure elucidation, *J. Antibiot.*, 47(1), 46–53.

Miles, E.A., Zoubouli, P., and Calder, P.C., 2005, Differential anti-inflammatory effects of phenolic compounds from extra virgin olive oil identified in human whole blood cultures, *Nutrition*, 21, 389–394.

Montedoro, G., Servili, M., Baldioli, M., and Miniati, E., 1992, Simple and hydrolyzable phenolic compounds in virgin olive oil: their extraction separation and quantitative and semi-quantitative evaluation by HPLC, *J. Agric. Food Chem.*, 40, 1571–1576.

Ogawa, A., Murakami, C., Kamisuki, S., Kuriyama, I., Yoshida, H., Sugawara, F., and Mizushina, Y., 2004, Pseudodeflectusin, a novel isochroman derivative from Aspergillus pseudodeflectus a parasite of the sea weed, Sargassum fusiform, as a selective human cancer cytotoxin, *Bioorg. Med. Chem. Lett.*, 14(13), 3539–3543.

Orlando, R., Franconi, M., Togna, A.R., Marra, C., and Togna, G., 2003, New olive oil polyphenol prevents the interaction of superoxide and nitric oxide, *31st National Congress of the Italian Society of Pharmacology*, Trieste, Italy, Book of Abstracts, p. 100.

Owen, R.W., Giacosa, A., Hull, W.E., Haubner, R., Wurtele, G., Spiegelhalder, B., and Bartsch, H., 2000a, Olive-oil consumption and health: the possible role of antioxidants, *Lancet Oncol.*, 1, 107–112.

Owen, R.W., Mier, W., Giacosa, A., Hull, W.E., Spiegelhalder, B., and Bartsch, H.. 2000b, Phenolic compounds and squalene in olive oils: the concentration and antioxidant potential of total phenols, simple phenols, secoiridoids, lignans and squalene, *Food. Chem. Toxicol.*, 38(8), 647–659.

Peng, J.P., Lu, F., and Ralph, J., 1999, Isochroman lignin trimers from DFRC-degraded *Pinus taeda*, *Phytochemistry*, 50, 659–666.

Perona, J.S., Cabello-Moruno, R., and Ruiz-Gutierrez, V., 2006, The role of virgin olive oil components in the modulation of endothelial function, *J. Nutr. Biochem.*, 17(7), 429–445.

Petroni, A., Blasevich, M., Salami, M., Papini, N., Montedoro, G.F., and Galli, C.. 1995, Inhibition of platelet aggregation and eicosanoid production by phenolic components of olive oil, *Thromb. Res.*, 78(2), 151–160.

Pignatelli, P., Pulcinelli, F.M., Lenti, L., Gazzaniga, P.P., and Violi, F., 1998, Hydrogen peroxide is involved in collagen-induced platelet activation, *Blood*, 91, 484–490.

Pignatelli, P., Pulcinelli, F.M., Celestini, A., Lenti, L., Ghiselli, A., Gazzanica, P.P., and Violi, F., 2000, The flavonoids quercetin and catechin synergistically inhibit platelet function by antagonizing the intracellular production of hydrogen peroxide, *Am. J. Clin. Nutr.*, 72(5), 1150–1155.

Praticò, D., Iuliano, L., Pulcinelli, F.M., Bonavita, M.S., Gazzaniga, P.P., and Violi, F., 1992, Hydrogen peroxide triggers activation of human platelets selectively exposed to nanoaggregating concentrations of arachidonic acid and collagen, *J. Lab. Clin. Med.*, 119, 364–370.

Ralph, J., Peng, J.P., and Lu, F.C., 1998, Isochroman structures in lignin: a new beta-1 pathway, *Tetrahedron Lett.*, 39, 4963–4964.

Rice-Evans, C.A., Miller, N.J., and Paganga, G.. 1996, Structure-antioxidant activity relationships of flavonoids and phenolic acids, *Free Radic. Biol. Med.*, 20(7), 933–956.

Romani, A., Mulinacci, N., Pinelli, P., Vincieri, F.F., and Cimato, A., 1999, Polyphenolic content in five Tuscany cultivars of *Olea europaea* L., *J. Agric. Food Chem.*, 47(3), 964–967.

TenBrink, R.E., Bergh, C.L., Duncan, J.N., Harris, D.W., Huff, R.M., Lahti, R.A., Lawson, C.F., Lutzke, B.S., Martin, I.J., Rees, S.A., Schlachter, S.K., Sih, J.C., and Smith, M.W., 1996, (S)-(-)-4-[4-[2-(isochroman-1-yl)ethyl]piperazin-1-yl]benzenesulfonamide, a selective dopamine D4 antagonist, *J. Med. Chem.*, 39(13), 2435–2437.

Togna, G.I., Togna, A.R., Franconi, M., Marra, C., and Guiso, M., 2003, Olive oil isochromans inhibit human platelet reactivity, *J. Nutr.*, 133(8), 2532–2536.

Tuck, K.L. and Hayball, P.J., 2002, Major phenolic compounds in olive oil: metabolism and health effects, *J. Nutr. Biochem.*, 13(11), 636–644.

Tzeng, S.H., Ko, W.C., Ko, F.N., and Teng, C.M., 1991, Inhibition of platelet aggregation by some flavonoids, *Thromb. Res.*, 64(1), 91–100.

Visioli, F. and Galli, C., 1995, Oleuropein protects low density lipoprotein from oxidation, *Life Sci.*, 55(24), 1965–1971.

Visioli, F., Bellomo, G., and Galli, C., 1998, Free radical-scavenging properties of olive oil polyphenols, *Biochem. Biophys. Res. Commun.*, 247(1), 60–64.

Visioli, F., Borsani, L., and Galli, C., 2000, Diet and prevention of coronary heart diseases: the potential role of phytochemicals, *Cardiovasc. Res.*, 47, 419–425.

Visioli, F., Grande, S., Bogani, P., and Galli, C., 2004, The role of antioxidants in the Mediterranean diets: focus on cancer, *Eur. J. Cancer Prev.*, 13(4), 337–343.

10 Mediterranean Diet and Olive Oil Consumption— Estimations of Daily Intake of Antioxidants from Virgin Olive Oil and Olives

Vardis Dilis and Antonia Trichopoulou

CONTENTS

SUMMARY

"Antioxidants" are molecules that prevent or delay the oxidation of susceptible compounds, thus conferring protection against the deleterious actions of "free radicals." It is believed that the traditional Mediterranean diet, being abundant in fruits, vegetables, red wine, and virgin olive oil, may, at least partly, owe its positive impact on human well-being to a high antioxidant potential. The effect of virgin olive oil on health is considered to stem from both its lipid profile and content in several minor constituents, many of which show antioxidant activity. The latter include phenolic compounds, hydrocarbons (mainly squalene), chlorophylls, carotenoids, and tocopherols. We estimated the intake of antioxidant compounds via olive oil and table olives by the Greek population. The calculations were based on literature data for the content of olive oil and table olives in antioxidant compounds, and on consumption data of more than 20,000 Greeks in the context of the Greek cohort of the European Investigation into Cancer and Nutrition (EPIC study). The calculated daily per-capita intake was found to be about 17 mg for phenolic compounds, 223 mg for squalene, and 12 mg for α-tocopherol. The elucidation of the overall content of the Mediterranean diet in antioxidant compounds may shed light on the biological interactions involved in the apparent protection that the traditional Mediterranean diet provides against chronic diseases.

10.1 INTRODUCTION

The traditional Mediterranean diet has been recognized as a healthy dietary pattern. Its health-promoting properties have been attributed mainly to the effect of the diet as a whole, rather than to specific foods or food groups it integrates (Trichopoulou et al., 1995; Willett et al., 1995; Trichopoulou et al., 2003). The Mediterranean diet incorporates a plethora of traditional foods and recipes. Among them, virgin olive oil holds a central position; it is used as the main added lipid during food preparation; it facilitates the ample consumption of plant foods in raw and cooked dishes; it represents a principal source of energy in the diet, an attribute that has been important in difficult times; and it has a very important cultural and economical role for populations surrounding the Mediterranean Sea. Consequently, olive oil comprises an indispensable part of the dietary and cultural traditions of the Mediterranean populations.

Besides triacylglycerols and a small percentage of free fatty acids, virgin olive oil also contains a variety of minor constituents amounting to about 1–2% of the oil (Visioli and Galli, 1998). Among them are hydrocarbons, tocopherols, carotenoids, chlorophylls, phytosterols, flavor compounds, and various polar phenolic constituents. These compounds are very important contributors to the oil's organoleptic properties and stability toward oxidation. They are derived from olive fruits that are processed only by physical means, while the production of most other plant oils includes solvent extraction and refining, procedures that cause their depletion of several important microcomponents.

It has been suggested that the beneficial impact of the Mediterranean diet on health may be attributed in part to its content in antioxidant compounds that are present abundantly in virgin olive oil, as well as in fruits, vegetables, and red wine (Willett, 1994; Trichopoulou and Lagiou, 1997; Trichopoulou et al., 1998; Trichopoulou et al., 1999). However, the extent to which antioxidants contribute to the overall impact of the diet on health has not yet been documented. Below we briefly review the antioxidant compounds present in virgin olive oil and their potential implications for human health. Moreover, we present estimates of their intake via olive oil and table olives in the Greek population based on data from the Greek cohort of the European Prospective Investigation into Cancer and Nutrition (EPIC) (Riboli and Kaaks, 1997).

10.2 PHENOLIC COMPOUNDS

The various phenolic compounds present in olives are believed to protect the plant from environmental stress. They contribute to the organoleptic profile of raw olives and consequently to that of virgin olive oil. Their concentration in the oil depends on various factors including cultivar, maturity, climate, rootstock, and agricultural practices (Ryan and Robards, 1998), as well as on the choice of extraction, separation, and quantification techniques (Visioli et al., 2002; Carrasco-Pancorbo et al., 2005; see also Chapter 3). The phenolic compounds exert their antioxidant activity by donating a hydrogen atom to the chain-propagating radicals formed during lipid peroxidation. Their role in photooxidation is rather limited (Psomiadou and Tsimidou, 2002b).

Most studies on the phenolic antioxidant properties of olive oil in humans concentrate on their effect on low density lipoprotein (LDL) and DNA oxidation, since these are believed to be key processes implicated in the development of atherosclerosis and cancer, respectively. The bioavailability as well as anti-inflamatory properties of certain phenolic compounds of olive oil have also been investigated (see Chapter 6). Their bioavailability was found to range widely depending on experimental conditions and the compound examined (Visioli et al., 2000; Miro-Casas et al., 2001a; Miro-Casas et al., 2001b; Vissers et al., 2002), but it can be very high. For example, hydroxytyrosol recovery in plasma and urine after ingestion of 25 ml virgin olive oil was about 98% (Miro-Casas et al., 2003). With respect to LDL protection, both Covas and colleagues (2006a) and Gimeno and colleagues (2007) found that intake of phenolic compounds via olive oil results in a significant increase in the phenolic content of LDL. This finding may be very important in conjunction with the inhibitory effect of olive oil phenolics on LDL oxidation (Visioli and Galli, 1994; Visioli et al.,

1995) and platelet aggregation (Petroni et al., 1995) in model systems. The protection conferred to LDL from oxidation, however, was not confirmed in two randomized trials on healthy nonsmoking or smoking volunteers (Vissers et al., 2001; Moschandreas et al., 2002). On the other hand, oxidized LDL levels of healthy subjects were reduced *in vivo* after consumption of a phenol-rich olive oil (Marrugat et al., 2004). In addition, intake of olive oil phenolic compounds was associated with a reduction in LDL oxidation levels of healthy males (Covas et al., 2006b) as well as patients with stable coronary heart disease (CHD) (Fito et al., 2005). Finally, studies have shown that virgin olive oil phenolic compounds significantly reduce the production of certain markers of inflammation that are involved in the atherosclerotic process (Leger et al., 2005; Visioli et al., 2005; Bogani et al., 2007; see also Chapters 6 and 8).

Human studies on the effect of olive oil phenolic compounds on DNA oxidation have produced diverse results. Daily intake of 25 ml olive oil has been reported to result in: (1) no effect on the excretion of etheno-DNA adducts, markers of lipid peroxidation and oxidative stress (Hillestrom et al., 2006); (2) reduction in DNA oxidation irrespective of the phenolic content of olive oil (Machowetz et al., 2006); (3) reduction in mitochondrial DNA oxidation associated with increasing phenol content of olive oil administered (Weinbrenner et al., 2004). Intake of a daily amount of 50 g olive oil with high phenolic content resulted in about 30% less DNA damage in postmenopausal women (Salvini et al., 2006).

10.3 SQUALENE

Squalene is a triterpenic hydrocarbon and an intermediate product of cholesterol biosynthesis. It accounts for at least 50% of the olive oil's nonsaponifiable fraction and for about 90% of its total hydrocarbon content (Psomiadou and Tsimidou, 1999). Squalene has been shown to act as an effective quencher of singlet oxygen (Kohno et al., 1995). It may confer a concentration-dependent moderate antioxidant activity by reducing the rate of oxidation in purified olive oil kept at 40 and 62°C (Psomiadou and Tsimidou, 1999). Absorption of squalene in humans was found to range within about 60–85% (Strandberg et al., 1990; Miettinen and Vanhanen, 1994). It accumulates primarily in skin tissue (Liu et al., 1976). It has thus been proposed that it may confer protection to the skin from lipid peroxidation caused primarily by UV light (Kelly, 1999). A tumor-inhibiting potential has also been attributed to squalene in animal as well as *in vitro* studies (Newmark, 1997).

10.4 PIGMENTS

Color is an important determinant of the organoleptic quality of virgin olive oil. The most important yellow pigments present are lutein and β-carotene, while chlorophylls are responsible for the oil's green coloring (Psomiadou and Tsimidou, 2001). The pigment content of virgin olive oil varies according to olive variety, geographical origin, environmental conditions, degree of olive ripeness, and extraction and storage conditions (Psomiadou and Tsimidou, 2002a; Psomiadou and Tsimidou, 2002b; Cichelli and Pertesana, 2004). The pigment profile has been proposed to serve as an indicator of typicality and authenticity of monovarietal olive oils (Gandul-Rojas and Minguez-Mosquera, 1996; Psomiadou and Tsimidou, 2001; Giuffrida et al., 2007).

Chlorophylls. Natural chlorophylls are among the most abundant pigments in nature. In chemical terms, they represent a group of magnesium-metallated tetrapyrroles. With respect to oxidation induced by light exposure (photooxidation), chlorophyll pigments show a prooxidant activity, contributing to the degradation of the organoleptic properties of olive oil. This is facilitated through the production of singlet oxygen species by transferring energy from light to triplet oxygen. In conditions that do not promote photooxidation, however, chlorophylls play a mildly protective (antioxidant) role on the stability of olive oil (Psomiadou and Tsimidou, 2002a, b). Chlorophyll tends to convert to derivatives after plant processing or ingestion (mainly pheophytin, pyropheophytin, and pheophorbide). It has been argued that these derivatives may have anticarcinogenic potential

(Negishi et al., 1997; Harttig and Bailey, 1998; Chernomorsky et al., 1999; Ferruzzi et al., 2002; de Vogel et al., 2005). Increased intake of heme iron from meat and reduced intake of chlorophyll from vegetables were significantly related to increased colon cancer risk among 120,852 Dutch men and women (Balder et al., 2006).

Carotenoids belong to tetraterpenes and are based on a 40-carbon isoprene unit backbone. Carotenoids containing only hydrogen and carbon are classified as carotenes, while when oxygen is also present, as xanthophylls. Carotenoids act as singlet oxygen quenchers against photosensitized oxidation by accepting energy from the singlet oxygen, as well as light filters (Psomiadou and Tsimidou, 2002b). Their contribution to olive oil autoxidation stability has been reported to be less significant than that of phenolic compounds and α-tocopherol (Aparicio et al., 1999). Although the consumption of foods rich in carotenoids has been linked to reduced heart disease risk in epidemiological studies, the overall evidence remains inconclusive (Kritchevsky, 1999). When the results of relevant studies were aggregated, supplementation with β-carotene was related to increased mortality (Bjelakovic et al., 2007). Further studies are needed to assess the impact of diets high in β-carotene, as contrasted to β-carotene supplementation, on the prevention of cardiovascular disease.

10.5 TOCOPHEROLS

The vitamin E group is chemically characterized as 6-hydroxy chroman derivatives bearing an isoprenoid unit. The group is represented by two types of compounds: four tocopherols (α, β, γ, and δ) and four tocotrienols (α, β, γ, and δ), that differ in the presence of double bonds in the isoprenoid unit of the latter type. Vitamin E is absorbed in the small intestine in the same way as dietary lipids (Hacquebard and Carpentier, 2005). Its major biological role is exerted through its antioxidant activity by conferring protection to unsaturated lipids from oxidation, including the inhibition of LDL oxidation. α-Tocopherol is the most abundant form of vitamin E in olive oil, and is equally important to hydrophilic phenols in olive oil stability during autoxidation. α-Tocopherol also plays an active role in photosensitized oxidation (Psomiadou and Tsimidou, 2002b).

A lower heart disease risk due to increased vitamin E dietary intake has been reported in a number of studies, but the effects obtained through vitamin E supplementation are not consistent (Gaziano, 2004; Knekt et al., 2004). In a recent meta-analysis, supplementation with vitamin E was associated with increased mortality (Bjelakovic et al., 2007). Further research is required toward the elucidation of the role of vitamin E (as for β-carotene) in cardiovascular and other chronic degenerative diseases.

10.6 ESTIMATION OF INTAKE OF ANTIOXIDANT COMPOUNDS VIA VIRGIN OLIVE OIL AND TABLE OLIVES BY THE GREEK POPULATION

Olives are processed to remove their natural bitterness, principally due to the secoiridoid oleuropein present in abundance in the raw olive fruit. The most economically important types of table olives in international trade include the Spanish-style green olives, the California-style black olives, and the Greek-style natural black olives (Romero et al., 2004). The main table olive cultivars commercially available in the Greek market include the Conservolea (green and natural black-type olives), Kalamon (special type of naturally black olives), and Chalkidiki (green-type olives) varieties (Blekas et al., 2002).

Data on the content of virgin olive oil and table olives in antioxidant compounds have not been consolidated. We have calculated the intake via virgin olive and table olives of the most important of these compounds in the Greek population (Table 10.1). Information on the content of virgin olive oil and table olives in antioxidant compounds was collected from the literature and evaluated on the basis of sampling procedures and method of analytical determination applied, as well as the geographical origin of the olive oils and table olives examined. Data on the consumption of

TABLE 10.1

Estimated Daily Intake of Antioxidant Compounds from Virgin Olive Oil and Table Olives by the Greek Population*[*]

Compound/Classes	Concentration in Virgin Olive Oil[a] (mg/kg)	Intake via Olive Oil (mg/day)	Concentration in Table Olives[b] (mg/kg)	Intake via Table Olives (mg/day)	Aggregated Daily Intake (mg/day)	Ref.
Phenolic compounds, total	232	12.2	404.5	4.5	16.7	Owen et al., 2000;[a] Blekas et al., 2002[b]
Hydroxytyrosol	14.4	0.8	315.1	3.5	4.3	Owen et al., 2000;[a] Blekas et al., 2002[b]
Tyrosol	27.5	1.4	61.6	0.7	2.1	Owen et al., 2000;[a] Blekas et al., 2002[b]
Secoiridoids, total	27.7	1.5	N	N	>1.5	Owen et al., 2000[a]
Lignans, total	41.5	2.2	N	N	>2.2	Owen et al., 2000[a]
Luteolin	N	N	27.8	0.3	>0.3	Blekas et al., 2002[b]
Squalene	4240	222.6	N	N	>222.6	Owen et al., 2000[a]
Chlorophylls, total	26.2	1.4	N	N	>1.4	Psomiadou and Tsimidou, 2001[a]
Pheophytin α	13.8	0.7	N	N	>0.7	Psomiadou and Tsimidou, 2001[a]
β-Carotene	2.1	0.1	3.2.2	Traces	0.1	Psomiadou and Tsimidou, 2001;[a] Lopez et al., 2005[b]
Lutein	1.2	0.1	N	N	>0.1	Psomiadou and Tsimidou, 2001[a]
α-Tocopherol	225	11.8	25.8	0.3	12.1	Psomiadou et al., 2000;[a] Hassapidou et al., 1994[b]
β-Tocopherol	0–9	0–0.5	Traces	Traces	0.5	Psomiadou et al., 2000;[a] Hassapidou et al., 1994[b]
γ-Tocopherol	0–40	0–2.1	5.9	0.1	0.1–2.2.2	Psomiadou et al., 2000;[a] Hassapidou et al., 1994[b]
δ-Tocopherol	4	0.2	Traces	Traces	0.2	Psomiadou et al., 2000;[a] Hassapidou et al., 1994[b]

[*] Based on a daily consumption of about 53 g of virgin olive oil and 11 g of table olives; N = not adequate information.

olive oil and table olives by the Greek population have been available through the Greek cohort of the European Prospective Investigation into Cancer and Nutrition (EPIC) (Riboli and Kaaks, 1997). The calculated daily per-capita intake was about 17 mg for phenolic compounds, 223 mg for squalene, and 12 mg for α-tocopherol. A limitation when calculating population intakes lies in the losses imparted by various preparation procedures and storage conditions applied to foods. Also, a fraction of the overall olive oil consumption is derived from refined olive oil, which contains lower quantities of certain minor compounds as compared to virgin olive oil. However, the majority of olive oil consumed in Greece is virgin olive oil.

10.7 COMMENTS

An early description of the Mediterranean diet reflected the nutritional habits of middle-aged men in the Greek island of Crete in the early 1960s (Keys, 1971; Nestle, 1995). At that time, the two main contributors of energy intake were olive oil and bread, contributing about 31 and 27% of the total energy intake, respectively (Keys et al., 1966). Olive oil contribution to energy corresponded to a daily intake of about 95 g. Table olives (mainly black olives) were consumed in rather small amounts (about 5 g of flesh per day) (Keys et al., 1966). The fact that the Cretan and other Mediterranean populations enjoyed one of the highest adult life expectancies and one of the lowest incidences of coronary heart disease in the world has been linked to the high olive oil consumption reported in these areas. Although Greek nutritional habits have been altered since the 1960s toward a more westernized dietary pattern, olive oil intake is still very high, the highest in the world according to the International Olive Oil Council, slightly exceeding 50 g/person/day (Naska et al., 2005; International Olive Oil Council, 2006).

The olive tree (*Olea europaea* L.) provides an excellent source of phenols. The major phenolic compound found in olive leaves is oleuropein (25 g/100 g of dry weight), followed by hydroxytyrosol (1.5 g/100 g of dry weight), flavone glucosides, and other phenols such as verbascoside and tyrosol (Benavente-Garcia et al., 2000). Other antioxidant compounds recovered from olive leaves are β-carotene and α-tocopherol (Tabera et al., 2004). Waste waters produced while extracting olive oil also represent a rich source of phenolic compounds with a total concentration similar to that of olive oil and processed olives. Hydroxytyrosol, tyrosol, elenolic acid, and derivatives, as well as luteolin and its 7-*O*-glucoside, have been reported to be the most important in Spanish, Italian, French, and Portuguese olive oil waste waters (Mulinacci et al., 2001). Furthermore, hydroxytyrosol, tyrosol, oleuropein, and ligstroside have been identified in olive tree wood (Perez-Bonilla et al., 2006). The increased demand for "natural" products provides a challenging area for the exploitation of phenolic compounds from *Olea europaea* L. by the contemporary nutraceutical industry.

It should be stressed, however, that emerging evidence suggests that several antioxidant compounds (e.g., β-carotene, vitamin C, vitamin E, polyphenols) may under specific circumstances exert prooxidant activity (Rietjens et al., 2002), catalyzed by transition metals and peroxidases (Yamanaka et al., 1997; Chan et al., 1999; Galati et al., 2002), especially when used in high doses (Lambert et al., 2007). Oleuropein, for example, showed a prooxidant activity in an experiment (Mazziotti et al., 2006), suggesting that its intake through commercial supplements should be done with caution. In this context, nutritional research suggests that the health effects from the intake of certain antioxidant micronutrients via foods are not always analogous to the effects reported by the intake of the same compounds in purified form (Kritchevsky, 1999; Bjelakovic et al., 2007). Consequently, supplementation with phenolic compounds isolated from *Olea europaea* L. should not be advised unless adequate evidence of a favorable effect on health when taken in a purified form is provided.

Antioxidants represent a broad category of compounds with diverse chemical structures and properties. Since they do not belong to a homogenous chemical group, the methods for their identification and quantification vary widely, hindering their collective determination in a food. They are defined in biological terms on the basis of the protection they confer to biological molecules (such as proteins, lipids, and DNA) from oxidation. The quantification of their biological potential in a food may be achieved *in vitro*, by determining the antioxidant capacity of the food matrix as compared to that of standards. Using the latter approach, however, the relative contribution of each of the entities to the overall antioxidant impact cannot be adequately assessed. An important issue that needs to be addressed in future studies concerns the determination of the magnitude of the contribution conferred by olive oil antioxidant compounds to the overall positive health impact of the Mediterranean diet. In this context, elucidation of the content of the Mediterranean diet in antioxidant compounds from olive oil as well as other sources seems essential. The latter task may contribute to understanding the biological processes involved in the apparent protection conveyed by the traditional Mediterranean diet against chronic diseases. Databases on the content of foods in certain microcompounds, such as the Database for the Flavonoid Content of Selected Foods (U.S. Department of Agriculture, 2007) and the BioActive Substances in Food Information System (BASIS Database) developed under the European Food Information Resource Network (EuroFIR, http://www.eurofir.net), could provide important tools toward this direction.

REFERENCES

Aparicio, R., Roda, L., Albi, M.A., and Gutierrez, F., 1999, Effect of various compounds on virgin olive oil stability measured by rancimat, *J. Agric. Food Chem.*, 47, 4150–4155.

Balder, H.F., Vogel, J., Jansen, M.C., Weijenberg, M.P., van der Brandt, P.A., Westenbrink, S., van der Meer, R., and Goldbohm, R.A., 2006, Heme and chlorophyll intake and risk of colorectal cancer in the Netherlands Cohort Study, *Cancer Epidemiol. Biomarkers Prev.*, 15, 717–725.

Benavente-Garcia, O., Castillo, J., Lorente, J., Ortuno, A., and Del Rio, J.A., 2000, Antioxidant activity of phenolics extracted from *Olea europaea* L. leaves, *Food Chem.*, 68, 457–462.

Bjelakovic, G., Nikolova, D., Gluud, L.L., Simonetti, R.G., and Gluud, C., 2007, Mortality in randomized trials of antioxidant supplements for primary and secondary prevention, *J.A.M.A.*, 297, 842–857.

Blekas, G., Vassilakis, C., Harizanis, C., Tsimidou, M., and Boskou, D., 2002, Biophenols in table olives, *J. Agric. Food Chem.*, 50, 3688–3692.

Bogani, P., Galli, C., Villa, M., and Visioli, F., 2007, Postprandial anti-inflammatory and antioxidant effects of extra virgin olive oil, *Atherosclerosis*, 190, 181–186.

Carrasco-Pancorbo, A., Carretani, L., Bendini, A., Segura-Carretero, A., Gallina-Toschi, T., and Fernandez-Gutierrez, A., 2005, Analytical determination of polyphenols in olive oils, *J. Separ. Sci.*, 28, 837–858.

Chan, T., Galati, G., and O'Brien, P.J., 1999, Oxygen activation during peroxidase catalysed metabolism of flavones and flavanones, *Chem. Biol. Interact.*, 122, 15–25.

Chernomorsky, S., Segelman, A., and Poretz, R.D., 1999, Effect of dietary chlorophyll derivatives on mutagenesis and tumor cell growth, *Teratogenesis Carcinogenesis Mutagenesis*, 19, 313–322.

Cichelli, A. and Pertesana, G.P., 2004, High-performance liquid chromatographic analysis of chlorophylls, pheophytins and carotenoids in virgin olive oils: chemometric approach to variety classification, *J. Chromatogr.*, 1046, 141–146.

Covas, M.-I., de la Torre, K., Farre-Albaladejo, M., Kaikkonen, J., Fito, M., Lopez-Sabater, C., Pujadas-Bastardes, M.A., Joglar, J., Weinbrenner, T., Lamuela-Raventos, R.M., and de la Torre, R., 2006a, Postprandial LDL phenolic content and LDL oxidation are modulated by olive oil phenolic compounds in humans, *Free Radical Biol. Med.*, 40, 608–616.

Covas, M.-I., Nyyssonen, K., Poulsen, H.E., Kaikkonen, J., Zunft, H.J., Kiesewetter, H., Gaddi, A., de la Torre, R., Mursu, J., Baumler, H., Nascetti, S., Salonen, J.T., Fito, M., Virtanen, J., Marrugat, J., and EUROLIVE Study Group, 2006b, The effect of polyphenols in olive oil on heart disease risk factors: a randomized trial, *Ann. Intern. Med.*, 145, 333–341.

De Vogel, J., Jonker-Termont, D.S.M.L., Katan, M.B., and van der Meer, R., 2005, Natural chlorophyll but not chlorophyllin prevents heme-induced cytotoxic and hyperproliferative effects in rat colon, *J. Nutr.*, 135, 1995–2000.

European Food Information Resource Network (EuroFIR), accessed July 2007, http://www.eurofir.net.

Ferruzzi, M.G., Bohm, V., Courtney, P.D., and Schwartz, S.I., 2002, Antioxidant and antimutagenic activity of dietary chlorophyll derivatives determined by radical scavenging and bacterial reverse mutagenesis assays, *J. Food Sci.*, 67(7), 2589–2595.

Fito, M., Cladellas, M., de la Torre, R., Marti, J., Alcantara, M., Pujadas-Bastardes, M., Marrugat, J., Bruguera, J., Lopez-Sabater, M.C., Vila, J., and Covas, M.-I, 2005, Antioxidant effect of virgin olive oil in patients with stable coronary heart disease: a randomized, crossover, controlled, clinical trial, *Atherosclerosis*, 181, 149–158.

Galati, G., Sabzevari, O., Wilson, J.X., and O'Brien, P.J., 2002, Prooxidant activity and cellular effects of the phenoxyl radicals of dietary flavonoids and other polyphenolics, *Toxicology*, 177, 91–104.

Gandul-Rojas, B. and Minguez-Mosquera, M.I., 1996, Chlorophyll and carotenoid composition in virgin olive oils from various Spanish olive varieties, *J. Sci. Food Agric.*, 72, 31–39.

Gaziano, J.M., 2004, Vitamin E and cardiovascular disease. Observation studies, *Ann. N.Y. Acad. Sci.*, 1031, 280–291.

Gimeno, E., de la Torre-Carbot, K., Lamuela-Raventos, R.M., Castellote, A.I., Fito, M., de la Torre, R., Covas, M.-I., and Lopez-Sabater, M.C., 2007, Changes in the phenolic content of low density lipoprotein after olive oil consumption in men. A randomized controlled trial, *Br. J. Nutr.*, doi: 10.1017/S0007114507778698.

Giuffrida, D., Salvo, F., Salvo, A., La Pera, L., and Dugo, G., 2007, Pigments composition in monovarietal virgin olive oils from various Sicilian olive varieties, *Food Chem.*, 101, 833–837.

Hacquebard, M. and Carpentier, Y.A., 2005, Vitamin E: absorption, plasma transport and cell uptake, *Curr. Opin. Clin. Nutr. Metab. Care*, 8, 133–138.

Harttig, U. and Bailey, G.S., 1998, Chemoprotection by natural chlorophylls in vivo: inhibition of dibenzo[a,I]pyrene-DNA adducts in rainbow trout liver, *Carcinogenesis*, 19, 1323–1326.

Hassapidou, M.N., Balatsouras, G.D., and Manoukas, A., 1994, Effect of processing upon the tocopherol and tocotrienol composition of table olives, *Food Chem.*, 50, 111–114.

Hillestrom, P.R., Covas, M.I., and Poulsen, H.E., 2006, Effect of dietary olive oil on urinary excretion of etheno-DNA adducts, *Free Radical Biol. Med.*, 41, 1133–1138.

International Olive Oil Council, accessed December 2006, World olive oil figures, http://www.internationaloliveoil.org.

Kelly, G.S., 1999, Squalene and its potential clinical uses, *Altern. Med. Rev.*, 4, 29–36.

Keys, A., 1971, Coronary heart disease in seven countries, *Circulation*, 41(s), 1–211.

Keys, A., Aravanis, C., and Sdrin, H., 1966, The diets of middle-aged men in two rural areas of Greece, *Voeding*, 27, 575–586.

Knekt, P., Ritz, J., Pereira, M.A., O'Reilly, E.J., Augustsson, K., Fraser, G.E., Goldbourt, U., Heitmann, B.L., Hallmans, G., Liu, S., Pietinen, P., Spiegelman, D., Stevens, J., Virtamo, J., Willett, W.C., Rimm, E.B., and Ascherio, A., 2004, Antioxidant vitamins and coronary heart disease risk: a pooled analysis of 9 cohorts, *Amer. J. Clin. Nutr.*, 80, 1508–1520.

Kohno, Y., Egawa, Y., Itoh, S., Nagaoka, S., Takahashi, M., and Mukai, K., 1995, Kinetic study of quenching reaction of singlet oxygen and scavenging reaction of free radical by squalene in n-butanol, *Biochim. Biophys. Acta*, 1256, 52–56.

Kritchevsky, S.B., 1999, β-Carotene and the prevention of coronary heart disease, *J. Nutr.*, 129, 5–8.

Lambert, J.D., Sang, S., and Yang, C.S., 2007, Possible controversy over dietary polyphenols: benefits vs. risks, *Chem. Res. Toxicol.*, 20, 583–585.

Leger, C.L., Carbonneau, M.A., Michel, F., Mas, E., Monnier, L., Cristol, J.P., and Descomps, B., 2005, A thromboxane effect of a hydroxytyrosol-rich olive oil wastewater extract in patients with uncomplicated type I diabetes, *Eur. J. Clin. Nutr.*, 59, 727–730.

Liu, G.C.K., Ahrens, E.H., Jr., Schreibman, P.H., and Crouse, J.R., 1976, Measurement of squalene in human tissues and plasma: validation and application, *J. Lipid Res.*, 17, 38–45.

Lopez, A., Montano, A., and Garrido, A., 2005, Provitamin A carotenoids in table olives according to processing styles, cultivars, and commercial presentations, *Eur. Food Res. Technol.*, 221, 406–411.

Machowetz, A., Poulsen, H.E., Gruendel, S., Weimann, A., Fito, M., Marrugat, J., de la Torre, K., Salonen, J.T., Nyyssonen, K., Mursu, J., Nascetti, S., Gaddi, A., Kiesewetter, H., Baumler, H., Selmi, H., Kaikkonen, J., Zunft, H.-J.F., Covas, M.-I., and Koebnick, C., 2006, Effect of olive oil on biomarkers of oxidative DNA stress in Northern and Southern Europeans, *FASEB J.*, 21, 1–8.

Marrugat, J., Covas, M.-I., Fito, M., Schroder, H., Miro-Casas, E., Gimeno, E., Lopez-Sabater, M.C., de la Torre, R., Farre, M., and members of SOLOS Investigators, 2004, Effects of differing phenolic content in dietary olive oils on lipids and LDL oxidation, *Eur. J. Nutr.*, 43, 140–147.

Mazziotti, A., Mazzotti, F., Pantusa, M., Sportelli, L., and Sindona, G., 2006, Pro-oxidant activity of oleuropein determined *in vitro* by electron spin resonance spin-trapping methodology, *J. Agric. Food Chem.*, 54, 7444–7449.

Miettinen, T.A. and Vanhanen, H., 1994, Serum concentration and metabolism of cholesterol during rapeseed oil and squalene feeding, *Amer. J. Clin. Nutr.*, 59, 356–363.

Miro-Casas, E., Farre-Albadalejo, M., Covas-Planells, M.I., Fito-Colomer, M., Lamuela-Raventos, R.M., and de la Torre, R., 2001a, Tyrosol bioavailability in humans after ingestion of virgin olive oil, *Clin. Chem.*, 47, 341–343.

Miro-Casas, E., Farre-Albadalejo, M., Covas, M.-I., Rodriguez, J.O., Menoyo Colomer, E., Lamuela Raventos, R.M., and de la Torre, R., 2001b, Capillary gas chromatography-mass spectrometry quantitative determination of hydroxytyrosol and tyrosol in human urine after olive oil intake, *Anal. Biochem.*, 294, 63–72.

Miro-Casas, E., Covas, M.-I., Farre, M., Fito, M., Ortuno, J., Weinbrenner, T., Roset, P., and de la Torre, R., 2003, Hydroxytyrosol disposition in humans, *Clin. Chem.*, 49, 945–952.

Moschandreas, J., Vissers, M.N., Wiseman, S., van Putte, K.P., Kafatos, A., 2002, Extra virgin olive oil phenols and markers of oxidation in Greek smokers: a randomized cross-over study, *Eur. J. Clin. Nutr.*, 56, 1024–1029.

Mulinacci, N., Romani, A., Galardi, C., Pinelli, P., Giaccherini, C., and Vincieri, F. F., 2001, Polyphenolic content in olive oil waste waters and related olive samples, *J. Agric. Food Chem.*, 49, 3509–3514.

Naska, A., Orfanos, P., Chloptsios, Y., and Trichopoulou, A., 2005, Dietary habits in Greece: the European Prospective Investigation into Cancer and Nutrition (the EPIC project), *Arch. Hellenic Med.*, 22, 259–269.

Negishi, T., Rai, H., and Hayatsu, H., 1997, Antigenotoxic activity of natural chlorophylls, *Mutat. Res.*, 376, 97–100.

Nestle, M., 1995, Mediterranean diets: historical and research overview, *Amer. J. Clin. Nutr.*, 61(s), 1313–1320.

Newmark, H.L., 1997, Squalene, olive oil, and cancer risk: a review and hypothesis, *Cancer Epidemiol. Biomarkers Prev.*, 6, 1101–1103.

Owen, R.W., Mier, W., Giacosa, A., Hull, W.E., Spiegelhalder, B., and Bartch, H., 2000, Phenolic compounds and squalene in olive oils: the concentration and antioxidant potential of total phenols, simple phenols, secoiridoids, lignans and squalene, *Food Chem. Toxicol.*, 38, 647–659.

Perez-Bonilla, M., Salido, S., van Beek, T.A., Linares-Palomino, P.J., Altarejos, J., Nogueras, M., and Sanchez, A., 2006, Isolation and identification of radical scavengers in olive tree (*Olea europaea*) wood, *J. Chromatogr. A*, 1112, 311–318.

Petroni, A., Blasevich, M., Salami, M., Papini, N., Montedoro, G.F., and Galli, C., 1995, Inhibition of platelet aggregation and eicosanoid production by phenolic components of olive oil, *Thrombosis Res.*, 78, 151–160.

Psomiadou, E. and Tsimidou, M., 1999, On the role of squalene in olive oil stability, *J. Agric. Food Chem.*, 47, 4025–4032.

Psomiadou, E. and Tsimidou, M., 2001, Pigments in Greek virgin olive oils: occurrence and levels, *J. Sci. Food Agric.*, 81, 640–647.

Psomiadou, E. and Tsimidou, M., 2002a, Stability of olive oil. I. Autoxidation studies, *J. Agric. Food Chem.*, 50, 716–721.

Psomiadou, E. and Tsimidou, M., 2002b, Stability of olive oil. II. Photo-oxidation studies, *J. Agric. Food Chem.*, 50, 722–727.

Psomiadou, E., Tsimidou, M., and Boskou, D., 2000, α-Tocopherol content of Greek virgin olive oil, *J. Agric. Food Chem.*, 48, 1770–1775.

Riboli, E. and Kaaks, R., 1997, The EPIC Project: rationale and study design. European Prospective Investigation into Cancer and Nutrition, *Int. J. Epidemiol.*, 26, S6–S14.

Rietjens, I.M.C.M., Boersma, M.G., de Haan, L., Spenkelink, B., Awad, H.M., Cnubben, N.H.P., van Zanden, J.J., van der Woude, H., Alink, G.M., and Koeman, J.H., 2002, The pro-oxidant chemistry of the natural antioxidants vitamin C, vitamin E, carotenoids and flavonoids, *Environ. Toxicol. Pharmacol.*, 11, 321–333.

Romero, C., Brenes, M., Yousfi, K., Garcia, P., Garsia, A., and Garrido A., 2004, Effect of cultivar and processing method on the contents of polyphenols in table olives, *J. Agric. Food Chem.*, 52, 479–484.

Ryan, D. and Robards, K., 1998, Phenolic compounds in olives, *Analyst*, 123, 31R–44R.

Salvini, S., Sera, F., Caruso, D., Giovanneli, L., Visioli, F., Saieva, C., Masala, G., Ceroti, M., Giovacchini, V., Pitozzi, V., Galli, C., Romani, A., Mulinacci, N., Bortolomeazzi, R., Dolara, P., and Palli, D., 2006, Daily consumption of a high-phenol extra-virgin olive oil reduces oxidative DNA damage in postmenopausal women, *Br. J. Nutr.*, 95, 742–751.

Strandberg, T.E., Tilvis, R.S., and Miettinen, T.A., 1990, Metabolic variables of cholesterol during squalene feeding in humans: comparison with cholestyramine treatment, *J. Lipid Res.*, 31, 1637–1643.

Tabera, J., Guinda, A., Ruiz-Rodriguez, A., Senorans, F.J., Ibanez, E., Albi, T., and Reglero, G., 2004, Countercurrent supercritical fluid extraction and fractionation of high-added-value compounds from a hexane extract of olive leaves, *J. Agric. Food Chem.*, 52, 4774–4779.

Trichopoulou, A. and Lagiou, P., 1997, Healthy traditional Mediterranean diet: an expression of culture, history and lifestyle, *Nutr. Rev.*, 55, 383–389.

Trichopoulou, A., Kouris-Blazos, A., Wahlqvist, M., Gnardellis, C., Lagiou, P., Polychronopoulos, E., Vassilakou, T., Lipworth, L., and Trichopoulos, D., 1995, Diet and overall survival in elderly people, *Br. Med. J.*, 311, 1457–1460.

Trichopoulou, A., Lagiou, P., and Papas, A., 1998, Mediterranean diet: are antioxidants central to its benefits? in *Antioxidant Status, Diet, Nutrition, and Health,* Papas, A.M., Ed., CRC Press, Boca Raton, FL, 107–118.

Trichopoulou, A., Vasilopoulou, E., and Lagiou, A., 1999, Mediterranean diet and coronary heart disease: are antioxidants critical? *Nutr. Rev.*, 57, 253–255.

Trichopoulou, A., Costacou, T., Bamia, C., and Trichopoulos, D., 2003, Adherence to a Mediterranean diet and survival in a Greek population, *N. Engl. J. Med.*, 348, 2599–2608.

U.S. Department of Agriculture, accessed July 2007, Database for the Flavonoid Content of Selected Foods, http://www.ars.usda.gov.

Visioli, F. and Galli, C., 1994, Oleuropein protects low density lipoprotein from oxidation, *Life Sci.*, 55, 1965–1971.

Visioli, F. and Galli, C., 1998, Olive oil phenols and their potential effects on human health, *J. Agric. Food Chem.*, 46, 4292–4296.

Visioli, F., Bellomo, G., Montedoro, G., and Galli, C., 1995, Low density lipoprotein oxidation is inhibited in vitro by olive oil constituents, *Atherosclerosis*, 117, 25–32.

Visioli, F., Galli, C., Bornet, F., Mattei, A., Patelli, R., Galli, G., and Caruso, D., 2000, Olive oil phenolics are dose-dependently absorbed in humans, *FEBS Lett.,* 468, 159–160.

Visioli, F., Poli, A., and Galli, C., 2002, Antioxidant and other biological activities of phenols from olives and olive oil, *Med. Res. Rev.*, 22, 65–75.

Visioli, F., Caruso, D., Grande, S., Bosisio, R., Villa, M., Galli, G., Sirtori, C., and Gallo, C., 2005, Virgin Olive Oil Study (VOLOS): vasoprotective potential of extra virgin olive oil in mildly dyslipidemic patients, *Eur. J. Nutr.*, 44, 121–127.

Vissers, M.N., Zock, P.L., Wiseman, S.A., Meyboom, S., and Katan, M.B., 2001, Effect of phenol-rich extra virgin olive oil on markers of oxidation in healthy volunteers, *Eur. J. Clin. Nutr.*, 55, 334–341.

Vissers, M.N., Zock, P.L., Roodenburg, A.J.C., and Leenen, R., 2002, Olive oil phenols are absorbed in humans, *J. Nutr.*, 132, 409–417.

Weinbrenner, T., Fito, M., de la Torre, R., Saez, G.T., Rijken, P., Tormos, C., Coolen, S., Farre-Albaladejo, M., Abanades, S., Schroder, H., Marrugat, J., and Covas, M.-I., 2004, Olive oils high in phenolic compounds modulate oxidative/antioxidative status in men, *J. Nutr.,* 134, 2314–2321.

Willett, W., 1994, Diet and health: what should we eat? *Science,* 264, 532–537.

Willett, W.C., Sacks, F., Trichopoulou, A., Drescher, G., Ferro-Luzzi, A., Helsing, E., and Trichopoulos, D., 1995, Mediterranean diet pyramid: a cultural model for healthy eating, *Amer. J. Clin. Nutr.*, 61(s), 1402–1406.

Yamanaka, N., Oda, O., and Nagao, S., 1997, Green tea catechins such as (-)-epicatechin and (-)-epigallocatechin accelerate Cu^{2+}-induced low density lipoprotein oxidation in propagation phase, *FEBS Lett.*, 401, 230–234.

11 Epilogue

Dimitrios Boskou

CONTENTS

11.1 MEDITERRANEAN DIET

The traditional Mediterranean diet is the dietary pattern found in the olive-growing areas of the Mediterranean region since the 1960s. Although different regions in the Mediterranean Sea have their own diets, several common characteristics can be identified; most of them stem from the fact that olive oil occupies a central position in all of the regions. It is therefore legitimate to consider these diets as variants of a single entity, the Mediterranean diet. Olive oil is important not only because of its several beneficial properties, but also because it allows the consumption of large quantities of vegetables in the form of cooked foods. The Mediterranean diet is characterized by high consumption of olive oil, vegetables, legumes, fruits, and unrefined cereals; regular but moderate wine intake, mostly during meals; moderate consumption of fish; low consumption of meat; and low to moderate intake of dairy products (The United Nations University, 2007).

The Mediterranean diet cannot fully explain the relatively good health of the Mediterranean people, as other factors may play a contributing role (see Chapter 2). However, it is highly likely that the diet is essential for the good health of the Mediterranean inhabitants.

The Mediterranean diet offers a healthy alternative approach to a low animal fat diet It is easily applied since it has an expanded range of options that could promote adherence over the long term. Besides, it provides no restriction on lipid intake as long as they are not saturated and are preferably in the form of olive oil.

11.2 PHENOLIC COMPOUNDS PRESENT IN OLIVE OIL

Phenolic antioxidants, widely distributed in the plant kingdom and abundant in our diet, are among the most talked about classes of phytochemicals today. They are broadly discussed as potential antioxidant prophylactics. Issues that have been studied in depth during the last decade are summarized as follows (Boskou, 2006):

- The levels and chemical structure of antioxidant phenols in different plant foods, aromatic plants, and various plant materials
- The probable role of plant phenols in the prevention of various diseases associated with oxidative stress such as cardiovascular and neurodegenerative diseases and cancer
- The ability of plant phenols to modulate the activity of enzymes, a biological action not yet fully understood
- The ability of certain classes of plant phenols such as flavonoids (also called polyphenols) to bind to proteins (flavonol–protein binding, such as binding to cellular receptors and transporters, involves mechanisms that are not related to their direct activity as antioxidants).
- The stabilization of edible oils, protection from formation of off-flavors, and stabilization of flavors
- The preparation of food supplements

The importance of antioxidant phenols also is seen in continuously emerging efforts to increase their levels in plants, to produce hydrophilic derivatives by enzyme modification of the structure and improving pharmacological properties to elucidate quantitative structure–activity relationships in various phenol classes, and finally to explore new effects.

Olive oil is one of the best sources of natural antioxidants and this fact further enhances olive oil's healthful reputation. Antioxidants are responsible for many health effects attributed to this valuable oil, but knowledge of the chemistry of minor products present in virgin olive oil and their properties, especially biological properties, is not yet complete. Much more research is needed to establish a credible basis for the health claims, to elucidate fully the biochemical relationships between structure and function, and to evaluate the effect on the human body of all the minor constituents. However, the data already available from biochemical and laboratory research as well as controlled intervention studies, combined with epidemiological studies, provide evidence for the health benefits of olive oil that seems to be convincing.

11.2.1 Chemistry, Antioxidant Activity, Biomarkers

Olive oil, especially virgin olive oil, contains a large number of structurally heterogenous compounds in small concentrations, such as aqualene, alpha-tocopherol, hydroxytyrosol, tyrosol, secoiridoids, phenolic acids, flavonoids, hydroxy-isochromans, pentacyclic triterpenes, and others, that are believed to be responsible for the beneficial effects on human health. The presence of these compounds in the oil is a further reason to recommend this oil as the main source of fat in the diet, in addition to the favorable fatty acid composition.

In evaluating various studies related to the biological properties of olive oil minor constituents, some data gaps on chemistry should be taken into consideration. Most of the studies in the past were set up using mainly oleuropein and hydroxytyrosol. We now know that free hydroxytyrosol is encountered in olive oil in small quantities and oleuropein in trace amounts; and that olive oil polar fraction is much more complex and that some minor components still remain unidentified. Today we know that olive oil polar fraction, very often characterized as olive oil "polyphenols," contains mainly secoiridoid aglycons, lignans, flavones, phenolic acids, hydroxy-isochromans, and elenonic acid (not a phenol but also a bioactive constituent), while other minor phenols are still recovered (Bianco, 2006). This diversity of phenolic content and the presence of other antioxidants should be kept in mind when experiments are set up to study antioxidant and other properties of olive oil phenols.

11.2.2 Levels

There is also a problem with levels of individual phenols. A typical example is **oleocanthal.** An excellent work was published in 2005 by a group of researchers (Beauchamp et al., 2005) indicating that the known aglycon, dialdeydic form of diacetoxy ligstroside aglycon, previously identified as one of the bitter compounds, is structurally related to ibuprofen. Taking as a starting point the irritating pungent sensation in the throat of this phenol the researchers synthesized it and proved experimentally that it has a similar biological effect as ibuprofen, a potent modulator of inflammation and analgesia.

Just like ibuprofen, both enantiomers of this aglycon (**oleocanthal**, also known as **p-HPEA-EDA**) cause dose-dependent inhibition of COX-1 and COX-2, cyclooxygenase enzymes catalyzing important steps in inflammation pathways related to arachidonic acid. The authors assumed that consumption of olive oil may help to protect against some diseases due to this activity of oleocanthal. However, taking into consideration the actual levels of oleocanthal in virgin olive oil, which are very low, it is more likely that other phenols or other minor compounds provide a total anti-inflammatory effect or other physiological functions.

For the moment there are only limited studies for Spanish and Italian oils that give some indication of the ranges and natural variability concerning the concentration of oleocanthal. It can be concluded from these studies that the levels of this aglycon and the expected intakes from daily consumption of olive oil are significantly lower. Thus the suggestion that the health effects of the Mediterranean diet are closely related to the intake of oleocanthal is open to discussion. Studies of bioavailability and biotransformation and measurement of the concentration of various aglycons, including oleocanthal, in plasma and urine after virgin olive oil consumption will probably provide more conclusive results.

11.2.3 Antioxidant Activity *In Vivo*

In the last two decades evidence has been accumulated supporting the notion that antioxidant content of olive oil contributes largely to its health benefits. Today, the hypothesized protection these antioxidants confer to biologically important molecules is evaluated mainly by measuring the oil's antioxidant capacity. There are many laboratory methods but it is recognized that more evidence is needed about the *in vivo* antioxidant activities of virgin olive oil in humans.

To evaluate the contribution of each antioxidant compound to the overall expected positive health impact, further studies are needed to fill the gap and understand better the link of health and constituents of the traditional Mediterranean diet.

Present-day methods of assessing antioxidant activity *in vivo* are based on measurements of malondialdehyde, lipid peroxides, circulating oxidized LDL, 8-oxo-deoxyguanosine in lymphocytes and urine, noninduced conjugation dienes, and isoprostane in urine and plasma.

As discussed in Chapter 6, biomarkers for oxidative damage must be selected on the basis of biomarker sensitivity and clinical significance. The sensitivity and specificity of some tests and measurements for lipid and LDL oxidation are currently questioned. Reliable markers should be considered that have been shown to be predictors for an oxidative stress-associated disease in large samples or in case-control studies, such as *in vivo* plasma-oxidized LDL or urinary F_2-isoprostanes. Besides oxidative damage markers, biomarkers related to oxidative stress-associated processes must be explored.

11.2.4 Analytical Methods

Standardized analytical methods are necessary to implement our knowledge of the chemical composition of olive oil and for setting out intervention or other studies that have to be controlled for the amounts of microconstituents. Improved analytical methodology is also needed to evaluate more objectively antioxidant capacity, to study the routes of degradation of phenols in different conditions, and to understand better the interactions between phenolic compounds and other minor constituents exerting an influence on olive oil oxidation.

11.3   VIRGIN OLIVE OIL AS A FUNCTIONAL FOOD

Virgin olive oil, the natural juice of the olive fruit, is a staple food for people living in countries surrounding the Mediterranean basin. The oil is now gaining popularity among consumers who in the past considered it only as part of an exotic dish. The popularity is mainly due to epidemiological data that provided the basis for the interest of the people. New consumers are trying to extract health benefits from the oil because of enthusiasm about the Mediterranean diet and the belief that there is a positive role of this diet and olive oil in the prevention of certain diseases and in particular of coronary heart disease.

Virgin olive oil can be characterized as a typical example of a "functional" because of its fatty acid composition and the presence of minor constituents, mainly phenols belonging to various chemical classes, and squalene (Stark and Madar, 2002). Accumulated evidence suggests that the oil may have health benefits that include:

Reduction of risk factors of coronary heart disease
Prevention of several types of cancers (breast, colorectal, prostate, others)
Modification of immune response, reduction of inflammation markers
Decrease of age-related cognitive decline

Considering the above and other properties, olive oil appears to be a real functional food whose components are expected to provide additional health benefits beyond basic nutritional needs.

11.4   FOOD SUPPLEMENTS AND FUNCTIONALIZATION OF FOOD

Oleuropein, a secoiridoid glucoside, and hydroxytyrosol, the free phenol obtained by various methods from olive leaves, olive pulp, or olive milling waste products, are now emerging as key antioxidants in many pharmacological tests and also as ingredients added to foods or food supplements. It has to be stressed, however, that solid evidence is lacking to indicate that phenolic-enriched products, possibly out of an original matrix, could be equally useful and it is not clear to what extent various preparations approximate the natural levels and the complex environment in which active molecules are found. Therefore, solid evidence of favorable effects on health when olive oil phenols are taken in a purified form should be provided

11.5   INTAKE OF ANTIOXIDANTS FROM OLIVE OIL AND OLIVES

The words *polyphenols* and *antioxidants* are today household words that can be seen on labels, advertisements, and websites. Estimations of daily antioxidant intake from the diet are now available in many countries. The Greek study discussed in this book gives a mean of 232 mg estimated intake of total phenols from virgin olive oil and table olive consumption. On the basis of this value, the approximately 23 g of oil recommended daily intake (U.S. Food and Drug Administration, 2004) add approximately 5 mg of polyphenols to diet.

These calculations, however, give rough figures because of the natural variability in olive oil and the methods of debittering table olives that influence significantly the level of phenols. Besides, since olive oil antioxidants do not belong to a homogenous chemical group, the methods for their identification and quantification vary widely, hindering their collective determination in a food. With current approaches the relative contribution of each of the entities to the overall antioxidant impact cannot be adequately assessed.

Lignans and enterolignans. Lignans are nutritionally important since they are transformd to enterolignans (enterodiol and enterolactone) that can potentially reduce the risk of certain cancers and cardiovascular diseases. Enterolignans are formed by the intestinal microflora after consumption of plant lignans (see also Chapter 7). Lignan mean intake was estimated to be of the level of 1.24 mg/day in the Netherlands. This intake is expected from the major food sources such as beverages, vegetables, nuts, seeds, bread, and fruit (Milder et al., 2005). From this point of view it is interesting to note that according to recent studies, pinoresininol is included in the list of entero-glycan precursors (Milder, 2005).

Pinoresinol and its derivatives (acetoxypinoresinol, hydroxypinoresinol) are major constituents of olive oil phenol fraction. Looking at olive oil as a source of lignans seems to be an interesting aspect, taking into consideration the high levels of the oil ingested in certain areas. Considering 40–50 mg/kg as the mean level of lignans in virgin olive oil, consumption of 23 g (2 tablespoons), the quantity that, as suggested by the U.S. Food and Drug Administration (2004), may reduce the risk of coronary heart disease, can provide approximately 1–1.5 mg of lignans per day .

Equally important may be calculations for the intake from olive oil of other bioactive compounds such as specific oleocanthal and secoiridoids and triterpenes.

11.6 ATHEROSCLEROSIS AND CANCER

Cardiovascular diseases (CVD) are considered as a group of multifunctional conditions associated with atherosclerosis, hypertension, and thrombosis. In Mediterranean countries, the incidence of atherosclerosis is different from that of occidental countries and this could be explained by the dietary pattern, as a number of studies have indicated an association between atherosclerosis and dietary fat, elevated serum cholesterol, and lipid levels. Recent research has emphasized the importance of microcomponents as modulators involved in the development of atherosclerosis. The protective effect of olive oil phenolic compounds on oxidative damage is established and this protective effect in humans is better displayed in situations with patients in which an enhanced oxidative stress status has been reported.

Some general questions that must be addressed in order to further clarify the real role of olive oil micronutrients on the thrombotic mechanism are doses ingested by the daily consumption of olive oil and metabolic disposition in humans and the mode of action of metabolites in blood. There is a scarcity of studies in which glucuronide and sulfate conjugates in biological samples were measured; and finally, the relative contribution of oleic acid, in comparison to minor constituents, on modulation of the hemostatic mechanism.

Cancer. Many studies were designed to evaluate the relationship between components of the Mediterranean Diet and cancer. These studies have provided supporting evidence indicating that olive oil is associated with decreasing cancer risk. Recent anticancer studies are associated with kinases, oncogenes, and tumor suppressor genes. However, the limitations of extrapolating the *in vitro* and animal results to human populations should always be taken into consideration. At the present time, the topic has not been sufficiently investigated to warrant categorically definite conclusions, but as noted in Chapter 7, experimental results collected so far indicate that there is a beneficial anticancer effect and this is a contribution of the specific action of oleic acid and minor constituents. They both exhibit properties influencing major structural and functional cell components. The effects studied so far are related to cell cycles, cell growth, progression, signaling, and apoptosis. Cancer research can be helped by specific studies, for example, investigation of olive oil phenols' angiogenic effect at a laboratory level and also trials to demonstrate activity in human subjects with surrogate markers for angiogenesis response.

Finally, it is interesting to note that all actions of olive oil compounds described are exerted without any cytotoxicity. This property may offer new possibilities for anticancer agents from a natural source that has been used as a food from time immemorial.

11.7   FLAVONES, LIGNANS, HYDROXY-ISOCHROMANS, OTHER PHENOLS, AND NONPHENOLIC MINOR CONSTITUENTS

Flavonoids and flavonoid-containing foods have been investigated for many biological properties including a selective inhibition activity against COX-2. However, it can be noted that data on olive oil are limited if compared to other plant sources. The same is true for lignans, hydroxy-isochromans, pentacyclic triterpene acids and alcohols, and newly discovered esters of tyrosol and hydroxytyrosol (Bianco, 2006).

Pentacyclic triterpenes are biologically active compounds and there is a plethora of publications related to their antitumoral and antinflammatory effects (vasorelaxant effects in aorta, modulation of the immune response, inhibition of cell proliferation, and others). Levels of these triterpenes in virgin olive oil are high enough for a biological effect but some forms of edible olive oil, such as olive residue oil, are very rich sources. The biological value of these olive oil grades should be reconsidered, keeping in mind that in addition to the presence of minor constituents they have the same fatty acid profile as virgin olive oil.

It is clear from the above that the contribution of olive oil to possible prevention of several human diseases is more likely to be due to the simultaneous presence of various active compounds or classes of compounds and to possible synergistic effects. Therefore, an important issue that needs to be addressed in future studies is the determination of the magnitude of the contribution of each active constituent to the overall positive health impact.

REFERENCES

Beauchamp, G., Keast, R., Morel, D., Lin, J., Pika, J., Han, Q., et al., 2005, Ibuprofen-like activity in extra virgin olive oil, *Nature*, 437, 45–46.

Bianco, A., Chiacchio, M., Grassi, G., Iannazzo, D., Piperno, A., and Romero, R., 2006, Phenolic components of *Olea europaea*: isolation of new tyrosol and hydroxytyrosol derivatives, *Food Chem.*, 95, 562–565.

Boskou, D., 2006, Sources of natural phenolic antioxidants, *Trends Food Sci. Technol.*, 17, 505–512.

Milder, I.J., Feskens, E.M., Arts, I.C.W., Bas Bueno de Mosquita, H., Holman, P.C.H., et al., 2005, Intake of lignans secoisolariciresinol, matairesinol, lariciresinol and pinoresinol in Dutch men and women, *J. Nutr.,*135, 1202–1207.

Stark, A.H. and Madar, Z., 2002, Olive oil as a functional food: epidemiology and nutritional approaches, *Nutr. Rev.*, 60, 170–176.

The United Nations University, 2007, *Bulletin*, 28, 2.

U.S. Food and Drug Administration, 11/01/2004, Announcement of the availability of a health claim for mono-unsaturated fat from olive oil and reduced risk of coronary heart disease (CHD), *Food Nutr. Bull.*, 28(2).

Glossary

Alperujo The solid by-product of the two-phase centrifugation method for olive oil extraction.

Beta-residue oil Pomace oil.

Astringent (positive attribute) A puckering sensation in the mouth created by tannins.

Bitter (positive attribute) A preferred characteristic, when it is not excessive. Usually obtained from green olives or olives turning color. Perceived on the back of the tongue.

Cake The residue remaining after the mechanical extraction of the oil from olives.

Centrifugation Rotary operation for separating the constituents of the paste or oily must by the differences in their density (International Olive Oil Council, IOOC).

Centrifugal system Processing system based on the use of a decanter for the separation of the liquid phase from the pomace.

Classic system The traditional batch method of olive processing using hydraulic plate presses.

Cold-pressing Process of extracting virgin olive oil by applying mechanical pressure to olive paste at a temperature of less than 25°C (IOOC).

Continuous system Processing of olives within a system that uses a horizontal centrifugal decanter.

Crude olive-pomace oil Oil obtained by treating olive pomace with a solvent.

Extra virgin olive oil Virgin olive oil having free acidity, as % of oleic acid up to 0.8, and the other characteristics according to regulations in force.

Fresh (positive attribute) Good aroma, fruity, not oxidized.

Fruity (positive attribute) Set of olfactory sensations characteristic of the oil, which depends on the variety and comes from sound, fresh olives, either ripe or unripe. It is perceived directly or through the back of the nose (retro-nasal).

Grass The taste of grass, seen in green olives or those crushed with leaves.

Green (positive attribute) A young oil, usually with a spicy-bitter taste.

Husk Residue solids after pressing of the pulp.

Lampante virgin olive oil Virgin olive oil not suitable for consumption with acidity more than 3.3% (expressed as oleic acid).

Malaxation The phase of mixing after crushing the olives in the centrifugation process, which promotes the coalescing of small oil drops.

Mediterranean Diet The traditional Mediterranean diet is the dietary pattern found in the olive-growing areas of the Mediterranea region in the 1960s. Although different regions in the Mediterranean basin have their own diets, several common characteristics can be identified, most of which stem from the fact that olive oil occupies a central position in all of them. It is therefore legitimate to consider these diets as variants of a single entity, the Mediterranean diet. Olive oil is important not only because of its several beneficial properties but also because it allows the consumption of large quantities of vegetables in the form of cooked foods.

The Mediterranean diet is characterized by high consumption of olive oil, vegetables, legumes, fruits, and unrefined cereals; regular but moderate wine intake, mostly during meals; moderate consumption of fish; low consumption of meat; and low to moderate intake of dairy products.*

Milling Processing of olives for the production of olive oil.

Natural olive oil Virgin olive oil.

Olive kernel oil The oil obtained from olive pomace.

---

* *Food and Nutrition Bulletin*, vol. 28, no. 2 © 2007, The United Nations University.

Olive oil Oil obtained by blending refined olive oil and virgin olive oil having free acidity, as % of oleic acid up to 1.0, and the other characteristics according to regulations in force.

Olive paste Paste produced by grinding the olives.

Olive pomace A by-product of olive processing containing fragments of skin, pulp, and kernel.

Olive pomace oil Blend of refined olive pomace oil and virgin olive oil for consumption.

Olive residue oil Oil obtained by blending refned olive residue oil and virgin olive oil having free acidity, as % of oleic acid up to 1.0, and the other characteristics according to regulations in force.

Orujo oil Spanish term, equivalent to sulfur olive oil.

Panel test Scoring of olive oil by a group of specially trained assessors under specified conditions.

Peppery A peppery bite in the back of the throat that can force a cough.

Pungent (positive attribute) "Picante" or biting tactile sensation characteristic of certain olive varieties or oil produced from unripe olives. Perceived in the throat (peppery).

Rancid (negative attribute) Flavor of oils that have undergone a process of oxidation and fragmentation of hydroperoxides into compounds with characteristic disagreeable odors such as aldehydes, ketones, alcohols, lactones, furans, esters, and others.

Refined olive oil Olive oil obtained from virgin olive oil refining that preserves its natural glyceridic composition, having free acidity, as % of oleic acid up to 0.3, and the other characteristics according to regulations in force.

Refined olive residue oil Olive oil obtained from crude olive residue oil by refining that preserves its natural glyceridic composition, having free acidity, as % of oleic acid up to 0.3, and the other characteristics according to regulations in force.

Remolido Repaso, second centrifugation oil.

Second centrifugation oil The oil obtained by centrifuging the paste from the two-phase decanters.

Traditional mill Classic system of extraction with hydraulic presses.

Unsaponifiable matter The whole of the products present in the substance analyzed that, after saponification with an alkaline hydroxide and extraction by a specified solvent, remains non-volatile under the defined conditions of the test.

Veiled virgin olive oil Cloudy virgin olive oil.

Virgin olive oil Virgin olive oil having free acidity, as % of oleic acid up to 2.0, and the other characteristics according to regulations in force.

Index

Milton Keynes UK
Ingram Content Group UK Ltd.
UKHW051951071024
449327UK00026B/2263